Praise for *The Ga*

"Every woman interested in her own health—not just those who want to conceive or to avoid pregnancy—needs a copy of this amazing book. Filled with solid information, thoughts of love, a fine feminist viewpoint, and great real-life stories, it is a feast of Wise Woman ways, guaranteed to empower everyone who reads it."
   —SUSUN WEED, author of *Wise Woman Herbal for the Childbearing Year*
   and *New Menopausal Years the Wise Woman Way*

"*The Garden of Fertility* bridges the facts of biology with feminine powers of daily observation. It encourages each of us to know how our reproductive systems work, and to use them well. It is an icon for medicine in the new century."
   —LARRY DOSSEY, M.D., author of *Healing Beyond the Body* and *Healing Words*,
   Executive Editor of *Alternative Therapies in Health and Medicine*

"Katie Singer has read widely and deeply. She offers this thoughtful, clear, informative discussion of Fertility Awareness in all of its ramifications, linking our personal health and womanly cycles to the greater world around us. Her book provides a basis for self-knowledge that enables us to understand our menstrual cycles and choose health care wisely."
   —THE BOSTON WOMEN'S HEALTH BOOK COLLECTIVE,
   authors of *Our Bodies, Ourselves for the New Century*

"This book's chapter on food and reproductive health succinctly presents the nutritional keys to creating regular, ovulatory cycles that are free from PMS, PCOS, progesterone deficiency, thyroid, and other gynecological problems—and that will ensure easy pregnancies and healthy children when they're desired. The keys that Katie Singer presents are the ones Dr. Weston A. Price discovered nearly a century ago in his remarkable studies of healthy, nonindustrialized peoples. At last, this information is available for contemporary women (and men) who want to create strong reproductive health through diet."
   —SALLY FALLON, author of *Nourishing Traditions*, President of the Weston A. Price Foundation

"This outstanding book teaches you how to interpret your menstrual cycle's signals and how to gauge your gynecological health, how to determine when you are fertile and infertile each month, what you can do at home to avoid or heal common problems, and what different health care systems provide when you need help. Katie Singer has done a brilliant job of integrating these complex subjects into one volume that is as delightful to read as it is comprehensive. If every woman read this book, I imagine that health care would be profoundly changed."
   —DAGMAR EHLING, D.O.M., author of *The Chinese Herbalist's Handbook*

The Garden of Fertility

A Guide to Charting Your Fertility Signals
to Prevent or Achieve Pregnancy—Naturally—
and to Gauge Your Reproductive Health

KATIE SINGER

AVERY
a member of Penguin Group (USA) Inc.
New York

Most Avery books are available at special quantity discounts for bulk purchase for sales promotions, premiums, fund-raising, and educational needs. Special books or book excerpts also can be created to fit specific needs. For details, write Penguin Group (USA) Inc. Special Markets, 375 Hudson Street, New York, NY 10014.

a member of
Penguin Group (USA) Inc.
375 Hudson Street
New York, NY 10014
www.penguin.com

Library of Congress Cataloging-in-Publication Data

Singer, Katie, date.
The garden of fertility : a guide to charting your fertility signals to prevent or achieve
pregnancy—naturally—and to gauge your reproductive health / Katie Singer.
p.   cm.
Includes bibliographical references and index.
ISBN 1-58333-182-4
1. Menstrual cycle.   2. Fertility, Human.   3. Natural family planning.   I. Title.
RG161.S55   2003   2003057943
612.6'62—dc22

Printed in the United States of America
1   3   5   7   9   10   8   6   4   2

BOOK DESIGN BY TANYA MAIBORODA

To Kyce Bello,
poet, herbalist, Fertility Awareness teacher, RN,
twenty-two-year-old
midwife to this book

To Andrus Brooke Pyeatt,
whose observations about the seasons
and all things fertile
daily fill my empty bowl

We know ourselves to be made from this earth.
We know this earth is made from our bodies. For we see ourselves.
And we see nature. We are nature seeing nature.

—SUSAN GRIFFIN

Contents

Acknowledgments

A COMMUNITY OF PASSIONATE PEOPLE created this book. Collecting and writing up the information has been my privilege. For their contributions, I give thanks:

To Donna Taylor, who generously teaches me Fertility Awareness with love, clarity, and infectious enthusiasm;

To Justina Trott, MD, Dorian Wilkes, Anne Robinson, and Delores Roybal, who gave me the green light to teach FA at Women's Health Services, making it one of the few nonprofit clinics in the United States to provide such classes;

To Suzannah Doyle, who dazzled me with her enthusiasm for using charts to gauge gyn health, then gave me her library;

To Dagmar Ehling, DOM, who weaves Chinese and Western meridians, regularly introduces me to new modes of healing, and gave this book (and me) indispensable research and support;

To Leah Morton, MD, whose friendship and ecological vision of health care encourage me deeply;

To Judy Norsigian, Jane Pincus, Wendy Sanford, and the rest of the team of women who created *Our Bodies, Ourselves*—without which I'd have had a very different life; and again to Wendy, whose editorial help on this book was crucial;

To Suzann Gage, L Ac, RNC, NP, and the Federation of Feminist Women's Health Centers—their book, *A New View of a Woman's Body,* was also one of my first teachers; and again to Suzann, whose original view of female reproductive anatomy makes this book *sing,* and who told me about Weston Price just when I began to teach Fertility Awareness;

To Toni Weschler, whose book, *Taking Charge of Your Fertility,* continues to break ground—along with her passion and generosity;

To Wendy VanDilla, ND, who helped teach me;

To Louise Rubin, web designer extraordinaire, whose desire to post www.gardenoffertility.com set this book in motion;

To Laura Wershler, who first named Fertility Awareness a life skill;

To Ilene Richman, coordinator of the Fertility Awareness Network, whose meticulous reading and keen insights improved this book more than I can say;

To the reference departments of the Santa Fe and Mesa Public Libraries; to Albert Robinson and Beth Salzman, librarians at St. Vincent Hospital, for indispensable, fabulous help;

To Sue Ek at the Billingses' US office, and all the Couple to Couple League folks who answer the phone, for their generosity and resourcefulness;

To Beth Kennard, MD, who edited the chapters on anatomy and gauging gyn health with the same humor and clarity that have delighted me since we were eleven, just beginning our lifelong conversation about menses, sex, and family relations;

To the numerous people who shined their lights on this book and also helped make the information here as accurate as possible: Nona Aguilar; Kyce Bello, RN; Bill Carey, PhD; Kaayla T. Daniel, PhD; Lakme Elior; Sally Fallon; Deborah Keller, ND; Katinka Locascio; Ann Lown; Geraldine Matus, PhD; Brooke Pyeatt; Sandra

Redemske; Stacey Malkan; Mary Martin, MD; Leah Shinbach, PA; Elisheva Simon; Bill Taylor, PhD; Susun Weed; Joyce Young, ND; and Sarah Young;

To Anou Mirkine, who created the fertility charts with humor and speed;

To Dyan Yoshikawa, who lent her graceful hand to the charts;

To Katey Branch and Alan Day, Donna and Bill Fishbein, Bob Levin, Sage Wheeler and Richard Pendleton, an anonymous individual, and an anonymous family—for their enthusiasm and faith;

To Dave Ewers, Steve Ewers, Rebecca Green, and Pauline Kenny, whose wizardry gives me computer use;

To Lisa Bloom, Deborah Dineen, Rebecca Green, Scott Markman, Kirin Narayan, Michael Nunnally, Virginia Pyeatt, Saz Richardson, Louise Rubin, and Anne Slepian—for friendship throughout the writing;

To Donna Downing, who read and clarified this book's first draft, and connected me;

To Cindy Spiegel, my fiction editor at Riverhead, who connected me;

To Laura Shepherd, whose grasp of this book helped focus me long before we had a contract;

To Dara Stewart, my editor at Avery, whose grace and clarity make publishing a pleasure;

To Betsy Amster, my literary agent, whose early insights helped me find the right tone and whose good cheer always gives me fuel;

To the farmers and ranchers and the wild land of northern New Mexico, which sustain me, body and soul;

To the women and men who've shared with me their stories, charts, and questions—and their delight in Fertility Awareness;

And to you, dear reader. I've long believed that readers bring much more to a book than the book brings to its readers. *The Garden of Fertility* is no exception.

WHEN A WOMAN COMES TO MY OFFICE AND says, "Something's wrong with my periods," I need to know what she means: How often is she menstruating? How heavy is her bleeding? Are her cycles ovulatory? How long is her luteal phase? Have these patterns changed since she started menstruating? The answers to these questions are essential to understanding her problem.

A woman's first step could well be to learn Fertility Awareness, a method usually known for preventing or achieving pregnancy, based on daily charting of the waking temperature and cervical fluid. While charts can be used to determine exactly when a woman is and is not fertile (and thereby to prevent or achieve pregnancy), women who chart their fertility signals also have a window into gauging their overall wellness.

From learning the basics of Fertility Awareness (which takes only a handful of hours to learn and about two minutes of daily attention to chart), a woman knows what's normal and not normal for her body. She knows the basic physiology of her menstrual cycle; she has a way to create a friendly relationship with her body, she's alert to her own rhythms and their connectedness to wider cycles. From reading her own charts, she knows whether she's ovulating, prone to miscarriage or hypothyroidism, pregnant, and more. These factors are all crucial for creating sound health. I know of no other tool or system that gives a woman such an ideal avenue to connecting with her own body, as well as a vocabulary for communicating effectively with her health-care provider.

The Garden of Fertility takes the method a step further than other books on the subject by presenting charting as a way for women to research their own menstrual cycles. The fertility charts in chapter 13 shift authority over women's health from physicians, academics, and pharmaceutical companies to individuals who know their own bodies. These charts create a new model for research. Indeed, there is unlimited potential for fertility charts to inform us about women's health without expense or invasiveness. Doctors and research institutes, heads up! This is clinical research.

The Garden of Fertility provides a foundation for anyone who wants to know and honor the body's wisdom. While it focuses on the reproductive system, Katie Singer's book has far-reaching implications about all aspects of health care. It shows how human health is linked with every living system on earth and how the menstrual cycle is a vital sign in that web.

For women who want to take responsibility for their own wellness and understand the body's rhythms and their connections to nature's wider cycles, Fertility Awareness is an essential life skill. I highly recommend that every doctor read this book before beginning to practice medicine; and that every woman read it before choosing a method of birth control, before trying to conceive, before going to a doctor for a gynecological exam.

—JUSTINA TROTT, MD, FACP
President of the American College of Women's Health Physicians

Introduction

IN JUNIOR-HIGH BIOLOGY ABOUT THIRTY
years ago, I looked under the microscope my teacher offered and struggled to figure out how the stuff on the slide was relevant to me. I'd just begun to menstruate,
and I wanted to know how my body worked. I wondered if other girls had strong
cramps and what they did to ease them. I wondered if menstruating meant that if
I had sex, I could get pregnant any day. Or was it just a few days each month? If it
was just a few days, which days were they?

Once I became sexually active, I got a diaphragm and then a cervical cap. I asked a doctor and a midwife if they knew a way I could learn to tell when I was fertile. Each of them shook their heads.

A Tangle

———

Years later, my boyfriend and I drove toward a cabin out of town to celebrate my birthday. "I've got another yeast infection," I said quietly.

"Well that's *lousy*," he said.

The *lousiness* wasn't that I was sick, but that we wouldn't be able to make love. Already that year I'd had several yeast infections because of irritation from the spermicide I used with my cervical cap.

How do I get out of here? I wondered. *Out of feeling like my birthday celebration is only about sex, out of birth control that makes me sick?*

Sex, fertility, love. Like the burning in my groin, they made a tangle too hot to touch.

Learning to Chart

———

Once I heard about Fertility Awareness (FA), also called Natural Family Planning (NFP), I decided to learn it. FA is based on a woman's daily charting of her waking temperature and cervical fluid. With Fertility Awareness, a woman can tell when she's fertile and infertile. To avoid pregnancy, couples postpone intercourse or use a barrier method on fertile days. To conceive, they know the best time to try.

Fertility Awareness is not the same as the (unreliable) Rhythm Method, which determines fertility by the patterns of *previous* cycles. FA gauges fertility as the woman's daily chart evolves. According to numerous studies, when its rules are followed, Fertility Awareness is virtually as effective as the Pill.

Through books and classes about Fertility Awareness, I finally learned the vocabulary of my menstrual cycle, the functions of different hormones, and how to determine when I am fertile and infertile. As I started to observe and record my fertility signals, I began to experience explosions of awe: I had never conceived or tried to, but from charting I could see bona fide proof of my fertility. My cycles had often been erratic, and now (from knowing when I ovulated), I could predict when my period would come. I was with a new man while I learned the method, and his interest in the method helped both of us appreciate my femaleness.

Brooke, my partner, realized that ever since he was a teenager, he'd woken every morning and asked, *When was the last time I had intercourse?* And, *Do I feel like masturbating?* (Based on surveys of men who've taken my classes, this is a pretty typical way for a man to start his day.) Once I started charting, Brooke had a new waking question: *Is Katie fertile?* (Other men report wondering, *What's my partner's temperature?*) As awareness of fertility patterns emerged, my feminine rhythm gently took the lead in Brooke's and my relating.

I began to see that the rhythm of masculine sexuality is essentially *on* all the time—essentially, men are fertile all the time. Meanwhile, because women are fertile, on average, only one-third of each cycle, feminine cycles seem to invite periodic rest from sexual intercourse.

Despite my feminist perspective, I came of age expecting that I should be available for sex all the time. I remember one three- or four-month period when I was physically able and wanting to have sex every day. Surely, I thought, my boyfriend and I would stay together if I could keep this up. Now, I wonder how my access to artificial birth control contributed to such thinking.

Indeed, sterilization, the Pill, Depo-Provera, the IUD, the diaphragm, the cervical cap, and condoms give women in heterosexual relationships the option of having fewer children than earlier generations. These methods allow choice about the course of our lives. However, artificial birth control is usually distributed without substantial information about how our bodies or the methods work.

I began to wonder what price we pay when we don't know this basic information about ourselves.

Charting my fertility signals, I felt more connected to myself, and to other women who understood their own cycles. Taking my temperature and observing my cervical fluid felt like rituals for contacting a rhythm larger than my own. Brooke and I found ourselves supported by the rhythm my charts offered. Why hadn't we learned this method before?

Trying to Become a Fertility Awareness Teacher

Because of my passion for the method, I began writing a story about its availability in northern New Mexico. One of the people I called was the director of a Natural

Family Planning clinic at an Albuquerque hospital. When the woman said she would be offering a course to train people to teach the method, I asked for an application.

"I could send you one," she said, "but I couldn't accept you."

I was stunned. "Why?" I asked.

"Because you're single and you have genital contact." If I was celibate or married, then her program could accept me.

This was spring 1997.

I wanted to understand this clinic's policy, which is common among Catholic programs wherein medical information is taught effectively and woven with moral messages. I wanted to understand why Fertility Awareness isn't more available, especially in secular communities. And I wanted the name of someone who could train me to teach the method. Indeed, the NFP clinic's policy raised numerous questions and propelled me on to a tour of conversations. I spoke with the director of medical affairs for Planned Parenthood, nurse practitioners in women's clinics, the medical journalist Nona Aguilar, and Suzannah Doyle, who wrote about the method for *Our Bodies, Ourselves.*

One of the first people I called was Kara Anderson, then Planned Parenthood's director of medical affairs. She explained that their practitioners rarely have more than twenty minutes with each client. "Most of the people who come to us have been sexually active for six months—without *any* birth control," Anderson said. "Our practitioners give each woman as much as they can."

If a Planned Parenthood client asks to learn Fertility Awareness (which is unusual), she's usually referred elsewhere—often to a teacher affiliated with a Catholic organization. "To learn this method well," Anderson said, "a woman needs to be in close touch with a teacher for three or four months. In many areas, Catholic organizations provide the method's only teachers. We simply don't have staff or finances available to offer it on a large scale, given the limited number of women who request it."

Anderson then succinctly articulated that Fertility Awareness can "enhance people's self-awareness, self-esteem, and communication skills. And these are things we want for all women."

I began to see that while learning Fertility Awareness is time intensive, once a woman owns a thermometer and knows the method, there's nothing to purchase again. I began to wonder how classes could be administered for a wide variety of people from a range of backgrounds.

My next call was to Laurie Holmes, a certified nurse-midwife who often dispenses birth control. "I've seen too many unwanted pregnancies with Fertility Awareness to feel entirely comfortable endorsing it," she said. "I bring it up, but people need time to learn it and stay with the daily charting. I think you need to be open to failure if you use it. I also find that people don't want abstinence."

I told Laurie, who, like most health-care practitioners, is not trained to use or teach FA, about the first woman I met who used it. She'd had two abortions by the time she was twenty-one, then vowed never again to have an unwanted pregnancy. After her second abortion, she chose FA for birth control; and 115 cycles later, she hadn't conceived again.

This woman taught herself the method from reading a book; and, indeed, it took her several months before she felt confident enough to engage in sexual intercourse. Now, though, this woman says, "I know when I'm fertile, and when I'm not. Artificial birth control feels too risky to me." After her abortions, learning how to read her cycles was a rite of passage.

Laurie Holmes found it exceptional that a woman would have the discipline to take her temperature every morning through her childbearing years.

I began to wonder if Fertility Awareness is not taught as well in the women's community as it is among Catholics (certainly it's less available) and how this might figure into practitioners' lack of faith in the method and people's capacity to commit to daily charting. Are the teaching methods, commitments, and self-control expressed in the Catholic community not available to others? Does the spiritual foundation that Catholic programs provide increase users' efficacy with the method?

The Couple to Couple League (CCL), one of several Catholic organizations dedicated to teaching Natural Family Planning, has 22,000 subscribers to its newsletter, *Family Foundations*. Founded in 1971, the CCL is staffed primarily by volunteers who perceive teaching as service; and it's therefore able to offer classes at a nominal fee. Indeed, the CCL is one of several groups that admirably meets the needs of practicing Catholics. Its publications include chart reviews, discussions of men's involvement with charting, the effects of breast-feeding on fertility, descriptions of the effects of various drugs on fertility signals, what to expect when coming off the Pill—and numerous prescriptions for living a moral life.

Currently, over 700 volunteer couples teach NFP through the CCL. These teachers are required to sign a principle statement advocating, for example, marriage and breast-feeding, and rejecting abortion, premarital sex, and homosexual behavior. While I appreciate the CCL's clear outlaying of their beliefs, their programs speak primarily to married, practicing Catholics who are open to the possibility of a child. Their literature is extensive (and available in Spanish); their teachers have been uniformly kind and generous—even while knowing I'm not Christian or married; and I often find beauty in their presentation of charting in a spiritual context. Alas, I'm not in concert with their basic tenet that there are a limited number of right and true ways to behave when it comes to sex and fertility. Learning Natural Family Planning through the CCL is not for everyone.

When I called Nona Aguilar, author of *The New No-Pill, No-Risk Birth Control* (Simon & Schuster, 1986), I described my frustration that I was not acceptable to the training program at the Albuquerque clinic. "Well," she said, respectfully, "I agree with that policy."

I leaned back in my chair. "Okay," I said. "I don't understand this. Please explain."

"Properly used," she began, "sex is about emotional and psychological union. In our culture, artificial birth control—which feminists have strongly advocated—has made sex a recreational activity. Sex certainly can be recreational, but its potential is to be transcendent. Sex is the life-bearing force of humankind. When lovemaking is recreational, it's a little like being color-blind during sunset over the Grand Canyon. Union becomes harder to experience, and that's a loss."

With Natural Family Planning, Aguilar continued, "issues of control and communication—which naturally arise in a sexual relationship—are strongly brought to the fore. The method can help support that exploration." And the container of marriage, she insisted, the commitment of marriage, supports the exploration.

Aguilar's thoughts stirred me deeply and encouraged me to revere Fertility Awareness more than before. Our conversations also strengthened my desire for classes that teach people how our bodies work and that offer opportunity for individuals to differentiate between their personal values around sexual issues and the prohibitions suggested by society. Properly trained, I felt that I could teach such classes, despite my not being celibate, despite my never having felt moved to marry.

Finally, I called the Boston Women's Health Book Collective. By then I doubted if I would ever meet someone who could or would train me to teach Fertility Awareness. I was given the number of Suzannah Doyle, who wrote about the method for the last several editions of *Our Bodies, Ourselves*.

Suzannah suggested that charting speaks to a tradition when women were in charge of their own health care. She impressed upon me that charts could be used to gauge gynecological health. She explained that Fertility Awareness teachers usually tell their clients that they have choices during their fertile phases: they can use barrier methods to prevent pregnancy, postpone intercourse, or enjoy sexual expression that doesn't include genital-genital contact. (She prefers to suggest that couples who don't want to conceive "postpone" intercourse—rather than abstain from it—during the woman's fertile phase.) "In any case," Doyle said, "since women are fertile only one third of their cycle, using birth control for two thirds of it—when a woman is naturally infertile—is a waste."

Doyle also confirmed that most of the scientists who've done research in this field have been male Catholic MDs. Until the 1980s, Fertility Awareness was only available from a Catholic perspective; when Doyle began learning FA, she couldn't have gotten the information she wanted from a women's clinic, either. Since then, a small number of nonreligious teachers (who usually learned the method through Catholic organizations) have offered classes throughout North America.

Now, the Fertility Awareness community is often divided between those who are pro-choice and pro-life. "I call myself *pre*-choice," Doyle said. "If people—including teenagers—know their fertility signals, they're more likely to make informed, responsible choices about sex." She also emphasized that each perspective serves a purpose and meets the needs of different populations.

Suzannah gave me the name of Wendy VanDilla, a colleague who could train me to teach Fertility Awareness. She also gave me her library on the subject, as she had moved on to a new career in music. I studied with Wendy, read voraciously, and attended a CCL workshop with Donna and Bill Taylor, internationally recognized authorities on lactational amenorrhea. I started teaching at the Santa Fe Community College, then began offering classes at Women's Health Services (WHS), an MD-staffed clinic founded in 1972 in Santa Fe. WHS is one of only a few secular, not-for-profit clinics in the country that offers classes in Fertility Awareness.

Using Charts to Gauge Gynecological Health

Later in 1997, because of menstrual irregularities, I went to see Dagmar Ehling, DOM (doctor of Oriental medicine), the author of *The Chinese Herbalist's Handbook*. I'd just begun teaching Fertility Awareness and brought my charts to her office. To my great joy, Dagmar could read them. In fact, she routinely requests that her women clients of childbearing age chart their waking temperatures. Dagmar had recently completed a postgraduate gynecology course for DOMs with Dr. Bob Flaws, who translates Chinese research (including studies on women's waking temperatures) into English for Blue Poppy Press. Blue Poppy's seminar had focused on using the waking temperature to gauge gynecological health; it did not include information about cervical fluid. Dagmar and I traded notes. We found ourselves eager for this information to be made available to health-care providers. In November 1999, we published "Gauging a Woman's Health by Her Fertility Signals: An Introductory Synthesis of Western and Chinese Medical Principles" in the peer-reviewed journal *Alternative Therapies*.

By this time, the first edition of Toni Weschler's groundbreaking book *Taking Charge of Your Fertility* had been published. Frequently referred to as the fertility bible, Toni's book initiated the movement to reform women's health by introducing Fertility Awareness to the mainstream. While many of my students were coming to class with charts that could not be found in textbooks, I found myself wanting clear guidelines—for women and health-care providers—about reading charts to gauge gynecological health. I wanted a repertoire of natural remedies for strengthening the menstrual cycle, and for women to hear each other's experiences with charting. I wanted to offer more information about using FA while breast-feeding. This book, which I see as a companion to Toni's, began to write itself.

Myths of Fertility

Thousands of years ago, women created the first calendars by marking the phases of the moon and their own menstrual cycles with tallies etched into objects like bison horns.[1] In *The Lunar Calendar,* publisher Nancy Passmore writes, "The origins of a wholistic view of the world lie in these early observations: *we are part of nature and nature is part of us.*"

Julius Caesar outlawed lunar calendars in 45 B.C.; the Council of Constantinople declared the concept of cycles heretical in the fifth century A.D.[2] Most calendars today largely ignore the lunar cycle. Some, such as the Jewish calendar, continue to be oriented to lunar and solar cycles.

I can't help but wonder how, over time, decreased awareness of lunar cycles has affected our awareness of fertility's cycles. So many people's ideas about fertility have been flat-out wrong. In 1672, for example, a researcher named Kerkring theorized that women "eject ova above all during the menses, or on being vehemently angry."[3] Some people still mistakenly believe that a woman ovulates only when she has an orgasm, or that pre-ejaculate doesn't contain enough sperm to cause a pregnancy. Our culture's general lack of information about reproductive physiology, coupled with the lack of effective ways to prevent unintended pregnancies, has meant that a lot of women have had more children than they wanted or could sanely handle. More recently, some pharmaceutical companies have created drugs that make monthly bleeding "optional"; and some gynecologists have proclaimed that suppressing periods "gets women to a more natural state."[4] (Personally, I don't see how suppressing menstruation is at all natural.) Meanwhile, many of us listen for the messages our bodies provide, and seek to live in concert with them.

A *Short* History *of* Fertility Awareness

In the 1920s, an Austrian surgeon and another in Japan simultaneously discovered that ovulation usually takes place fourteen days before the onset of the next period. With this discovery, the first scientific study in modern times of a natural system of family planning began. Called the Calendar or Rhythm Method and based on information from a woman's past cycles, it helped women with predictable cycles to prevent pregnancy. Women with irregular cycles still had no way to determine when they were fertile.

In the 1960s, Drs. John and Evelyn Billings, Australian physicians, found that healthy women have a standard cervical mucus pattern that parallels hormonal changes. During a woman's fertile phase, glands in the cervix secrete mucus, which can keep sperm alive for up to five days; at ovulation, this same fluid helps sperm travel toward a mature egg in a fallopian tube. During infertile days, the cervix's dry secretions create a hostile environment for sperm to survive.

The Billingses realized that women could observe their mucus patterns and identify their own fertile and infertile times. They began offering workshops worldwide to teach the Ovulation Method to couples wanting a natural way to either avoid or achieve pregnancy. The Sympto-Thermal Method of Fertility Awareness was born when charts of cervical fluid were combined with charts of the waking temperature.

According to numerous studies, *if its rules are followed,* Fertility Awareness is as effective as the Pill in preventing pregnancy. The method has also helped countless couples to conceive, and it can be used to help gauge gynecological health.

Why isn't Fertility Awareness widely known? Plenty of folks have heard of the Rhythm Method, and that it's ineffective; many people confuse the two. Few health-care providers know about FA, while they do know about the Pill. And usually, those who teach Fertility Awareness are in touch with each other informally, without institutional support. As our society has become more health conscious and more interested in addressing our concerns (including reproductive concerns) without pharmaceuticals, Fertility Awareness has become more popular.

A Community of Charters

A short time after I began teaching Fertility Awareness to prevent or achieve pregnancy, the women in my classes started using their charts to conduct research on their own health. They observed how long it took to ovulate after they'd been on hormonal contraceptives. One woman charted her signals for nearly two months with an IUD (which she'd had inserted five years before) and then continued charting after it was removed. Others noticed how different diets affected their monthly cycles. None of these women are doctors, and yet their research gave me something I could share with new students in similar situations. As women continue charting and asking keen questions about their own health and health care, they come to understand their bodies and the ecosystems within which they live with increased strength and fullness.

From these women's observations, I've come to understand how consumption of organic butter, my thyroid, hazardous waste in our oceans, my menstrual cramps, and my relationship with my partner are all connected!

I'm dreaming now: of adolescents knowing how their reproductive systems work before they become sexually active and before they choose a method for preventing pregnancy; of women *and* men being as aware of our fertility as we are of our sexuality; of Fertility Awareness classes as available as the Pill and fertility-enhancing drugs; of alliances between those who provide health-care education in women's and Catholic communities; of alternative and allopathic medical students learning how to read fertility charts; of medical research on fertility signals; of every person intimately knowing the sacredness of their procreative powers.

I CALL THE INFORMATION PRESENTED IN chapters 1 through 6 the core material of Fertility Awareness. I consider knowing it a basic life skill. Information presented in the other chapters is no less important, but understanding the core material is necessary to reap full benefit of these other aspects of Fertility Awareness.

PART

1

Fertility Awareness

*Those who contemplate the beauty of the earth find
reserves of strength that will endure as long as life lasts.
There is symbolic as well as actual beauty in the
migration of the birds, the ebb and flow of the tides, the
folded bud ready for the spring. There is something
infinitely healing in the repeated refrains of nature—
the assurance that dawn comes after
night, and spring after the winter.*

—RACHEL CARSON
The Sense of Wonder, 1965

1. A Woman Is Like the Earth: Reproductive Anatomy and Physiology

LIKE THE EARTH'S SURFACE, A WOMAN of childbearing age cycles through phases of cooling and heating, which in turn create moistening and drying, which in turn create a fertile environment for life to evolve. Rocks, glaciers, plants, and animals (including humans) all evolve in concert with these processes. In the same way that a meteorologist predicts weather by observing patterns of heating and cooling and moistening and drying at the earth's surface, a woman of childbearing age can observe her body's fertility signals and know whether or not she's ovulating, when she's fertile and infertile, if she's prone to ovarian cysts or miscarriage, if she's pregnant, and more.

The first step is learning reproductive anatomy (the parts of the body) and physiology (what the parts do).

The Female Reproductive System

The female reproductive system operates in a cyclical rhythm. Until puberty, a girl is not fertile. Once she begins to menstruate, she's entered her childbearing years; and she's potentially fertile until menopause, when reproduction is no longer possible. Unlike most species (female orca whales are another exception), human females can live for decades after their biological fertility has ended.

During the childbearing years, each menstrual cycle moves a woman through infertile, fertile, and again infertile phases. Like the earth's seasons, women move through a dry-infertile phase, then a moist-fertile phase, and again a dry-infertile phase. To observe your own fertility, the first step is learning reproductive anatomy.

The *uterus* is a sterile muscle, about the size of a lemon and shaped like an upside-down pear. There are no bacteria in the uterus so that it can provide a hospitable environment for a baby. This lack of bacteria also renders it vulnerable to sexually transmitted infections. The neck of the uterus, the *cervix*, projects into the vaginal canal. The cervix's opening is called the *os*. This is the area that's swabbed during a pap smear to test for cervical cancer. Menstrual blood also passes through this opening. During childbirth, the os dilates ten centimeters.

The cervix is filled with glands, called *crypts*, which produce cervical fluid. Inside the crypts, cervical fluid can keep sperm alive for up to five days. I've known some Fertility Awareness teachers to call these recesses in the cervix "the sperm hotel." Cervical fluid also filters out impaired sperm and provides a conduit for sperm to travel at ovulation from the cervix to the ripe egg in the fallopian tube.

On each side of the top of the uterus, there's an *ovary*, a gland that contains *follicles;* follicles are unripe eggs held in sacs. By the time a female fetus is just four months old, she's already made all of the follicles that she will ever produce. At birth, a baby girl's ovaries hold about one million follicles. By the time menstruation begins, half of these follicles will have dissolved. By midlife, it becomes more difficult to stimulate a follicle to release an egg and for a released egg to be penetrated by sperm.

Fallopian tubes also extend from each side of the top of the uterus. Conception takes place in a fallopian tube, which also transports the fertilized egg to the uterus for pregnancy.

The vaginal canal stretches from the cervix to the lips of the vagina. The lips are also called the *labia*. When a woman is aroused, the walls of her vagina secrete arousal fluid, sort of like sweat, so that she is lubricated well and intercourse will not be painful.

Just above the vaginal opening, under a small hood where the labia join, is the *clitoris*. This small knob contains a woman's most sensitive sexual nerves.

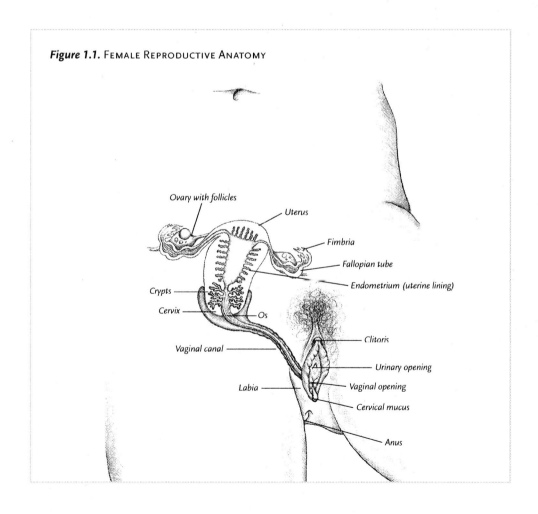

Figure 1.1. FEMALE REPRODUCTIVE ANATOMY

Ovary with follicles

Uterus

Fimbria

Fallopian tube

Endometrium (uterine lining)

Crypts

Cervix

Os

Clitoris

Vaginal canal

Urinary opening

Labia

Vaginal opening

Cervical mucus

Anus

The Menstrual Cycle

To begin a menstrual cycle, the pituitary gland sends a hormonal message to the ovaries. *Hormones* are essentially messengers that travel through the blood to direct organs to carry out specific functions. The word *hormone* comes from the Greek words *horma*, which means "impulse," and *horman*, which means "to urge on."

Throughout the cycle, the pituitary gland secretes *follicle-stimulating hormone (FSH)*, which encourages follicles in both ovaries to mature. During each cycle, about a dozen follicles are given the impulse to ripen. As they mature, these follicles produce *estrogen*.

While follicles are maturing and emitting estrogen, the woman is in her *follicular phase*. Also called the preovulatory phase, it typically begins a few days after menstruation and ends at ovulation. During this part of the cycle, estrogen is dominant.

Estrogen has several key functions:

- It stimulates the production of cervical fluid, which can keep sperm alive for up to five days.
- It cools the woman's temperature. Likewise, when a man is maturing sperm—which happens to be *all the time* from puberty on—the testicles are a couple of degrees cooler than the rest of his body. This is why the testicles hang outside a man's trunk, which is warmer. While we are maturing eggs and sperm, humans prefer a cooler temperature.
- It softens the cervix, raises its location in the vaginal canal, and opens the os—in order to receive sperm more readily.
- It builds a new endometrial lining in the uterus in preparation for a possible pregnancy.
- And, as the meaning of its Greek root, *ois-tros*, suggests, estrogen makes many women "mad with desire" at this phase in the cycle.

When one egg within a follicle reaches maturity (10 percent of the time, two eggs simultaneously reach maturity, which is how fraternal twins are conceived), rising estrogen levels signal the pituitary gland to send out *luteinizing hormone (LH)*. LH causes the ripe egg to burst out of its follicle, and out of the ovary. The *fimbria* (the fallopian tube's fingers) then reach out and grab the egg. This process is called *ovulation* (see figure 1.2). Even if two or more eggs are released, the hormonal sequence that results in ovulation occurs only once each cycle.

A ripe egg (about the size of the period at the end of this sentence) can live in the outer third of the fallopian tube for twelve to twenty-four hours. If there are sperm in the woman's cervix or if the couple has intercourse while an egg is alive in a fallopian tube, the sperm will swim up through the uterus and the fallopian tube, where they will try to fertilize the egg. It is not known how sperm sense that a ripe egg is available, but they can reach it in as little as thirty minutes. Fertilizing the egg is called *conception*.

If there are no sperm present in the cervix, and if the woman has no unprotected sexual intercourse while the egg is alive, then the egg will simply dissolve.

It's important to note that being fertile is not the same as ovulating. A woman is fertile when she has cervical fluid that can keep sperm alive; ovulation refers to the release of a mature egg and its twelve to twenty-four hour lifespan in a fallopian tube.

Before I describe what happens to a fertilized egg, let's go back to the follicle, which is now an empty sac, still residing in the ovary.

After ovulation, the follicle changes its name and its job. Now it's called the *corpus luteum,* and it emits the hormone *progesterone.* After ovulation, the menstrual cycle enters the *luteal phase.* Named for the corpus luteum, this postovulatory phase is dominated by progesterone.

When I hear "progesterone," I think *pro-gestation.* This hormone has several functions:

- It dries up cervical fluid. If you do become pregnant, progesterone helps form a sticky "mucus plug" over your cervix to keep bacteria from entering the uterus. This keeps your baby's environment sterile until birth.
- It warms your body temperature, because a fetus requires a slightly warmer temperature while it develops.
- It closes the os and hardens and lowers the cervix.
- It helps the new layer of your uterus become spongy, so that if you do conceive, the fertilized egg has bloody tissue in which to implant. If you don't conceive, the blood and tissue are released at menstruation.
- It also helps facilitate easy menstruation and ease the transition to menopause.

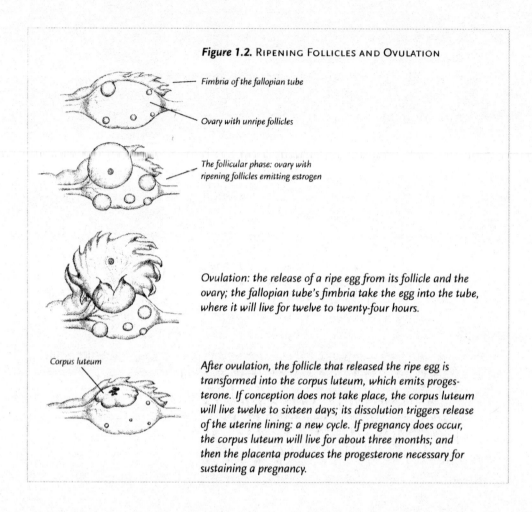

Figure 1.2. RIPENING FOLLICLES AND OVULATION

Fimbria of the fallopian tube

Ovary with unripe follicles

The follicular phase: ovary with ripening follicles emitting estrogen

Ovulation: the release of a ripe egg from its follicle and the ovary; the fallopian tube's fimbria take the egg into the tube, where it will live for twelve to twenty-four hours.

Corpus luteum

After ovulation, the follicle that released the ripe egg is transformed into the corpus luteum, which emits progesterone. If conception does not take place, the corpus luteum will live twelve to sixteen days; its dissolution triggers release of the uterine lining: a new cycle. If pregnancy does occur, the corpus luteum will live for about three months; and then the placenta produces the progesterone necessary for sustaining a pregnancy.

Progesterone is activated after ovulation whether you conceive or not. Typically, the corpus luteum will live (and emit progesterone) for twelve to sixteen days. If you don't become pregnant, the corpus luteum will die. As a result, your temperature will drop, and you won't have enough progesterone to sustain your uterine lining: menstruation will begin within a day or two.

Once about two hundred sperm reach the fallopian tube, they begin a cooperative project of softening the egg's enzymatic shell—so that one sperm can penetrate and fertilize the ripe egg.

If the egg is fertilized, *cilia* (whiplike cells that line the tube) take about five days to move the *conceptus* (the fertilized egg) down the tube to the uterus. Preg-

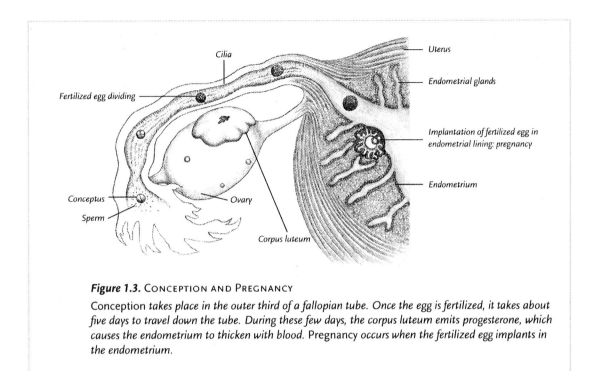

Figure 1.3. CONCEPTION AND PREGNANCY

Conception *takes place in the outer third of a fallopian tube. Once the egg is fertilized, it takes about five days to travel down the tube. During these few days, the corpus luteum emits progesterone, which causes the endometrium to thicken with blood. Pregnancy occurs when the fertilized egg implants in the endometrium.*

nancy occurs when the conceptus implants in the uterine lining (see figure 1.3). *Human chorionic gonadotropin (HCG),* the only hormone healthy men and women don't have in common, is then secreted by the fertilized egg itself; HCG instructs your body to nourish the growing fetus. Urine tests for determining pregnancy look for the presence of HCG. If pregnancy does occur, the corpus luteum will continue to emit progesterone for three months; and then the placenta takes over progesterone production.

To learn what happens to the menstrual cycle when a woman is on the Pill, see page 129 in chapter 7. Also, to see images of normal cycles and how the Pill affects them, www.fertilityawareness.net posts photographs of the cervixes of women who aren't on the Pill, and one who is.

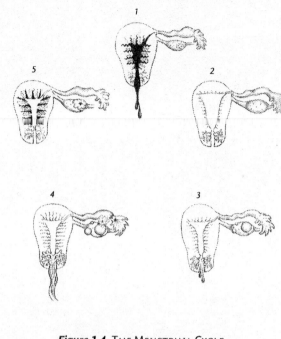

Figure 1.4. THE MENSTRUAL CYCLE

1. Menstruation begins when the corpus luteum dissolves and the previous cycle's uterine lining is released.

2. Typically, after her period, a woman has a few days of lowered hormonal activity. No mucus is produced and temperatures are low.

3. The follicular phase. About a dozen follicles (sacs holding unripe eggs) are given the impulse to mature and emit estrogen, which causes production of cervical fluid. (CF can keep sperm alive for up to five days.) Estrogen also cools a woman's basal temperature and signals the cervix to open, soften, and rise in the vaginal canal. It also signals the uterus to build a new, bloody lining. The follicular phase typically lasts seven to ten days. In some conditions, it can last for months or years.

4. Luteinizing hormone (LH), secreted by the pituitary gland, causes a ripe egg to burst from its follicle and the ovary. This is ovulation. Mucus may be very slippery at ovulation, or it may already have begun to dry up. The ripe egg will live in the tube for twelve to twenty-four hours.

5. The luteal phase. Here the corpus luteum emits progesterone, which makes the endometrium spongy, in case conception has occurred. (A spongy uterine lining is required for implantation—pregnancy—to be successful.) Progesterone also causes mucus to dry up; the temperature to warm up; and the cervix to close, become firm, and lower in the vaginal canal. If, after twelve to sixteen days, pregnancy has not occurred, the corpus luteum dissolves and a new cycle begins.

The Male Reproductive System

At puberty, the *pituitary gland* sends a hormonal message to a boy's *testicles* (male reproductive glands, which are protected inside a sac called the *scrotum*) to begin producing *testosterone*. With the activation of this hormone, the larynx becomes longer and the voice deepens; facial and body hair appear; the shoulders become broader; and production of sperm begins. Starting in adolescence, in the testicles' seminiferous tubules, a healthy man produces one thousand sperm per second— twenty-four hours a day, seven days a week. (As my grandmother would have said, this explains *a lot* of things.)

Men tend to produce more sperm during the winter, because sperm prefer a cooler temperature while they're maturing. It therefore follows that a man who bikes in tight shorts to the hot tub every day throughout the summer after work baking pizza might find himself with a low sperm count!

While sperm production and the ability to cause a pregnancy can continue until a man dies, age and decreased testosterone levels typically cause sperm production and the ability to have an erection to decrease. Also, because of environmental toxins, sperm counts are now decreasing at an alarming rate of 2 percent per year in men of all ages. But essentially, beginning at puberty, men are fertile *all the time.*

Once they're produced, sperm are matured and stored in the *epididymis,* a duct that is also held in the scrotum. The maturation process takes about two months: sperm produced at the beginning of January wouldn't be ejaculated until the beginning of March. Just before orgasm, sperm move from the testicles through the *vas deferens,* tubes that carry sperm to the urethra. Fluid is collected from the *prostate gland,* the *Cowper's glands,* and the *seminal vesicles* and then mixes with the sperm to create *semen,* which is then ejaculated through the urethra. Semen is chemically similar to cervical fluid, and it also provides nourishment to help keep sperm alive (see figure 1.5).

In a healthy man, each ejaculation contains between 250 and 350 million sperm. Typically, it takes thirty-six hours to replenish a man's sperm count.

With a vasectomy, the vas deferens are cut to prevent sperm from being ejaculated. Sperm are still produced and matured after a vasectomy, but they're prevented from being released through the penis. If a man has had a vasectomy, the amount of his ejaculate will still look the same: even 350 million sperm are not discernible to the naked eye.

Sperm are measured by their numbers, their ability to swim (motility), and their shape (morphology). If a man has a low sperm count, he should have it tested again a few weeks later, because sperm counts can fluctuate significantly in a short period of time.

It's also important to note that the *pre-ejaculate,* emitted during arousal, can contain enough sperm to cause a pregnancy or transmit a *sexually transmitted infection (STI).* And of course some STIs, such as herpes and human papilloma virus, are transmitted through mucous membranes (skin), not ejaculate or pre-ejaculate.

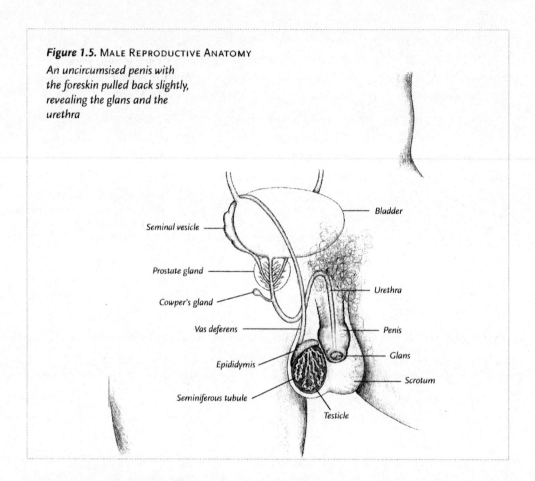

Figure 1.5. MALE REPRODUCTIVE ANATOMY

An uncircumsised penis with the foreskin pulled back slightly, revealing the glans and the urethra

Bladder

Seminal vesicle

Prostate gland

Cowper's gland

Urethra

Vas deferens

Penis

Epididymis

Glans

Scrotum

Seminiferous tubule

Testicle

COMPARATIVE ANATOMY:

1. The testicles are analogous to what in a woman?
2. Cervical fluid is similar to what in a man?
3. The vas deferens are like what in a woman?
4. The scrotum is similar to a woman's what?
5. The glans of the penis is analogous to what in a woman?
6. What is the only hormone that healthy men and women don't have in common?

Answers:

1. The ovaries—they're even similar in shape and size.
2. Seminal fluid. Like cervical fluid, it protects and nourishes sperm.
3. The fallopian tubes. Both male and female tubes are conduits through which sperm or a ripe egg must pass for pregnancy to occur.

SEMINAL IDEAS

To maintain health, how often should a man ejaculate?

Different cultures have different ideas. According to Chinese theory, while a woman's energy is actually strengthened by having orgasms, ejaculation depletes a man's body of *qi* (pronounced *chee*)—life force or essence.[1]

To determine how many days it takes to restore *qi* between ejaculations, Chinese theory suggests that a man multiply his age by two tenths.[2] Thus, a forty-year-old man (40 x .2 = 8) would space his ejaculations at least eight days apart; a twenty-year-old man (20 x .2 = 4) would space his ejaculations at least four days apart.

If a man is irresistibly aroused before the minimum amount of time has passed for his *qi* to be restored between ejaculations, non-ejaculatory sex is recommended. Some tantric practices teach men how to experience orgasm without releasing seminal fluid.

Meanwhile, some Christians believe that withholding ejaculate is a sin. This belief comes from the story of Onan in Genesis: when his older brother died, Onan was called to marry his widow, Tamar, to help her bear a son and continue the family's lineage. While he agreed to marry Tamar and to make love with her, Onan withdrew his penis before he ejaculated, and "spilled his seed" on the ground. Displeased, the Lord caused Onan to die.

To some Christians, this story shows that God expects us to be truthful to whatever we agree to do; and Onan's withholding ejaculate during lovemaking was like withholding his heart. Catholics who practice Natural Family Planning believe that if a couple seeks to avoid pregnancy, then condoms, non-ejaculatory sex, and/or sex that excludes intercourse (at any time during a woman's cycle) prevent them from giving themselves fully to their marital agreement—and these practices are thereby discouraged.

The extreme differences in these theories make me think there are as many ideas about what constitutes healthy sex (including healthy ejaculation) as there are people and cultures.

4. The labia. The scrotum and the labia evolve from the same cells, have a similar texture, and serve to protect the genitals.
5. The clitoris (although the clitoris has six thousand nerve endings, about twice as many as the penis).
6. Human chorionic gonadotropin (HCG), which signals pregnancy.

A New Language for Thinking About Fertility

As I began talking to other women who charted their fertility signals, I heard a new way of thinking and speaking about fertility. For example, since learning Fertility Awareness, the term *birth control* stopped making sense to me, because I don't know anyone who can control her body or her reproductive system. I can be *aware* of my body, *aware* of my fertility. I can be committed to strengthening my relationship to my body, to observing how it responds to different foods, environments, and lifestyle choices. I can chart my cervical fluid and waking temperature to know when I'm fertile and infertile—and then choose whether to have intercourse during my fertile phase. For me, this isn't birth control; it's Fertility Awareness.

I've also thought a lot about the word *menstruation*. Its Indo-European root, *me*, means "to measure." Moon, month, menopause, semester, and diameter all have the same root. From the beginning of time, women have measured their lives by their menstrual cycles or their lack of cycles. Knowing our anatomy and physiology can deepen our appreciation of our bodies and the wider cycles in nature.

The Hebrew word for menstruation, *niddah*, means "solitude." Far from the common understanding that Jewish laws were created to separate men from women who are menstruating because they're "unclean," the rabbis' intent was to guarantee women solitude every cycle.[3] In this way, a spirit of respect and courtship was encouraged, even in long marriages. Some Native Americans have a similar tradition: during menstruation, women separate themselves from the rest of their community and reside in a special tent. Through separation, the strong, dreamy powers of a menstruating woman are honored and revered.

OH, TO BE A RAT

- Some female butterflies, moths, and beetles appear to choose their mates based on the male's ability to provide healing plants. Before mating, as a sort of nuptial gift, the male offers herbs to his potential mate; and the female judges him by the strength of the plants' smells. She'll use the herbs for her own protection and also insert them into her eggs to protect them from predators and infection.[4]
- Female elephants are fertile for four days every four years; they communicate their fertility through vibrations made by their feet. After two years of gestation, mother elephants give birth after a few minutes of pushing. *Musth,* a state of heightened sexual and aggressive activity in adolescent male elephants, can be tamed by introducing older males to the population.[5, 6]
- Mantises, relatives of cockroaches, reproduce when the female beheads and eats her mate during copulation; in some of the mantises' two thousand species, this is the only way for the male to pass on his sperm.[7]
- Goats, rabbits, cats, marmots, rodents, and horses commonly terminate unwelcome pregnancies by resorbing very young fetuses into their bodies. Resorptions often occur with the arrival of a new adult male into the community, or perhaps because of the lack of resources for feeding a newborn.[8]
- Except humans, mammals routinely eat their placentas after birth.[9]
- After a female emperor penguin lays a one-pound egg, her male partner takes it into a pouch in his feet and incubates it for two to three months while he fasts. The mother goes off to the sea with other females in search of food; she often returns on the day of her chick's birth.[10]
- Rats reproduce in litters of six to twelve at a time as many as seven times each year.[11] After contractions lasting a few seconds, a mother rat pulls her babies out with her own mouth.[12]

As dancers, healers, and saints all know, when you turn your
attention toward even the simplest physical process—breath,
the small movements of the eyes, the turning of a foot midair—
what might have seemed dull matter suddenly awakens.

—SUSAN GRIFFIN
The Book of the Courteous

2. How to Observe and Chart Your Fertility Signals

YOUR FERTILITY SIGNALS OFFER A WAY TO tell you where you are in your menstrual cycle; they provide a way to read your body's hormonal shifts. If the first step toward knowing how to determine when you're fertile and infertile is learning reproductive anatomy, observing and charting your fertility signals every day is the second step.

Charting can expand your vocabulary and your conversation with your body. Like any language, it may take time to learn. Most women need at least two or three cycles to chart their signals confidently. If you're breast-feeding or coming off of hormonal contraceptives, it can take much longer.

Your Primary Fertility Signals

A woman has three primary fertility signals:

- Cervical fluid (and vaginal sensation).
- Basal body temperature.
- Cervix changes.

Cervical fluid (CF) is also called *cervical mucus,* or simply *mucus.* It's the stuff many women notice on their underwear—and may not know how to interpret. *Vaginal sensation* refers to the quality of wetness or dryness at the labia, the vaginal lips.

The *basal body temperature (BBT)* is a woman's waking temperature after at least three hours of rest. The BBT is cooler before ovulation and warmer after ovulation.

The *cervix* tends to be soft, open, and high in the vaginal canal when a woman is fertile; it tends to be firm, closed, and low in the vaginal canal during infertile phases.

For most women, charting mucus and the waking temperature gives enough information for using Fertility Awareness effectively. If you are breast-feeding or coming off the Pill or another hormonal medication, you may need to chart your cervix changes as well.

Once you get the hang of it, charting takes about two minutes of daily attention.

Cervical Fluid

When I first heard that Fertility Awareness meant charting my cervical mucus, I felt sure I wouldn't be able to do it right. I just didn't believe I could read my own secretions accurately enough to know when I'm fertile and infertile. I'm happy to say I proved myself wrong.

Cervical fluid is produced in the cervix's crypts with the help of estrogen. CF has four functions:

- It provides nourishment for sperm to live up to five days.
- It filters out abnormal sperm.
- Its alkaline quality protects sperm from the vagina's acidity.

• It provides a conduit for sperm to swim up through the uterus and fallopian tube at ovulation.

After the period, typically there's no CF. Then it progresses from a tacky quality to a creamy, then slippery, egg white–like texture. Then it returns to a dryer quality.

You will need to observe your cervical fluid three times a day. *Before* urinating, wash your hands. (Urinating can obscure your mucus reading.) Take a sample of cervical fluid by wiping the tip of your clean finger just inside your vagina. Some women prefer to sample their mucus with a folded square of toilet tissue. Just be sure to take your sample from the same place throughout the cycle.

Feel the sample before you look at it. (If you take your sample with toilet tissue, you still need to feel the CF with your fingers.) Is there anything there? If nothing's there, you could say that you're dry. If you're wondering how you could have "nothing there," have you ever tried for a sample of mucus in your nostril and found "nothing there"? Noticing dryness just inside the lips to your vagina is a similar observation.

If you do observe CF, the *consistency* might be sticky, milky, creamy, like egg white, or stretchy. Sticky is like the tacky paste you used in first grade. Creamy is like hand lotion. Egg white is like the whites of an egg you'd find in your fridge. (See figure 2.1 for an illustration of different consistencies of cervical fluid.)

You also want to notice if your cervical fluid is white, clear, or streaked.

If your mucus is yellow or greenish, has an odor, and/or doesn't change throughout the cycle, you should see a health-care provider about the possibility of a vaginal infection.

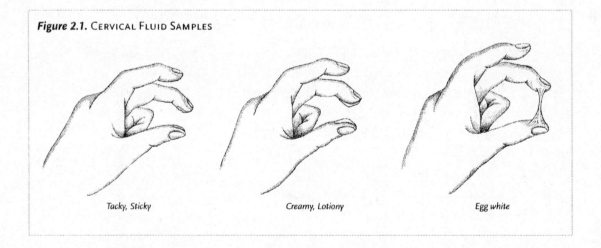

Figure 2.1. CERVICAL FLUID SAMPLES

Tacky, Sticky   Creamy, Lotiony   Egg white

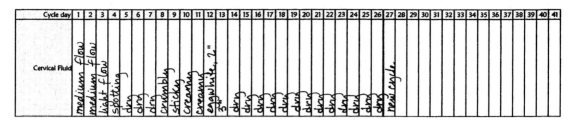

Cycle day	1	2	3	4	5	6	7	8	9	10	11	12	13	14	15	16	17	18	19	20	21	22	23	24	25	26	27	28	29	30	31	32	33	34	35	36	37	38	39	40	41
Cervical Fluid	medium flow	medium flow	light flow	spotting	dry	dry	crumbly	sticky	creamy	eggwhite, 2"	3"	dry	dry	dry	dry	dry	dry	dry	dry	dry	dry	dry	dry	new cycle																	

Figure 2.2.

To chart your mucus, write down your wettest sample from the day. This woman observed two inches of egg white on Day 12. On Day 13, when she observed three inches of egg white, she simply wrote 3".

At the end of the day, write down on your chart a description of the wettest sample of your mucus. For example, if your CF sample was dry in the morning, then creamy at noon, and tacky in the evening, at the end of the day you would write *creamy* (the wettest of these samples) on your chart. If you've got egg white that stretches to two inches, you could write *egg white, 2"*. For shorthand, you could write *2"*. For an example, see figure 2.2.

Some women describe their mucus as crumbly, milky, goopy, or bouncy. You need descriptions that make sense to you.

You can also describe the amount of mucus you observe: Is it scant or abundant?

Vaginal Sensation

Again, vaginal sensation refers to the quality of wetness or dryness at your vaginal lips. Typically, the labia are dry after the period, moist or wet before ovulation, and dry after ovulation. Wiping yourself with toilet tissue after urinating, you may notice that the lips of your vagina feel wet or moist—though you're not aroused. Or the sensation may be dry (though you've just urinated). Becoming familiar with your vaginal sensation is mainly about awareness. Essentially, you need to know if it's dry or wet.

Without needing to touch, most of us are aware if our nose's internal sensation is moist or dry. Charting your vaginal sensation requires becoming similarly alert to the moistness at your vaginal lips.

At the end of the day, record the wettest sensation from the day. *W* = wet or moist. *D* = dry. See figures 2.3 and 2.4 for some typical charts of mucus and vaginal sensation.

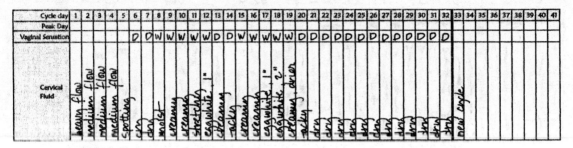

Figure 2.3.

On Day 12, her vaginal sensation was wet and she observed an inch of eggwhite. On Day 13, her vaginal sensation was dry, and the wettest mucus she observed was creamy.

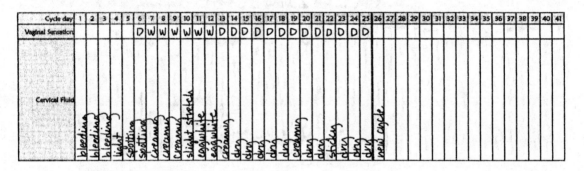

Figure 2.4.

This woman did not observe any dry days after her period. On Day 7, her vaginal sensation was wet, and she observed creamy mucus.

Factors That Can Affect Your Reading of Mucus or Vaginal Sensation

Sometimes, cervical fluid (specifically, the kind that's slippery, stretchy, egg white–like) and arousal fluid can look and feel the same. But arousal fluid is produced by the vaginal walls; its job is to lubricate the vagina so that intercourse isn't painful for the woman. It can't keep sperm alive or perform CF's other functions.

How do you tell the difference between arousal fluid and mucus? Once you're aroused, you can't tell from feeling or looking at it. So it's necessary to check your CF throughout the day.

Also, your mucus or vaginal sensation *might* be obscured if you:

- Take antihistamines (CF could be dryer than normal).
- Take cough syrup (CF could be runnier than normal).
- Swim in a chlorinated pool (CF could be dryer than normal).

- Have a vaginal infection (CF could be yellow, greenish, or like cottage cheese).
- Take the fertility drug Clomid (it can dry up mucus).

Women who take the Pill or other hormonal forms of birth control will not show a build-up in their cervical fluid pattern throughout their cycle—unless the drug isn't working properly.

If you are coming off the Pill, you may not notice a change in your CF for several cycles: it might be creamy, creamy, creamy for months. This is because progestin (synthetic progesterone) from the Pill thickens mucus so that sperm can't swim to a ripe egg (in the event of ovulation); and it can take a while for your cervix to resume healthy production of mucus. While I've seen women coming off the Pill return to a healthy CF pattern within a cycle or two, it typically takes at least three or four cycles.

If you are exclusively breast-feeding (not feeding your baby anything but your own milk), you may have a dry sensation and no mucus for as long as eighteen months or more. Once the baby sleeps through the night and/or begins drinking other fluids or eating solids, your mucus (and ovulatory cycles) will probably return. (See more about breast-feeding and Fertility Awareness in chapter 4.)

You can bleed and produce cervical fluid at the same time, *but you won't be able to read your cervical fluid when you're bleeding or spotting.* On days that you bleed or spot, in the section normally slated for CF, write down the color and quality of your blood (red, clotted, or perhaps dark brown and dryish). Also, write down the amount (heavy flow or perhaps spotting). Some physicians can use these observations to make a diagnosis about your health.

One more note about cervical fluid: some women's mucus doesn't change from day to day. It's always sticky, or just plain dry. It's never like egg white. Two weeks of this kind of mucus is called a *basic infertile pattern,* or *BIP.* A BIP is common in women who are not ovulating—perhaps because they are coming off the Pill, breast-feeding, or premenopausal. If you observe a BIP, please read the special section starting on page 43 in the next chapter.

Sage, twenty-four. It took me a long time to figure out when I'm dry and when I'm wet. It just wasn't obvious to me at first. Once I finally could tell the difference, after about four cycles, I started working as a nurse. During an eight-hour shift, I often have no chance to go to the bathroom—or check my mucus. Then I figured out that if I wear black underwear, I can see it, right there at the end of the day on my pants—unless it's a dry day.

KEGEL EXERCISES

If you have semen and/or spermicide in your vagina after intercourse, they can obscure your reading of your cervical mucus. Doing Kegel exercises can expel them. Kegel exercises are vaginal contractions: you slowly squeeze and release the pubococcygeal (pronounced pubo-cock-sa-gee-ul) muscle, which holds up your pelvic floor and can stop the flow of urine.

To tone your vaginal muscles, start by *slowly* squeezing and releasing the walls of your vagina for about ten pulses; try holding the contraction for five to ten seconds before you release it; try a few quick pulses. Gradually increase to about five sets of Kegel exercises each day.

You can do Kegel exercises while working at your computer, on the subway, while meditating or washing dishes, you name it.

Kegel exercises were developed in the 1940s by a gynecologist, Arnold Kegel, to help women who had bladder-control problems. People soon discovered that these exercises helped nourish women's and men's entire genital systems. Most known for helping women who are preparing for or recovering from childbirth, Kegel exercises can also be used by women to increase libido and the ability to experience orgasm, to prevent problems with incontinence, and to encourage lubrication before intercourse; and by men to strengthen their prostate gland, fertility, and sexual potency.

Basal Body Temperature (BBT)

The BBT is the body's temperature on waking, taken before activity begins.

To chart your BBT, you'll need a digital thermometer that will retain your last recorded temperature until you read it. Basal mercury thermometers are rarely available now. (If you do own one, it shouldn't measure above 100 degrees.)

- Place your thermometer on your nightstand, within easy reach and away from heat.
- Take your temperature every day when you wake up, ideally at the same time. If you take it at a markedly different time one day, record the time on the chart. (Typically, the temperature will rise about one tenth of a degree every half hour.)

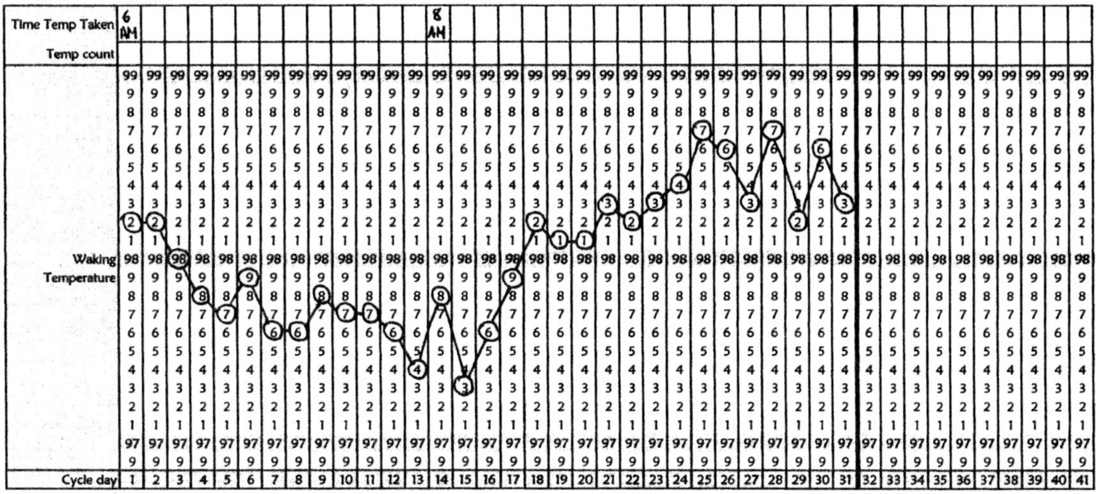

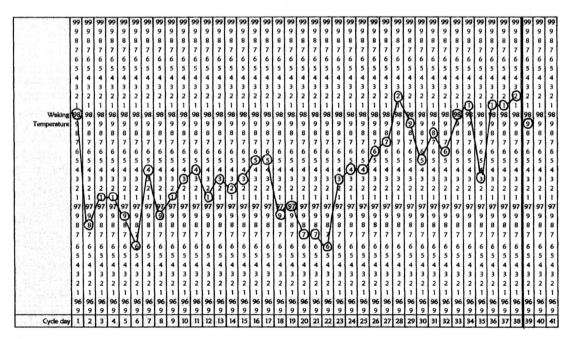

Figure 2.5.

This woman's temperature on Day 6 is 97.9; on Day 21, it's 98.3. On Day 14, this woman took her temperature at a different time than usual, so she marked the time on her chart.

Figure 2.6.

A sample BBT chart for a woman with low temperatures.

- Take your temperature in the same place (orally or under your arm) with the same thermometer throughout a cycle. Do not take it vaginally—women have accidentally inserted the thermometer into their urethra.
- Take your temperature before you eat, drink, make love, have a bowel movement, or climb stairs.
- You don't need to read or chart your temperature until you go to bed. If you keep the thermometer away from heat, it will retain an accurate reading.

Many women wake up early in the morning needing to urinate—then stay restlessly awake, waiting to use the bathroom until seven (or whenever they normally wake up) in order to get an accurate BBT. Practicing Fertility Awareness shouldn't mean suffering over a full bladder! Likewise, I'd rank a baby's cries above an accurate temperature reading—and encourage you to do the best you can to get a daily reading at a consistent time, as close as possible to the time you normally wake up.

If for some reason you want a second reading of your temperature, when using a digital thermometer you need to wait at least five minutes between readings for the second one to be accurate.

Your waking temperature can be affected by drinking alcohol the night before, sleeping embraced with a partner or child, sleeping with an electric blanket or on a heated waterbed, illness, restless sleep, traveling (especially between different time zones), and/or taking your temperature at a different time than usual. Typically, the BBT won't be affected by sleeping with extra blankets or in a room that's cooler or warmer than usual. If you think your temperature has been affected by one of these things—or something else—mark it on your chart (see figure 2.5 for a sample BBT chart).

Some women's waking temperatures are lower than 97.0 degrees. If yours are, you can use a chart that includes lower temps (see figure 2.6). Blank charts—for women with regular and low temperatures—can be found at the end of this book and on my website, www.fertilityawareness.net.

Cervix Changes

For most women, charting cervix changes is not necessary for effective use of Fertility Awareness. Charting these changes can be especially helpful when you're breast-feeding, coming off the Pill, or approaching menopause. At these times, mucus may be difficult to discern, and you may not be ovulating regularly, if at all. Observing your cervix can give you extra information so that you can more accurately determine when you're fertile. (And again, how to determine when you're fertile is explained in the next chapter. How to encourage healthy, ovulatory cycles is explained in part 2.)

Charting your cervix changes can also give helpful information if you're having difficulty conceiving.

For many women, the cervix is an "uncharted" body part. It may take a while to observe your cervix comfortably and to get the information you need for your chart. The more familiar you are with your cervix changes, the easier it will be to make use of them when you want the extra information this signal provides.

And the next time you have a pap smear, ask your practitioner for a mirror so you can *see* your cervix!

Wait until your period has ended to feel your cervix. Also, because it tends to be higher when you first wake up and may open slightly after a bowel movement, you might wait a half hour after waking and/or after you've had a bowel movement to check it. Check once a day, at about the same time, in the same position— perhaps before or after your morning shower. Squatting is the most effective position, since it pushes the cervix closest to the vaginal opening.

Wash your hands well, and insert your clean middle finger (with a trimmed nail) into your vaginal canal until you feel something like the tip of your nose. Find your cervix at the end of your vaginal canal, perhaps a little to the left or the right. The cervix's angle tends to be straight at ovulation and more tilted on infertile days.

You're checking for three things: the cervix's texture, the os's opening, and the cervix's location.

The texture might feel firm, like the tip of your nose, with a slight indentation or opening at the os. Or it might feel soft like your tongue.

The os could be closed, partly open, or fully open. If you've delivered a child vaginally, your os will be slightly more open and flatter than a woman who has not.

The cervix's location also changes throughout a typical cycle: it can be low, midway, or high in the vaginal canal.

The next chapter explains how to interpret these differences to determine when you're fertile and infertile.

To record your observations of your cervix's texture, use the letters *F, M,* or *S* to

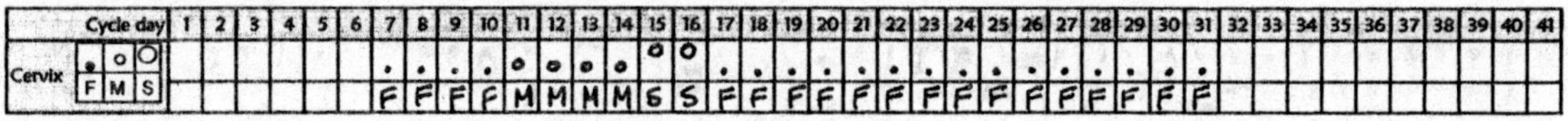

Cycle day	1	2	3	4	5	6	7	8	9	10	11	12	13	14	15	16	17	18	19	20	21	22	23	24	25	26	27	28	29	30	31	32	33	34	35	36	37	38	39	40	41
Cervix F M S							•	•	•	•	○	○	○	○	Ⓞ	Ⓞ	•	•	•	•	•	•	•	•	•	•	•	•	•	•	•										
							F	F	F	F	M	M	M	M	G	S	F	F	F	F	F	F	F	F	F	F	F	F	F	F	F										

Figure 2.7.

A chart of cervix changes might look like this: On Days 7 through 10, her cervix is low, firm, and closed. On Days 11 through 14, it's slightly higher, medium soft, and slightly open. On Days 15 and 16, it's high, soft, and open. On Days 17 through 31, it's again low, firm, and closed.

mean firm, medium, or soft. To record the os's opening and location, mark a closed or open circle low, midway, or high in the space provided on your chart (see figure 2.7).

Becoming familiar with your cervix can take practice. Changes are usually most obvious before and after ovulation.

Edie, thirty. In college, I read about a Catholic high school that was severely criticized for teaching Natural Family Planning. At the time, I thought it was very weird that a school would teach teenagers about their fertility. But now that I can read my own signals, I think it's awesome. I'm shocked that I was twenty-five and had had a child before I'd touched my cervix and learned that the goop I get every cycle is healthy cervical fluid.

In 1984, the Federation of Feminist Women's Health Centers published a fabulous book, *A New View of a Woman's Body*, featuring drawings by Suzann Gage (who also illustrated *this* book) and color photographs by Sylvia Morales of different women's cervixes throughout their cycles. These amazing photos show the cervixes of a twenty-nine-year-old lesbian who uses no birth control; a forty-six-year-old woman who's had one abortion and one birth; and a nineteen-year-old on the Pill. They can be seen on the Federation's website, www.womenshealthspecialists.org (in the self-help section), and on my website, www.gardenoffertility.com (in the section on female reproductive anatomy).

Also, www.woomb.org (click on "Behavior of the Cervix") has an animated video of mucus changes throughout the cycle. This site is posted by Australian physicians John and Evelyn Billings, who developed the Ovulation Method—Natural Family Planning by observing cervical fluid changes only.

Each of these is really worth a look!

Secondary Fertility Signals

Cervical fluid, the basal body temperature, and cervix changes are primary fertility signals. Most women can expect to observe these signals in a uniform way, and studies of CF and the BBT have created dependable rules for determining fertility and preventing pregnancy. Secondary signals include mittelschmerz (midcycle pain), saliva, spotting, breast tenderness, acne, and interest in sex. Secondary signals are commonly experienced, but not uniformly enough for them to determine dependably when you are fertile and infertile.

With mittelschmerz, for example, you might feel a dull ache or even a sharp pain near your ovaries around the time you ovulate. Researchers don't know for sure what causes either of these sensations, or why some women experience it and others don't. Some women observe mittelschmerz just before their primary signals indicate ovulation; others feel it afterward. The feeling might last a few minutes or a few hours. Some women mark the times when they experience mittelschmerz in the miscellaneous section of their chart.

Fertility indicators, available online or over the counter, also measure secondary signals. Some of them measure your estrogen levels by saliva: you lick a tiny acrylic slide on a microscope shaped like a lipstick, let it dry, then observe your sample by lighting the slide. If it looks like ferns (like the leaves of the potted plant), you're fertile. If the sample is just a bunch of bubbles, you're not fertile. Some ovulation indicators test your urine for luteinizing hormone.

Honestly, I've never known a Fertility Awareness teacher who found these gizmos to line up with her primary signals. Eventually, technology may advance for more accurate on-the-spot readings. For now, though, I certainly wouldn't trust them for anyone wanting to prevent pregnancy. I'm also hesitant to recommend these testers because they don't teach women how their bodies work; they teach how to read the tester.

Midcycle spotting, which tends to happen more frequently in long cycles, might be caused by a drop in estrogen just before ovulation. Some women consider it a secondary signal of ovulation. (Midcycle spotting or bleeding can also indicate problems, such as fibroids, endometriosis, and cervical or uterine cancer. If you are at all concerned, check with your doctor.) Other secondary fertility signs that some women experience around ovulation include abdominal bloating, increased energy, breast tenderness, and heightened senses.

One of my favorite stories about a secondary signal is from a woman who didn't ovulate for six months. On the day she ovulated, while wearing her usual T-shirt and jeans, five men invited her to bed! Indeed, a fertile woman is especially radiant. Male dogs all know when a neighborhood female is in heat—because of her smell. I'm sure that women also have nonverbal, subconscious ways of communicating when we're fertile—and that men can receive the signals. In fact, I know some couples who consider the man's interest in sex as a secondary fertility signal: when he's *very* interested, she's probably fertile.

How to Chart Your Own Research

The miscellaneous section at the bottom of the chart is for you to observe the things that are relevant to you. It can help you research your own health. I've known women who keep track of whether they eat sugar, exercise, feel depressed, have headaches, are interested in sex, take medication, receive acupuncture, you name it—to see if any of these might correlate with hormonal changes during their cycle. I've known women who observe the moon's phases in this section or their secondary fertility signals.

Some women check or color-code the boxes. Others rank how much sugar they eat (for example) on a scale from one to ten. It's your section to observe what you want to research!

Susie, nineteen. I decided to keep track of each day I go swimming, drink alcohol, or have restless sleep. It took only a few weeks for me to notice that I drank whenever I hung out with my old boyfriend, and that I had restless sleep on those nights I drank—or the next ones. I might not have thought about this if I hadn't been charting; but this way, I had concrete evidence and a clear message that hanging out with this guy wasn't good for me.

Charting Basics, Line by Line

Fertility Cycle
This refers to the number of cycles you have charted. If this is the second cycle that you're charting, put a number 2 here.

Start Date:

This is the date your menstrual period begins.

 # Days in Luteal Phase:

This refers to the number of days in your postovulatory phase. (You'll learn how and why to calculate this when you learn the rules for preventing or achieving pregnancy and for gauging gynecological health.)

 # Days This Cycle Length:

Refers to the number of days from the start of one cycle until the last day of that cycle. If, for example, you begin a new period on Day 1 and again on Day 32, your cycle would be 31 days long.

Cycle Day:

Day 1 is the day your menstrual period begins; Day 2 is the second day of your cycle; and so on.

Date:

Refers to the actual date—as in March 23. Some people circle the dates that fall on Saturdays and Sundays to locate the weekend easily.

Intercourse:

Check this column on the days you have unprotected intercourse. You can mark a *C* if you have intercourse with a condom, a *D* if you use a diaphragm, and a *P* for play that doesn't include genital-genital contact. (And while you're learning the method to prevent pregnancy, you may want to postpone genital-genital contact until you know how to discern when you're fertile and when you're not. Learning to read your mucus is much easier when it's not obscured by semen, spermicide, or lubricant.)

Temp Count:

This line is used to confirm ovulation by your temperature. The next chapter explains how.

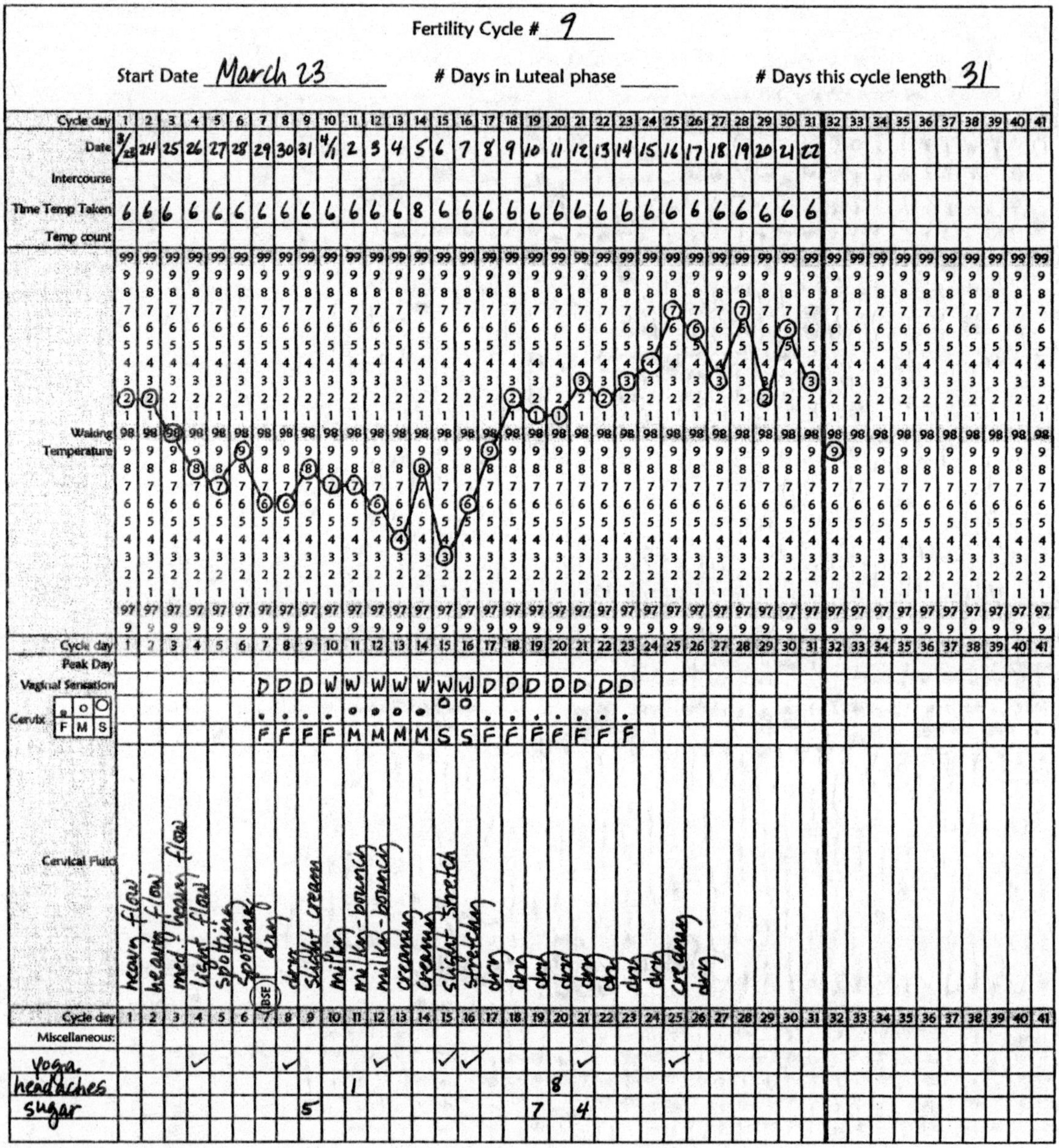

Fertility Cycle # 9

Start Date **March 23**   # Days in Luteal phase _____   # Days this cycle length **31**

Cycle day	1	2	3	4	5	6	7	8	9	10	11	12	13	14	15	16	17	18	19	20	21	22	23	24	25	26	27	28	29	30	31
Date	3/23	24	25	26	27	28	29	30	31	4/1	2	3	4	5	6	7	8	9	10	11	12	13	14	15	16	17	18	19	20	21	22
Intercourse																															
Time Temp Taken	6	6	6	6	6	6	6	6	6	6	6	6	6	8	6	6	6	6	6	6	6	6	6	6	6	6	6	6	6	6	6

(Waking Temperature graph — temperatures plotted on a scale from 97 to 99°F)

	1	2	3	4	5	6	7	8	9	10	11	12	13	14	15	16	17	18	19	20	21	22	23	24	25	26	27	28	29	30	31
Vaginal Sensation							D	D	D	W	W	W	W	W	W	W	W	D	D	D	D	D	D	D	D						
Cervix (dots)							•	•	•		•	•	•	•	○	○															
Cervix F/M/S							F	F	F	F	M	M	M	M	S	S	F	F	F	F	F	F	F	F							

Cervical Fluid notes: heavy flow, heavy flow, med.? heavy flow, light flow, spotting, spotting, dry (BSE), dry, slight cream, milky, milky–bouncy, milky–bouncy, creamy, creamy, slight stretch, stretchy, dry, dry, dry, dry, dry, dry, dry, dry, creamy, dry

Miscellaneous	1	2	3	4	5	6	7	8	9	10	11	12	13	14	15	16	17	18	19	20	21	22	23	24	25	26	27	28	29	30	31
yoga			✓				✓			✓			✓	✓			✓			✓											
headaches											1								8												
sugar								5											7	4											

Figure 2.8.

This woman has charted all of her primary fertility signals. She is also observing how yoga and sugar affect her cycle.

Waking Temperature:

Here you indicate your basal body temperature by circling the appropriate numbers. If your temperature is 98.0 (as it is on Day 3 in Figure 2.8), circle 98; if your temperature is 97.8 (as it is on Day 4 in Figure 2.8), circle the number 8 above the (gray) 97. Draw lines between your temperatures (connecting the dots) to make it easier to read your chart. If you take your temperature at a significantly different time than you usually do, be sure to mark the time on your chart. (See figure 2.5 on p. 24 for an example.) To mark the end of one cycle and the start of a new one, circle your temperature on the day that bleeding begins, but don't connect it to the previous day's temperature.

Peak Day:

This line is used to confirm ovulation by your cervical fluid. The next chapter explains how.

Vaginal Sensation:

Here's where you indicate the sensation at your vaginal lips. Mark *W* for moist or wet, *D* for dry.

Cervix:

Recording information about your cervix changes takes two lines. In each day's top box, draw a closed or open circle to show the openness of your cervix; place this circle low, midway, or high in the box to indicate your cervix's location in your vaginal canal. In the box below this circle, write an *F* if your cervix's texture was firm that day, *M* for medium, or *S* for soft.

Cervical Fluid:

Here you can record your blood flow and color (heavy, medium, light, or spotting; red or brown). After your period, write down dry when you observe no mucus throughout the day. When you do observe CF, record your wettest sample from the day—sticky, creamy, egg white, or stretchy.

BSE:

BSE stands for Breast Self-Exam. Day 7 of each cycle is a good day to examine your breasts, since you're least likely after your period to have lumps caused by progesterone. While most lumps are benign, if you have one that does not dissolve with your new cycle, get it checked by your health-care practitioner. Become familiar with your breasts and use "BSE" on your chart as a reminder to check them monthly. Once you've checked, you can circle BSE on your chart.

Miscellaneous:

This section is for observing whatever you consider relevant—perhaps the days you exercise, eat sugar, or experience headaches. For example, write "yoga" on the line at the left and then check each day that you practice it.

Remember, you don't have to wait for your next period to begin charting. Say your last period started ten days ago. You can check your mucus and vaginal sensation and begin charting them on Day 10. Get yourself a thermometer, take your temperature on the morning of Day 11, and you're on your way. Depending on where you are in your cycle, you may be able to use this first chart to determine several aspects of your gynecological health.

Many women find that the hardest part of charting is getting into the habit of it. Once you're in the habit, it's easy to continue. Call on a girlfriend who's also learning FA (or who already practices it). Writing down your questions can also engage you with the method. If you want to use your charts to prevent pregnancy, I can't encourage you enough to double-check your interpretation of them with a teacher. (See "How to Find a Teacher" on p. 231 for more information.)

For Women in Special Circumstances

If you are coming off the Pill, consider the first day of withdrawal bleeding (during your week off the Pill) as Day 1; then begin charting as usual.

If you've recently stopped using the Pill, Depo-Provera, an IUD, or a fertility-stimulating drug like Clomid, it may take a few cycles or more for your fertility signals to be restored to their natural pattern. If you've recently given birth, had a miscarriage or an abortion, or you're breast-feeding, it may also take your body a while to resume regular, ovulatory cycles. Or, you might return quickly to a healthy, discernible pattern. As your hormones readjust, you might also notice new challenges surfacing in places like your emotional balance, your skin, your relationship with your partner. These are all challenges to know yourself more deeply. Be patient and gentle with yourself!

Charting your signals can be a fascinating pleasure. For some women, however, it's a frustration. If you find that's the case, give your charts a rest and focus on nurturing yourself in other ways.

If you are taking medication (prescription drugs, herbs, homeopathic remedies, etc.), check with your practitioner to see how your fertility signals might be affected. Toni Weschler's *Taking Charge of Your Fertility* and *The Art of Natural Family Planning* by John and Sheila Kippley both include information about the effects of various drugs on fertility signals.

Martha, fifty-two. I charted my fertility signals through my childbearing years even though I didn't need to prevent pregnancy, and I wasn't trying to become pregnant, either. I'm a lesbian. I wanted to know what was going on with my body, and Fertility Awareness gave me a foundation for that.

Louise Lacey, author of Lunaception. I read my charts like they were sheets of music. Better than any photograph, they represented the "real" me.

Learning Fertility Awareness

When I teach Fertility Awareness, I break the class into four sections. The information you've read so far (on reproductive anatomy and how to observe and chart your fertility signals) is covered in the first class. In the second class, we go over the rules for preventing pregnancy and how to enhance your chances of conceiving. In the third class, we go over the rules again, using the tests in the appendix; and I also talk about how to use charts to gauge gynecological health. The last class presents options for addressing nutritional and emotional concerns that come up for people who chart; and people often share the personal observations they've made since practicing Fertility Awareness.

For most people, absorbing the amazing information about how our bodies work (which you've just read in these first two chapters) is a lot to take in. Getting started with charting, rereading these chapters, sharing the info with your partner and/or a girlfriend, writing in a journal what it's like to understand your reproductive system—all these things can deepen your understanding.

When you feel comfortable with the vocabulary of the menstrual cycle and you've had a good week or two to chart, go on to the next chapter—about preventing pregnancy. If you want to conceive, I recommend reading this chapter as well, because it explains how to determine when you're about to ovulate and how to confirm that you *have* ovulated.

For the record, I usually space my classes three to four weeks apart so that people have plenty of time to raise questions as they learn the method. Of course, the beauty of learning from this book is that you can do it at your own pace and refer back to the basic information as often as you need.

To feel confident about my ability to prevent pregnancy,
I need to know when I'm fertile and when I'm not.
Artificial birth control is too risky for me. Charting
my fertility signals is the only way.

—CARRIE
thirty-five years old, 126 charted cycles
(and no pregnancy)

3. The Rules for Using Fertility Awareness to Prevent Pregnancy

ACCORDING TO NUMEROUS STUDIES, FERtility Awareness is virtually as effective as the Pill in preventing pregnancy *if you follow the rules*. Following the rules means charting your signals every day, understanding the rules, and using them conscientiously.

Fertility Awareness teachers like to repeat, *When in doubt, don't*. Risking an undesired pregnancy and worrying that you might have had sex on a fertile day is not effective use of the method. Being confident in your understanding of the rules is a necessary part of FA's effectiveness. While you're learning, make love without genital-genital contact, or use a barrier method. Most people take several cycles before they are confident in their understanding of the rules and able to use the method.

Fertility Awareness is known as the cooperative method for preventing pregnancy. If both partners fully understand how to read a fertility chart, then the responsibility of postponing intercourse or using a barrier method during the fertile phase becomes a joint venture. Practicing FA brings questions about sexuality, health, gender, and family to the fore; it creates an arena for talking directly about these matters and shows how they're intimately connected with your fertility. Learning the method requires focused attention, patience, and cooperation.

A woman I know who just began learning Fertility Awareness told her lover that if she became pregnant unintentionally, she'd keep the baby. This startled her partner and made him doubt the method's effectiveness. For me, the conversations that follow these kinds of differences are part of the beauty of using Fertility Awareness.

To learn the method well, reread this chapter several times, then take the tests in the appendix (pages 238 to 251) to confirm what you know and to answer your questions. Ask your partner to take the tests, too; and talk your answers through with an FA teacher until you are clear.

FA is not for everyone. If the daily discipline of charting (and sometimes postponing intercourse or using a barrier method) isn't for you right now, acknowledge it and don't use this method to prevent pregnancy. Pat yourself on the back for knowing your limitations and acting on them.

No method is 100 percent effective in preventing pregnancy. Women have become pregnant while on the Pill, Depo-Provera, and Norplant; while using a diaphragm, a cervical cap, an IUD, a condom. Women have become pregnant after having their fallopian tubes tied and after their partners have had vasectomies. I even know of a woman who got pregnant unexpectedly at fifty-three, three years after her last period.

And still, Fertility Awareness can have a bad reputation, because many people trust drugs and devices more than a woman's observations of her own body's signals. If you use this method to prevent pregnancy, you have responsibility to yourself and to the method to chart diligently and to understand and follow the rules as well as you'd want anyone behind a wheel in your neighborhood to know how to drive a car.

Here then are the rules. And a reminder: being *infertile* means that unprotected intercourse will not lead to pregnancy. Being *fertile* means that unprotected intercourse can lead to pregnancy.

During the Menstrual Period

Most women will not conceive if they have intercourse during the menstrual period. *However!* It is possible to become pregnant as a result of sex during your period. It happens like this: while you're still bleeding or spotting, your follicles could be mature enough to produce estrogen—which causes your cervix to produce cervical fluid. When you're bleeding or spotting, you can't tell whether you have cervical fluid present.

Say you have intercourse on Day 4, while you're still bleeding—and, unbeknownst to you, you also begin producing mucus (which can keep sperm alive for up to five days) during Day 4. Menstrual blood, cervical fluid, and sperm can all live happily together in the cervix—until you ovulate (say) five days later, on Day 9, with sperm on the ready for travel to your ripe egg.

The only rule for determining whether you're fertile while menstruating is based on *past* cycles. You need to have had a clear temperature shift that confirmed ovulation in your previous cycle. You also need to know the exact length of your past twelve cycles:

- If your last twelve cycles have all been twenty-six days or longer, you can consider yourself infertile during your period's first five days.
- If any of your last twelve cycles have been twenty-five days or less, you can only consider yourself infertile during your cycle's first three days.

If you've ever had a short cycle and are definitively not open to a pregnancy, don't take the risk. Also, premenopausal women should always consider the period potentially fertile, since hormonal changes during the years approaching menopause can result in dramatically early ovulation.

Gauging When You Are Fertile and Infertile by Cervical Fluid

Typically, after the menstrual period, a woman will observe a dry vaginal sensation and no mucus for several days. (Mucus, cervical fluid, and CF all refer to the same stuff. If you need clarification of what "dry vaginal sensation and no mucus" means, reread chapter 2.) Without CF, sperm cannot survive for longer than four hours.

THE RHYTHM METHOD VS. FERTILITY AWARENESS

The Rhythm Method is based on a math formula that determines a woman's fertility by her previous cycles. The formula comes from the idea that most women begin menstruating about fourteen days after they ovulate: the luteal (postovulatory) phase is usually about two weeks long. In the 1930s, after two surgeons independently discovered this information, a Dutch physician created a formula so that women could approximate their fertile time. (You can read more about this in "The Many Names of Fertility Awareness," on page 225 in the appendix.)

Called the Rhythm Method, this initial formula proved ineffective for most women because most women's cycles are not consistently predictable. The follicular (preovulatory) phase is especially unpredictable. A woman might ovulate on Day 10 in one cycle and Day 20 in another. The luteal phase is more predictable, because it won't last longer than sixteen days unless the woman is pregnant (or she has a rare, luteal cyst). But it, too, can still vary from cycle to cycle. Indeed, many factors can affect the regularity of a woman's cycles: illness, travel, diet, stress, or lifestyle changes. While many of us are taught to expect twenty-eight-day cycles (fourteen days before ovulation, fourteen days after ovulation), few women have them. And many women's cycles change from month to month. Because it's based on past cycles, the Rhythm Method can lead to an unintended pregnancy *or* incorrect timing of intercourse for a desired pregnancy.

With Fertility Awareness, you're charting your fertility signals every day so that you can discern when you are and aren't fertile day by day. To use this method effectively, a predictable "textbook cycle" isn't required. Charting your signals—and knowing how to interpret your charts—is what makes Fertility Awareness effective.

Typically, after two or three dry days, vaginal sensation becomes moist, and cervical fluid begins building up. Often, the mucus begins with a tacky texture. From there it usually builds to a creamy consistency; then it becomes stretchy, like egg white.

The presence of wet vaginal sensation *or* any cervical fluid after menstruation signals that your follicular (fertile) phase has begun. Follicles (containing unripe eggs) are now maturing and emitting estrogen. Estrogen stimulates the production of mucus, which can keep sperm alive for up to five days. *As soon as you ob-*

serve a moist vaginal sensation or the presence of CF after your period, you are potentially fertile.

In a "textbook" cycle, the cervical fluid will build to a slippery texture—like egg white—just before ovulation; and then it will transition to a dryer texture. Vaginal sensation will also dry up after ovulation. Typically, these will both stay dry through the end of the cycle.

Of course not all cycles are "textbook." For example, mucus can show up during or immediately after the period.

After Menstruation and Before Ovulation Rules

Unintended pregnancies usually result from sex that happens before ovulation, in the fertile, preovulatory phase. They can be avoided if you know how to recognize that you're fertile. Once you confirm that ovulation has occurred and your egg(s) are dead and gone, you can make love without risk of becoming pregnant—until your next cycle begins. But let's go back to the days after your period, before you've ovulated.

If your vaginal sensation is moist and/or if you have cervical fluid present in the days immediately after your period, then you do not have an infertile phase before you ovulate. This typically happens in women with shorter cycles. (See figure 3.3.)

After menstruation, if you observe dry sensation and no cervical fluid three times throughout the day, you are considered infertile after 6 P.M. of that day.

The following day (whether or not you had intercourse the night before), you need to observe your vaginal sensation and cervical fluid again to determine whether you are fertile or infertile. If, once again, you observe dry sensation and no mucus three times throughout the day, you are again infertile after 6 P.M. of that day.

What's the reasoning behind this rule? Without mucus, the vagina creates an acidic environment that is hostile to sperm. Without mucus, sperm can't live longer than thirty minutes to four hours. Studies show that if you've been dry all day and you have intercourse after 6 P.M. on that day, your risk of conceiving is less than 2 percent (see figure 3.1).

If you do have intercourse in the evening of a dry day, Kegels after intercourse can expel the semen—so that it doesn't obscure your mucus readings on the following day. (See p. 22 for a description of how to do Kegels.)

Again, any wet sensation or cervical fluid after the period (and before ovulation) signals that you are fertile: you've got mucus that can keep sperm alive until you ovulate. You have entered your fertile phase. You need to consider yourself fertile until your chart confirms that you have ovulated and that your egg or eggs are dead and gone. Here are three charts that show how to determine whether you're fertile after your period, before you ovulate.

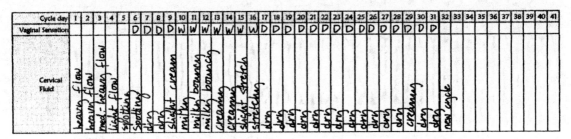

Figure 3.1.

After the period and before ovulation, this woman observed dry sensation and dry CF on Days 7 and 8. She is safe for intercourse on these days after 6 P.M.

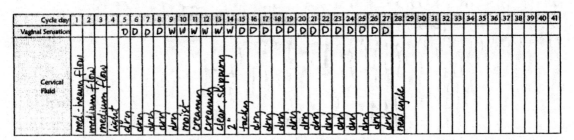

Figure 3.2.

This woman is infertile after 6 P.M. on Days 5 through 8. Her fertile phase begins on Day 9, because her vaginal sensation is wet on Day 9.

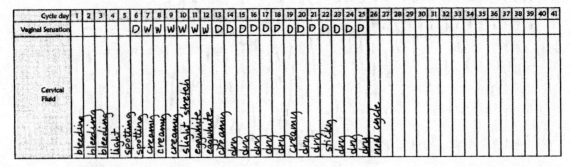

Figure 3.3.

This woman does not have any dry days after her period. She therefore needs to consider herself fertile until she can confirm ovulation.

Ovulation and the Peak Day Rule

To use cervical fluid to confirm that you've ovulated, you first need to identify your *Peak Day*. The Peak Day is the *last* day of moist vaginal sensation or wet mucus, and it signals that ovulation is about to take place. The Peak Day is not your *wettest* day, but the *last* day of wetness before a drying pattern begins. You can't identify your Peak Day until the *next* day, when your CF starts to dry up.

While the Peak Day typically signals that ovulation is about to take place, the release of your egg(s) can actually take place plus or minus two days from your Peak Day.

Say you observe cervical fluid that builds up from tacky, to creamy, then egg white; then you have a day of moist vaginal sensation and no mucus followed by a day of dry sensation and tacky mucus. The day you had moist sensation would be called your Peak Day.

Mark the Peak Day with a *P* on your chart. Mark the following day (when you transition to dryer vaginal sensation and mucus) with a *1*. Subsequent dryer days are marked *2, 3,* and *4*. You are considered infertile after 6 P.M. on the fourth day of mucus that's dryer than it was on your Peak Day.

You need to wait four days after the Peak Day before you have intercourse, because it's possible that you won't begin to ovulate until two days after your peak. At ovulation, you can release two eggs within twenty-four hours of each other (as with fraternal twins), and each of these eggs can live a maximum of twenty-four hours. This adds up to four days after the peak (see figure 3.4).

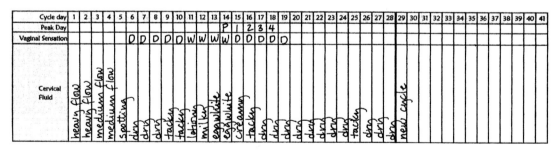

Cycle day	1	2	3	4	5	6	7	8	9	10	11	12	13	14	15	16	17	18	19	20	21	22	23	24	25	26	27	28	29	30	31	32	33	34	35	36	37	38	39	40	41
Peak Day														P	1	2	3	4																							
Vaginal Sensation						D	D	D	D	D	W	W	W	W	D	D	D	D	D																						
Cervical Fluid	heavy flow	heavy flow	medium flow	medium flow	spotting	dry	dry	tacky	tacky	lotiony	milky	eggwhite	eggwhite	creamy	tacky	dry	dry	dry	dry	dry	dry	tacky	dry	dry	new cycle																

Figure 3.4.

This woman's postovulatory infertile phase begins after 6 P.M. on Day 18.

Note that tacky mucus before ovulation typically signals that you're fertile. After ovulation, tacky mucus can be infertile—if it's dryer than Peak Day mucus. Here's a ranking of mucus variations in terms of dryness to wetness:

- Dry.
- Tacky or sticky.
- Creamy or lotiony.
- Egg white or slippery.

So, if you've got egg white followed by a day of creamy mucus with a dry sensation, the day of egg white would be your Peak Day. (See figure 3.4.)

If, however, a day with egg white was followed by a day of creamy mucus and a

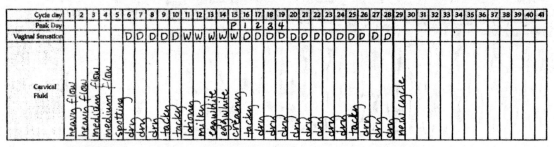

Figure 3.5.

This woman's mucus has begun drying up on Day 15. But because Day 15 is her last day of wet vaginal sensation, it's her Peak Day. Her postovulatory infertile phase begins on Day 19, after 6 P.M.

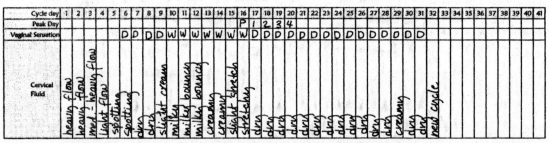

Figure 3.6.

This woman's Peak Day is Day 16. Her postovulatory infertile phase begins on Day 20, after 6 P.M.

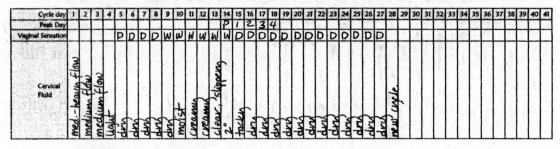

Figure 3.7.

This woman's Peak Day is Day 14. Her postovulatory infertile phase begins on Day 18, after 6 P.M.

wet sensation, and then the next day you had tacky mucus with a dry sensation, the day of creamy mucus and wet sensation would be your peak. (See figure 3.5.)

Split Peaks

Sometimes, your cervical fluid may show a "split peak." In this case, your body prepares to ovulate, and your CF builds up, but you don't ovulate. After drying up, you begin producing mucus again. You'll know you haven't ovulated during a false peak because your temperature won't rise and stay high for at least three consecutive days. (See the section about using the waking temperature to confirm ovulation, beginning on page 45.)

With a *split peak,* your mucus builds up again—possibly several times—until you finally do ovulate. (It's also possible to bleed without ovulating after a split peak or peaks—this would be called *withdrawal bleeding,* not a menstrual period.) Split peaks are common among women with long cycles, including those who are breast-feeding or coming off the Pill. They can also happen when you're under stress. If they occur more than once a year because of stress, you may be at risk for ovarian cysts: essentially, you've got follicles developing, but not enough hormonal activity to cause ovulation. In any case, the possibility of a split peak is an excellent reason to chart every day *and* to observe your waking temperature to confirm ovulation (see figure 3.8).

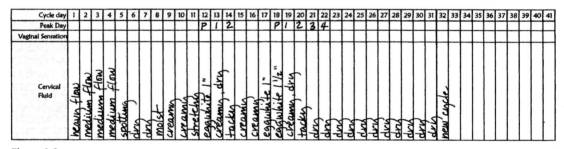

Figure 3.8.

Here's a chart of a split peak. This woman is infertile after 6 P.M. on Days 6 and 7. Her fertile phase begins on Day 8. She has a false peak on Day 12. Her true peak is on Day 18. Her postovulatory infertile phase begins on Day 22, after 6 P.M.

Anovulation and the Basic Infertile Pattern (BIP)

If your mucus pattern isn't typical (progressing from dry to sticky, to creamy, to an egg white peak, then to dryer mucus), you may be challenged to discern when you're fertile and not fertile. You may be ovulating infrequently, or not at all. While charting can still provide valuable information about your gynecological health (read more in chapter 6), using the method to prevent pregnancy can be frustrating. If you are ovulating, you can use the temperature to determine when you're in your postovulatory, infertile phase. In any case, you need to consider yourself potentially fertile until you can prove otherwise. To prevent pregnancy, you can make love without genital-genital contact, or use a barrier method (condoms, diaphragm, cervical cap) until regular, ovulatory cycles resume.

How do you prove infertility by CF? Your mucus will show what's called a *basic infertile pattern* (BIP). You'll observe cervical fluid that doesn't change. It'll be dry or sticky—or some combination of these—and you won't observe egg white. Your vaginal sensation will be dry; and you won't observe a temperature shift.

To determine your BIP, you need to observe your mucus for two weeks. During this time, ideally, you abstain from intercourse to prevent semen or spermicide from obscuring your observations.

Once you establish your basic infertile pattern, you can apply the following two rules to prevent pregnancy:

1. You are safe for unprotected intercourse during the evening of each day your mucus is dry or sticky (as it appears in your BIP).
2. If you observe a change in your BIP, locate your Peak Day (the *last* day of wet mucus); and consider yourself fertile until the evening of the fourth consecutive day after your peak. (See figure 3.9.)

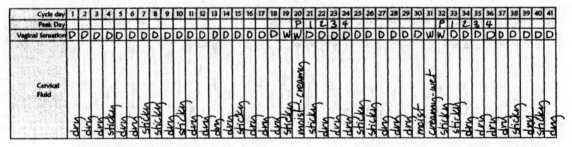

Figure 3.9.

This woman is establishing her BIP Days 1 through 14. Her vaginal sensation is continuously dry, and her CF is either dry or sticky during these two weeks. When she observes wet sensation or moist mucus, she considers herself fertile, and waits for four days after her Peak Days before considering herself infertile again. This woman is safe for intercourse on the evenings of Days 15 through 18, 24 through 29, and 36 through 41.

If your BIP is always moist or wet, you need to consider yourself fertile. Your cervix can be observed as a cross-check to confirm your observations of mucus and vaginal sensation.

Women who don't ovulate are often very motivated by their charts to strengthen their gynecological health—perhaps through diet, a change in night-lighting, exercise, or pace. (Part 2 offers many suggestions for addressing anovulation.) And even the most motivated of women may feel very frustrated. Be gentle with thyself!

Using the Basal Body Temperature (BBT) to Prevent Pregnancy

Before ovulation, while follicles emit estrogen, your body is cooler. After ovulation, your temperature will rise and remain high. (After releasing its egg, the follicle transforms into a corpus luteum and emits progesterone, a warming hormone.) In a healthy cycle, your basal temperatures will remain warmer until your corpus luteum dies and a new menstrual cycle begins.

Before ovulation, the waking temperature cannot tell you when you're fertile or infertile. You still need to take your basal body temperature (BBT) every day—so that you can compare low and high temperatures and confirm that ovulation has taken place. Daily recording can also provide valuable information about your overall health.

Confirming Ovulation by the BBT

Throughout your cycle, you'll observe small rises and falls of your temperature. To use your BBT to confirm that you've ovulated and are no longer fertile in a cycle, you need a cluster of low temps in relation to a cluster of high ones that *stay* high. You need a line—called a *coverline*—that separates your lower, preovulatory temperatures from your higher, postovulatory ones.

To draw your coverline:

- First look for a rise in temperature (at least two tenths of a degree higher than any of your last six temperatures).
- Put your finger on the low temperature before the rise.
- Starting with this first low temp before the rise, count back six temps.
- Locate the highest of these six temperatures.

- Draw a line one tenth of a degree above the temperature that is the highest of this cluster of six: this is your coverline. Its location will probably change from cycle to cycle.

You're considered infertile after 6 P.M. on the evening of your third *consecutively* high temperature above your coverline. You need to wait for *three consecutive* high temperatures above your coverline because you might not ovulate until twenty-four hours after the rise. Then, 10 percent of the time, women release two eggs at ovulation. Say each of these two eggs lives twenty-four hours. If the first egg wasn't released until twenty-four hours after the rise, and you had two eggs living twenty-four hours each, you'd be fertile for three days after the rise in temperature.

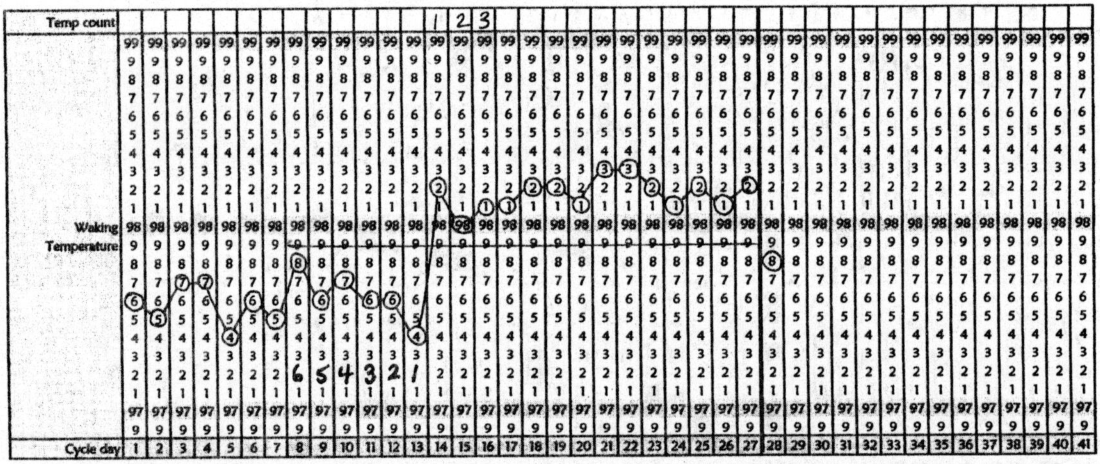

Figure 3.10.

She has a rise in temperature on Day 14. To draw her coverline, put your finger on her temperature on Day 13. Counting Day 13 as your first temperature, count back six (to Day 8). The highest of these six low temperatures is 97.8 degrees. Her coverline is therefore at 97.9 degrees.

To determine when the infertile phase begins, you need to count three consecutive temperatures above the coverline. Here, Days 14, 15, and 16 are consecutively above the line. Her postovulatory infertile phase begins on Day 16, after 6 P.M.

In figure 3.11, notice the rise between Days 13 and 14. If, on Day 13 you begin counting back six temperatures and draw a coverline at 97.9 degrees (one tenth of a degree above the highest of the cluster of six low temperatures [Day 9]), then Days 15 and 16 fall *below* the line, and Day 17 falls right *on* it. In this chart, a coverline at 97.9 degrees doesn't work: it doesn't separate the follicular and luteal phases.

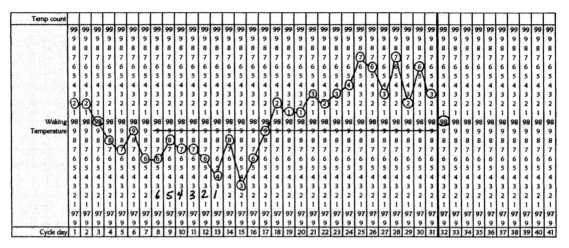

Figure 3.11.

Still trying to locate a working coverline on the same chart (see figure 3.12), on Day 18, there's another rise in temperature. On Day 17, begin counting back six temperatures, and locate the highest of these (97.9). Draw a line at 98.0 degrees (one tenth of a degree higher than 97.9). Days 18, 19, and 20 are consecutively above the line! Her postovulatory infertile phase begins on Day 20, after 6 P.M.

You can discount one of your six temperatures before the rise if it appears significantly different from the other five. Say you had a restless night and woke with an unusually high BBT—if it's just one unusually high temp, you can cross it out (see figure 3.13).

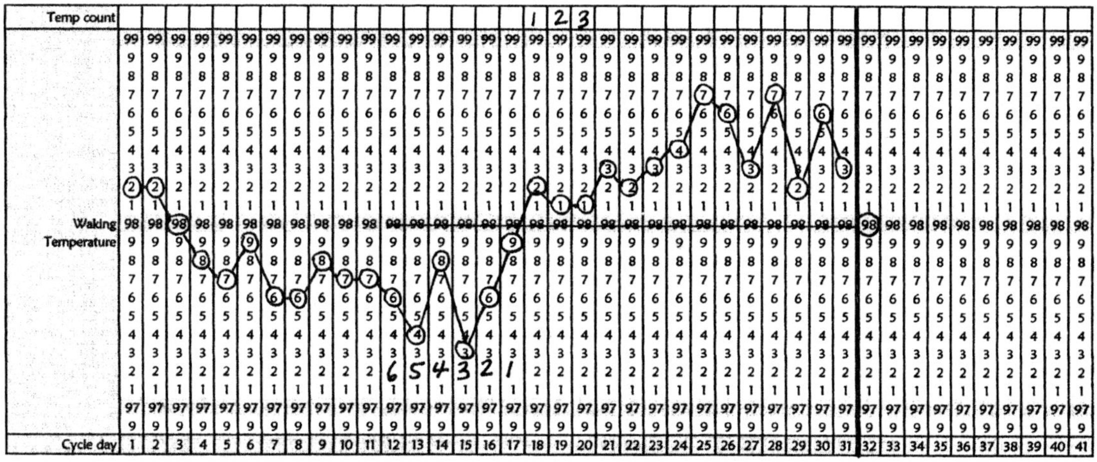

Figure 3.12.

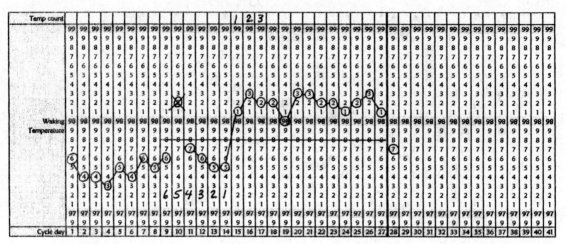

Figure 3.13.

Because this woman's temperature on Day 10 is significantly different from the other five before her temperature shift on Day 15, it can be discounted when she draws her coverline.

(18)

Determining Pregnancy by the BBT

The luteal (postovulatory, progesterone-dominant) phase typically lasts twelve to sixteen days; then a new cycle begins. If your luteal phase is eighteen days long (if you have eighteen high temperatures after ovulating and no period), then you're probably pregnant. You need eighteen days because it's possible that you don't conceive until a second egg is released two days after ovulation; add those two days plus sixteen

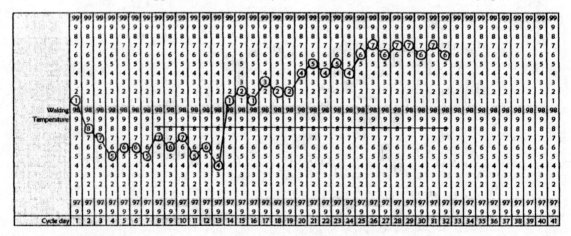

Figure 3.14.

This women's temperature chart confirms that she is pregnant on Day 31, when she has eighteen temps above her coverline.

(the maximum length of the luteal phase unless you're pregnant), and you get eighteen. The only exception to this rule is a corpus luteum cyst, which is very rare.

Figure 3.14 is a pregnant woman's chart. Note that after ovulation, every five to six days, her temperature goes up a degree or two, creating three levels of temperatures. This "tri-phasic" shift, due to the effect of HCG, the pregnancy hormone, is typical (but not necessarily present) with pregnancy. She can confirm that she's pregnant on Day 31. If this woman's temperature dropped and she began bleeding on (say) Day 33, that would signify a miscarriage—not a "late period."

WAKING LATE, WAKING EARLY

If you take your temperature at a different time than usual (say you sleep late, or wake early), mark the unusual time on your chart. Typically, the basal temperature goes up one tenth of a degree every half hour. Noting the time on your chart could help explain an aberrant temperature. However, adjusting temperatures can cause trouble. I recently spoke with a woman who began a new job (and waking an hour and a half earlier) mid-cycle. She added three tenths of a degree to each temperature, drew a coverline based on the adjustment, didn't include a split peak in her calculations, and became pregnant unintentionally. Be alert that a temperature taken at an unusual time may not be reliable.

Cervix Changes

Most of the time, cervix changes aren't necessary for determining when you're fertile or infertile. But when you're breast-feeding, coming off the Pill, wanting to conceive, or approaching menopause, this signal can be very helpful.

When you're fertile, the cervix is soft and high in the vaginal canal, and the os is open. When you're not fertile, the cervix is firm and lower in the vaginal canal; and (except when you're menstruating) the os is closed.

If, before ovulation, your CF and vaginal sensation are dry but your cervix is open, soft, or high—consider yourself potentially fertile. In the preovulatory phase, the cervix's signal of potential fertility overrides the infertility signaled by dry mucus and dry vaginal sensation (see figure 3.15).

While studies of the effectiveness of using only the cervix changes to determine fertility have not been conducted, it's still an excellent signal to chart regularly. At times when you ovulate irregularly, familiarity with your cervix could be especially appreciated.

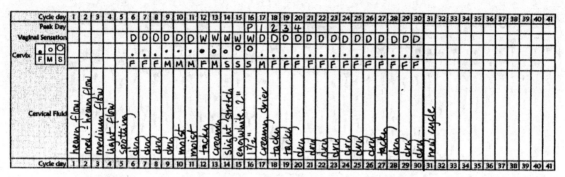

Figure 3.15.

This woman's cervical fluid and vaginal sensation were dry Days 6 through 9, suggesting that she could consider herself infertile after 6 P.M. on each of these days. However, because her cervix was slightly high and soft on Day 9, she needed to consider herself potentially fertile beginning on that day. Her cervix's signal of potential fertility overrides the dryness of mucus and vaginal sensation: her fertile phase therefore begins on Day 9.

Using a Barrier Method with Fertility Awareness

While some couples find that postponing intercourse during the woman's fertile phase enhances their relationship, others choose to use a barrier method (a diaphragm or cervical cap with spermicide, or a condom) on fertile days and enjoy intercourse throughout her cycle. While your risk of pregnancy due to barrier-method failure increases in this way (since you're using the barrier only during fertile days), if you chart and know when you're fertile, you can still enjoy barrier-free lovemaking for almost two thirds of your cycle.

To use a barrier effectively:

- Follow the rules for Fertility Awareness during the period described on page 37. Don't use a diaphragm or cervical cap while you're bleeding, since you don't want to keep blood at your cervix for the six to eight hours required for the diaphragm or cap to destroy sperm.
- Chart your basal temperature every day.

- After the period, you're safe for unprotected intercourse after 6 P.M. of dry days.
- Once you observe wet cervical fluid or wet vaginal sensation, your fertile phase has begun. Either postpone intercourse or use a barrier until you can confirm by your temperature that you've ovulated. Since your CF readings can be obscured after intercourse with spermicide present, you don't need to continue observing it, though you do need to continue charting your temperature.
- When you can confirm ovulation with three consecutive temperatures above your coverline, you can make love without a barrier for the rest of the cycle (see figure 3.16).

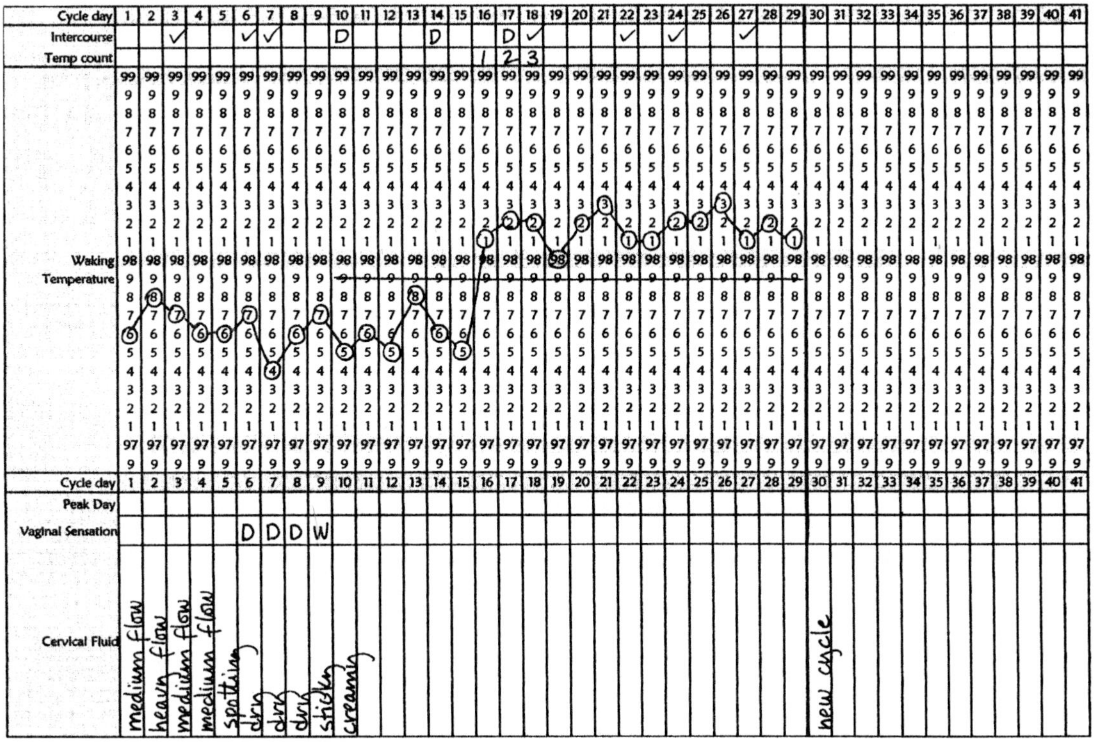

Cycle day	1	2	3	4	5	6	7	8	9	10	11	12	13	14	15	16	17	18	19	20	21	22	23	24	25	26	27	28	29	30	31	32	33	34	35	36	37	38	39	40	41
Intercourse		✓			✓	✓				D				D			D	✓			✓			✓			✓														
Temp count																1	2	3																							

Waking Temperature grid (99 down to 97) with coverline and plotted readings; Peak Day row blank.

Cycle day	1	2	3	4	5	6	7	8	9	10	...	41
Vaginal Sensation						D	D	D	W			

Cervical Fluid (handwritten): medium flow, heavy flow, medium flow, medium flow, spotting, dry, dry, sticky, creamy ... new cycle

Figure 3.16.

This woman had intercourse without a barrier (or risk of pregnancy) on Day 3, while she was still menstruating. After her period, her CF and vaginal sensation were dry on Days 6 through 8, making her safe for unprotected intercourse on those days after 6 P.M. Her fertile phase began on Day 9, when her mucus was sticky and her vaginal sensation was wet. On Days 10, 14, and 17—when she was in her fertile phase—she wore a diaphragm while making love. She was able to confirm ovulation by her temperature on the evening of Day 18; after 6 P.M. on that day, the couple could resume barrier-free intercourse.

- Check your chart on the days you have intercourse. On the days you use a barrier method, mark a *D* in this column for "diaphragm," a *CC* for "cervical cap," or a *C* for "condom."
- If you use a diaphragm or cervical cap, have it fitted during your fertile phase, since the cervix changes shape throughout the cycle, and you want it to fit when you're fertile.

Points to Remember

- Once a mature egg is released by the ovary and drawn into the fallopian tube, the egg can live for twelve to twenty-four hours. It can then be fertilized by the sperm that cervical fluid has kept alive in the cervix. So, you're fertile *before* you ovulate because your cervical fluid can keep sperm alive *until* you ovulate. You can have sex on Monday, and not conceive until the following Friday—if that's when you ovulate.
- Pre-ejaculate contains enough sperm to cause a pregnancy and/or an STI.
- The riskiest time for an unintended pregnancy is in the days after your period and before you ovulate. Once you confirm that your egg(s) from one cycle are dead and gone, you can have intercourse all day long and not get pregnant (until your new cycle begins).
- Cervical fluid and BBT patterns don't always line up exactly. If yours don't, postpone intercourse or use a barrier method until you've confirmed ovulation by both signals.
- If you make assumptions based on past cycles ("I've ovulated on Day 17 for five cycles in a row, and so I'm safe for intercourse until Day 11 without checking my mucus"), nature can be unforgiving. Every cycle is new.
- When in doubt, consider yourself fertile.

Sample Charts for Preventing Pregnancy

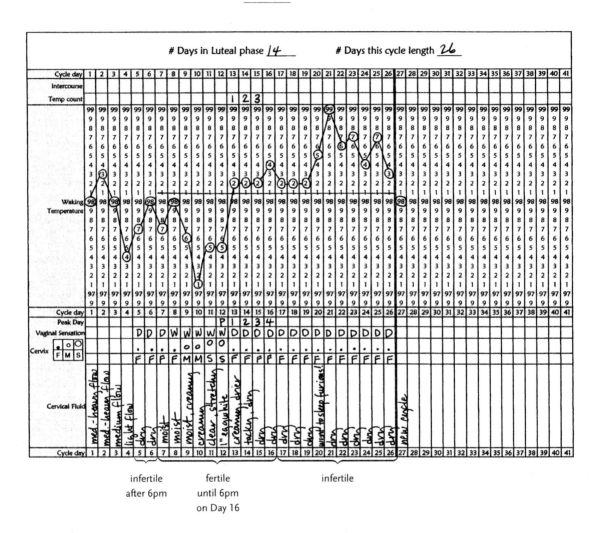

Figure 3.17.

She's infertile after 6 p.m. on Days 5 and 6. Her fertile phase begins on Day 7. Her Peak Day is Day 12. By her mucus, her postovulatory infertile phase begins at 6 p.m. on Day 16. Her coverline is at 98.1. By her temp count, her postovulatory infertile phase begins at 6 p.m. on Day 15. For maximum effectiveness, she should go by her more conservative signal and wait until 6 p.m. on Day 16 to consider herself infertile.

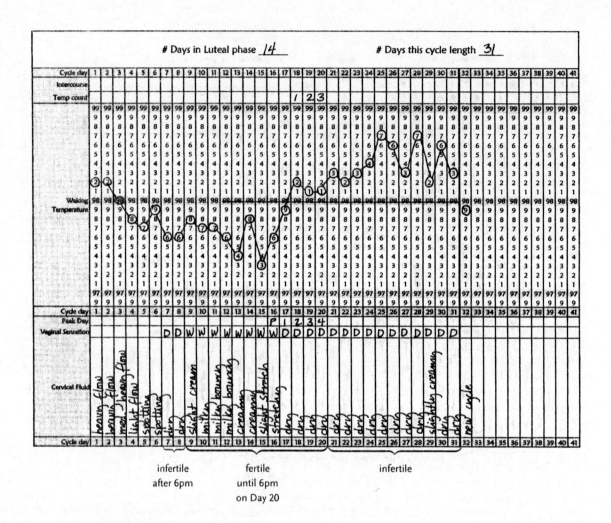

Figure 3.18.

This woman is infertile after 6 P.M. on Days 7 and 8. Her fertile phase begins on Day 9. Her Peak Day is Day 16. By her mucus, her postovulatory infertile phase begins at 6 P.M. on Day 20. Her coverline is 98.0. By her temp count, her postovulatory infertile phase begins at 6 P.M. on Day 20: her CF and temperature match up exactly.

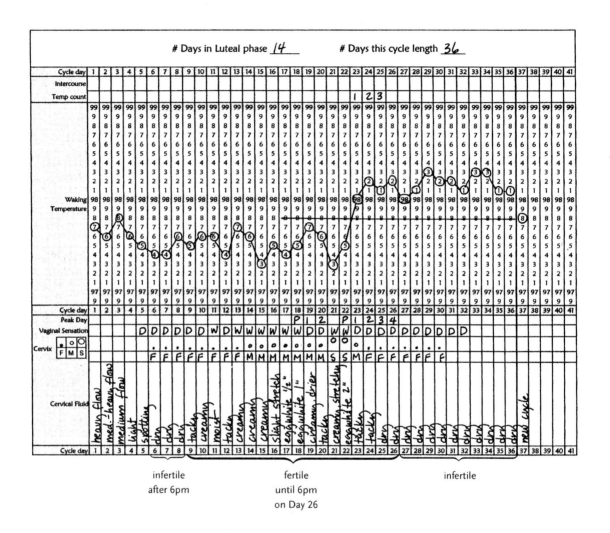

Figure 3.19.

This woman is infertile after 6 P.M. on Days 6, 7, and 8. Her fertile phase begins on Day 9. She has a false peak on Day 18. Her true Peak Day is Day 22. By her CF, her postovulatory infertile phase begins at 6 P.M. on Day 26. Her coverline is at 97.8. By her temp count, her postovulatory infertile phase begins at 6 P.M. on Day 25. For maximum effectiveness, she should go by her more conservative signal and wait until after 6 P.M. on Day 26 to consider herself infertile.

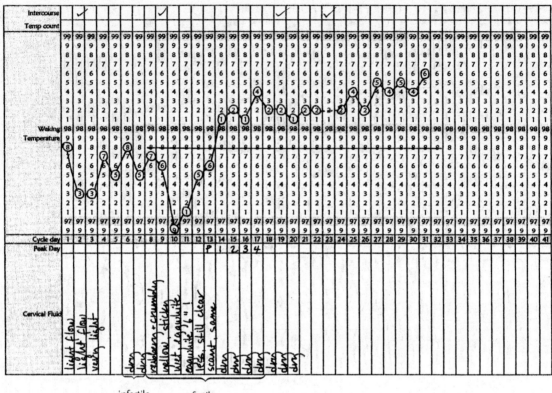

infertile
after 6pm

fertile
until 6pm
on Day 17

Figure 3.20.

On Day 8, Linda observed "rubbery, crumbly" cervical fluid and therefore entered her fertile phase. Day 13 was her Peak Day, because she had "scant, still clear" CF, and then transitioned to dryer CF on Day 14. (Again, the Peak Day is the last day of wet sensation or wet mucus; it indicates that ovulation is imminent.) By her CF, Linda's postovulatory infertile phase begins at 6 P.M. on Day 17. Her coverline is 97.8. By her temperature, her postovulatory infertile phase begins at 6 P.M. on Day 16. She most likely ovulated between Days 13 and 14. Linda had intercourse on Day 9, a fertile day. On Day 31, with 18 high temperatures after ovulation, Linda could confirm pregnancy. Be it known: mucus really can keep sperm alive for up to five days!

Wanting Intercourse During Your Fertile Phase

For much of history, people have been keenly aware of nature's seasons. Many cultures have festivals that celebrate the dark of the winter, spring blossoms, and fall harvests. They've also created guidelines to honor the cyclical nature of human relationships and fertility. Ecclesiastes, the biblical verses that begin "There is a time for everything, and an appropriate moment for all that one desires to do," include the line "A time to embrace and a time not to embrace." Menstruation has often been perceived as a time for solitude, when a woman separates from her partner and the rest of her community. In some cultures, women celebrate this inward focus with each other, without men or children.

It's no coincidence that the women's liberation movement that began in the 1960s coincided with the arrival of the Pill. Finally, women had a seemingly easy way to limit their number of children while they focused on their education and work outside of home—and continued to express themselves sexually. Two generations of women have now grown up with the Pill. Taking this drug is often perceived as "natural." The expectation of having intercourse every day has also become normal to our thinking, along with fresh fruit through all seasons.

I wonder if we pay a price for these perceptions. On the Pill, a woman's reproductive system essentially shuts down, and she becomes available for sex all the time without the consequence of pregnancy. This is male fertility rhythm. Besides its effects on a woman's health and that of her offspring, I wonder how the Pill affects our thinking—about our desires; about what constitutes healthy sex; about our connectedness to nature's seasons.

When you begin practicing Fertility Awareness, all of these questions may surface. Many couples find that their desire to make love is strongest when the woman is fertile. If you want to avoid or postpone pregnancy, how do you deal with that?

Many people find it helpful to begin with an appreciation of nature's cycles. From there, you can abstain completely during the fertile phase. You can make love without genital-genital contact. Some couples use barrier methods such as a condom, diaphragm, or cervical cap (with spermicide). Talking with your partner about what's right for you—which may change from cycle to cycle—is one of the juiciest and most necessary aspects of practicing Fertility Awareness. The method is probably most satisfying and effective when you and your partner know how to read your charts accurately, and when you're in agreement about how to respond sexually to your fertile phase.

The unintended pregnancies I hear about usually happen when couples are newly in love, when the woman is coming off the Pill or Depo-Provera, when one or both parties are ambivalent about having a child, when the tenacity of a relationship is being tested, or when women are approaching menopause. All these scenarios require scrupulous charting and following of rules. When a woman tells me she knows intuitively when she's fertile, I can practically see her hormones jumping up and down: now they've got the chance to show her just how unpredictable they can be.

Chart your fertility signals every day and keep your conversation with your partner alive!

Leah Morton, MD. *Charting your fertility signals is a great first step toward health, because it's a daily method for questioning and understanding your body. It's an immense responsibility to have a body—and then to use Fertility Awareness to prevent pregnancy.*

Fertility Awareness is a science. It's not an improvisation where you adapt the recipe to make your fertility be as you want. It requires you to bow down to nature. If you don't observe your signals and follow the rules every day, nature will correct your sloppiness: if you don't pay attention, nature will prevail.

I've heard FA be criticized because it doesn't protect people from sexually transmitted infections (STIs). Actually, a woman who observes her cervical fluid is much more likely to notice if her vaginal secretions are foul-smelling or colored. And neither the Pill nor the IUD is in any way able to prevent STIs. Only condoms can do that.

Ondrea, twenty-three. *As soon as I met Tom, when I was twenty, we had an amazing physical connection. Just holding hands could send us into waves of sweet feelings. After a few weeks, we moved in together. All of a sudden we were sharing a dog, a bathroom, and groceries.*

We had sex every day. I wanted to please Tom, and because I was on the Pill, I was available that much. Ninety percent of the time, I really enjoyed making love. Sometimes, I just wanted to get it over with. Sometimes Tom could get me to feel like I wanted it.

After two years, we took a Fertility Awareness class, because my mother didn't like me being on the Pill. I was fuming when we walked out of the class: we wouldn't be able to have intercourse every day unless we used condoms?! *But Tom's very health conscious, and*

A SUMMARY OF FERTILITY AWARENESS RULES
FOR PREVENTING PREGNANCY

During the Menstrual Period

Because you can have mucus while you are menstruating or spotting (and not be able to see or feel it), consider the period a fertile time. Once you've had twelve consecutive ovulatory cycles that are twenty-six days or longer, you are safe Days 1 through 5.

Dry Day Rule

After the period (and before ovulation), you are considered infertile after 6 P.M. if you have been dry all day. The following day, you need to be dry all day again to be considered infertile after 6 P.M.

In a dry vaginal environment, sperm cannot survive longer than four hours. The absence of cervical fluid also shows that estrogen levels are too low for ovulation to occur.

Once CF appears, you are fertile: unprotected intercourse may lead to pregnancy.

Peak Day Rule

The last day of wet mucus or wet vaginal sensation is called the Peak Day, and it indicates that you are about to ovulate. You are considered infertile after 6 P.M. on the fourth consecutive day of cervical fluid that is dryer than it was on your Peak Day.

Four days of drying up are needed to confirm that your egg is dead and gone: it's possible that you don't begin ovulating until forty-eight hours after the peak, and 10 percent of the time women release two eggs—each living a maximum of twenty-four hours.

Temperature Shift Rule

When you see a rise in temperature, count back six low temperatures and draw a coverline one tenth of a degree above the highest of them. You are considered infertile after 6 P.M. on the third consecutive day that your waking temperature is above your coverline.

With ovulation, the follicle is transformed into a corpus luteum that releases progesterone and warms you up. While a rise in temperature usually indicates that you *have* ovulated, it's possible that you don't ovulate until twenty-four hours after the rise; and two eggs can live twenty-four hours each—requiring a total of three days of high temperatures to confirm that your egg is dead and gone.

continued

he said, "I love learning things with you. Let's try it." I was really taken by his interest. Actually, I don't think I would have gone off the Pill without his support.

For the first two weeks, we had no sex. I ovulated in my first cycle off the Pill, which thrilled me. I had a taste of connecting to my body.

I got a cervical cap. For about a week, it was great. We went back to sex every day. Then I got a raging yeast infection (probably a reaction to the spermicide), followed by an intense bladder infection. For a whole month, we had almost no sex. We started to break apart. I began asking myself, What connects us besides sex?

My body was screaming at me to claim my own space. I decided to take a job out of town for two months. When my infections cleared up, we got condoms without spermicide. In the two weeks before I left, we had raging fights. Tom felt angry when I wore clothes he considered sexy out of the house. He didn't want me taking the job. The strange thing was, we were still having great sex.

Then one night when I knew I was fertile, the condom broke. The next day, I took the emergency contraceptive pill, which made me more furious. I was sick of putting junk in my body.

Out of town, I kept charting. I loved knowing what was going on with my cycles and having my own space. I started to see that I mingle pretty deeply with a man when I have intercourse. If I do it every day without a break, I get enmeshed.

A haze lifted when I went off the Pill. I started discovering myself. Now, if I want sex with Tom, I ask, What does my chart say? And, What do I feel? Those two things aren't always compatible, but I've learned to honor them both. I like that my sexuality is mine to decide and that it's connected to my fertility, which feels bigger than me somehow.

Jack, thirty. I was dubious about the method at first. It took effort to learn, and we live in a society that likes to solve problems by popping pills. In the past I would've agreed that birth control is the man's responsibility as much as the woman's, but I didn't have a way to take that responsibility. Now, at the end of the day, I read Jenny's thermometer, ask her about her mucus, and record these on her chart.

Fertility Awareness helps me know what's going on with Jenny, biologically and emotionally. I've also discovered that my interest in sex increases significantly when she's fertile. I would never have noticed this if I hadn't been doing our record keeping. Because we're faced with our fertility and our desires every day (and the need to talk them through), charting gives us a kind of intimacy that goes beyond sexual intimacy.

Inez, thirty-four. I learned Fertility Awareness from a book—I loved the info and practically devoured the book. But during the first two months I charted (and kept rereading), we didn't have intercourse. I just didn't feel confident that I understood the rules. When I finally found a teacher who could answer my list of questions, that was a happy day! Now my sister's learning the method. I love hearing her questions and the answers to the ones I don't know. I look forward to the day when FA is so common that you can go to the grocery store, run into friends, and hear your questions discussed.

Bruce, thirty-eight. If I'm spending a lot of time with a woman, whether I consciously feel it or not, I'm affected by what's happening in her body. If she's on the Pill (which manipulates her hormones—no two ways about it), then somehow the chemistry between us is affected. I've only been with one woman who used Fertility Awareness, and even though we broke up almost ten years ago, I still think about the method. I still prefer it to anything else I've experienced. With FA, just knowing how her body works made my partner a lot more comfortable with herself and freer to express herself genuinely. I'd also say that the method encouraged our imagination during fertile times. And when she entered her infertile phase, it was cause for celebration!

Mia, twenty-seven. I got pregnant right after I met Richard. I mean right away. We got married and I gave birth all in a whirl. After our son was born four years ago, I went on the Pill. I've been off it and charting for three cycles, and already I can see that Richard and I are most interested in each other when I'm fertile. I'm not ready for another child now. I've also learned that kissing can turn me on so much that I lose confidence in my ability to stop making love. We're considering not kissing while I'm fertile, to see if that's a *viable option. It sounds crazy, but I want to try it. We're talking about all of this—it's intensely hard and worth it.*

Nadine and Gordon, MDs. *We read a little about the Sympto-thermal Method in med school, but it certainly wasn't dwelled on. We assumed the menstrual period to be an infertile time. About a year after we'd each begun practicing family medicine, we made love on Day 5 of Nadine's cycle, while she was still bleeding. To our surprise, she became pregnant.*

Our daughter is nineteen now, a great joy in our lives. We're happy to say that she and her boyfriend took a Fertility Awareness class while they were still in high school. And we think the education of physicians ought to include comprehensive information about Fertility Awareness!

In the formative human past, a baby would have unrestricted access to its mother's breast, nursing on demand through the day and night. When the child's demand for maternal milk declined . . . this change would send a signal to the mother's reproductive system that it was safe to resume normal fecundity without the danger of having to "metabolize for three."

—PETER ELLISON
On Fertile Ground

4. Fertility Awareness While Breast-feeding

HISTORICALLY, IN NON-WESTERNIZED cultures, spacing children at least three years apart has been considered ideal for the health of the mother, the children, and the community as a whole.[1, 2] The means for sustaining a woman's infertility for at least two years after giving birth includes a combination of breast-feeding, keeping the mother and baby close throughout the day (by carrying the baby in a sling), and sleeping in darkness. With the introduction of infant formulas, strollers, the Pill, and barrier methods of contraception, knowledge about fertility while breast-feeding has waned. Most mothers—even grandmothers—aren't able to tell their daughters how to delay or encourage return to fertility, nor how to determine when it is in fact returning. Few medical training programs include this information, which women need whether they want to avoid, postpone, or receive a new pregnancy.

As more mothers who likely weren't nursed themselves choose to breast-feed their own children, questions about returning to fertility postpartum also increase. I often share my clients' excellent questions with Donna Taylor, a mother of four breast-fed children. For twenty-five years, Donna and her husband Bill have taught Natural Family Planning with the Couple to Couple League (CCL), an international group of largely Catholic volunteers who teach the method. Bill is a biomedical engineer, and the Taylors coauthored a study on lactational amenorrhea funded by the National Institutes of Health (NIH). It's thanks to people like the Taylors (and their mentor Sheila Kippley, who cofounded the CCL in 1971 with her husband, John, and authored *Breast-feeding and Natural Child Spacing*), that the wheel of information about breast-feeding and fertility doesn't have to be invented again.

Before I proceed with this chapter, I'll say that its information is designed for people who are already familiar with reproductive anatomy and using Fertility Awareness to prevent pregnancy (discussed in chapters 1 through 3). Learning this method at the same time you're establishing a relationship with your baby may be especially challenging. And, if you're game to learn it, I'm delighted to share this information. I'd also encourage you to meet with a qualified teacher to clarify your understanding of the rules while nursing.

That said, let me explain how hormones are affected during breast-feeding, and clarify a few terms.

The Hormones of Breast-feeding

Whether or not your baby nurses, milk production is first triggered by giving birth. Continued milk depends on your baby's sucking and your letdown (releasing) of milk. Typically, once breast-feeding begins, the more frequently your baby nurses, the more milk you'll produce.

During pregnancy, *prolactin* (think pro-lactation), a hormone produced by the pituitary gland, stimulates the breast to develop for nursing. After birth, the baby's sucking increases prolactin's production, which in turn causes milk production (see figure 4.1).

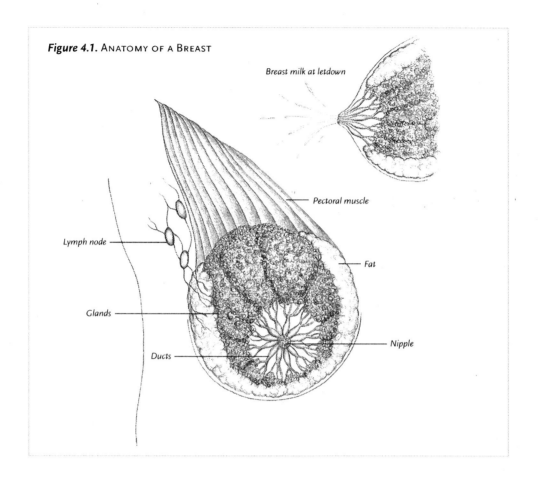

Figure 4.1. ANATOMY OF A BREAST

Breast milk at letdown

Pectoral muscle

Lymph node

Fat

Glands

Nipple

Ducts

Elevated levels of prolactin are associated with suppressed production of the hormones that are required for ovulation. In simple terms, your baby's frequent sucking will tend to delay your return to ovulatory cycles; less frequent nursing— or not nursing at all—will tend to speed up your return to ovulatory cycles (with sufficient progesterone for sustaining a new pregnancy).

Oxytocin—sometimes called "the love hormone"—triggers orgasm, uterine contractions during labor, contractions that return the uterus to its prepregnant size in the first few days after birth, and letdown of milk. Oxytocin also promotes bonding between the mother and baby. Pitocin, a drug that is sometimes given to women to stimulate labor, is a synthetic version of oxytocin.

It sure dazzles me to see how fertility and sexuality (and love, which is also activated while nursing) are so intimately connected!

Defining Frequent Breast-feeding

Many contemporary mothers define themselves as "frequent" nursers when they breast-feed their babies every two to three hours during the day, and perhaps once during the night. Surprisingly, this style of nursing may not be enough to create *lactational amenorrhea*, the absence of menstrual cycles while nursing. While researchers still don't know exactly how breast-feeding inhibits ovulation, frequency seems to be key.[3] Prolactin levels, a woman's metabolic load (rate of energy used for organs and muscles to function), and a feedback system between the hypothalamus and pituitary glands and suckling are also considered part of the picture.

How frequently, then, do you need to nurse to create the unambiguous infertility that some women achieve for years after giving birth? Anthropological studies may provide the answer. Zinacanteco Indians in Mexico nurse their babies about twice per hour.[4] !Kung San women of Botswana nurse, on average, every thirteen minutes.[5] The amount of milk these mothers feed their babies is actually equal to that of North American women, and the number of minutes they nurse throughout a twenty-four-hour period (which varies depending on the baby's age) is also about the same. The difference is in the frequency of feedings.

Dr. Bill Taylor says that the time to establish "unambiguous infertility"—characterized by dry mucus and dry vaginal sensation—is in your baby's first few months. To create lactational amenorrhea, Dr. Taylor suggests nursing once or twice per hour during the day and two to three times or more at night during your baby's first two to three months. A feeding might last thirty seconds—or much longer. Once dryness is established, women can usually nurse less frequently and still continue with unambiguous infertility.

Anthropologist Meredith Small reports that nursing wherein babies have continuous access to the breast (including at night) seems to foster quiet, sated babies and tightly knit families and communities; bottle-feeding, nursing at infrequent intervals, parents and babies sleeping in separate rooms, and strollers encourage emotional distance and social independence. Dr. Small suggests that women "nurse on cue" when their babies reach for the nipple. (The term *nursing on demand* may encourage an unfriendly attitude about eating and mothering.) Her book, *Our Babies, Ourselves,* also reports that nipple soreness, insufficient amounts of milk, and insufficient fat in the mother's milk can all be caused by feeding intervals that are too far (two to three hours) apart—and that increased feedings can appease each of these situations.[6]

The mothers who traditionally nurse one to four times each hour also, typically, do not nurse in isolation. They return to their work grinding corn, tending rice paddies, or participating in meetings after their babies are born; they carry their babies in slings while they work. What's a North American mother to do? Perhaps we need more acceptance of nursing in public, more acceptance of nursing mothers at the workplace, wardrobes that allow for graceful nursing, and a comfortable sling for every new mom!

What to Expect from Different Styles of Nursing

Exclusive breast-feeding means giving your baby nothing but your own milk from your breast; frequent nursing, including at night; pacifying the baby at your breast, rather than with a rubber pacifier; and feeding without a schedule. These behaviors will likely dry up your cervical fluid and also keep you from ovulating or menstruating. Sheila Kippley calls these behaviors *ecological breast-feeding* when they're combined with a daily nap (taken with your baby) and when you sleep with your baby for easy night nursings.

If you nurse once or twice per hour during the day and two to three times or more at night, expect to attain dry mucus (a sign of lactational amenorrhea) once your afterbirth fluids have stopped—about six weeks after birth. (Some doctors, unaware that vaginal dryness is normal during lactational amenorrhea, may prescribe estrogen creams to encourage moistness. Donna Taylor says, "These creams can foul up your fertility signals.")

- If you are exclusively breast-feeding, you can have intercourse in the first eight weeks after giving birth, and your risk of a new pregnancy will be almost nil. I have heard of breast-feeding women who bled as soon as five and a half weeks postpartum, but these were probably breakthrough bleeds—not true menstrual periods preceded by ovulation. Breast-feeding women whose fertility signals return earlier than expected may be nursing at intervals spaced too far apart (in their baby's first few months) to establish lactational amenorrhea. They may not be nursing through the night and/or sleeping in total darkness.

- If you continue with *exclusive* breast-feeding for your baby's first six months, your risk of becoming pregnant is less than 2 percent.
- After six months, a nursing mother has about a 60 percent chance of ovulating before her menstruation resumes.

According to Sheila Kippley, "About 70 percent of ecologically breast-feeding mothers in the United States experience their first menstruation between nine and twenty months postpartum." Kippley and Bill Taylor and his colleagues have found that the average return of menstruation for ecologically breast-feeding mothers is between fourteen and fifteen months.

Partial breast-feeding means giving your baby water, formula, and/or a pacifier in addition to nursing. If your baby is left with sitters and/or sleeps through the night (without nursing), that's also characteristic of partial breast-feeding. With partial breast-feeding, fertility can return as quickly as with bottle-feeding or as late as three to four months after birth, depending on how frequently you nurse and whether you take a daily nap with your infant or practice the family bed. Donna Taylor says, "If you leave your baby with a sitter for the weekend, you might ovulate."

Pumping your milk if you are away from your baby is nutritionally sound; but because your baby won't be sucking from your breast, that could encourage ovulatory cycles to return more quickly. The effects of pumping on return to fertility have not been studied. Donna Taylor knows a mother who pumped her milk while she worked full-time, nursed her baby frequently in the evenings and at night, practiced the family bed (slept with her baby), and did not return to fertile cycles for a year. I know another woman who returned to work when her child was three and a half months old and did not have menses until her child was almost two— she also pumped her milk at work and practiced the family bed.

If you bottle-feed your baby, ovulatory cycles typically return three to ten weeks after birth.

Solid foods tend to be introduced when the baby is about six months old. As you continue to nurse on cue, breast-feeding can supplement all that your baby eats and drinks. Some women who nurse toddlers (at nap time, at night, or more frequently) continue to stay dry and unambiguously infertile; many begin ovulating while breast-feeding continues.

Preventing Pregnancy While Breast-feeding

When to Chart Your Fertility Signals

While you observe dry vaginal sensation and dry CF, you do not need to chart. You *do* need to be on the lookout for wet vaginal sensation and/or wet cervical fluid. Once these arrive, begin charting your mucus and vaginal sensation along with your waking temperature and cervix changes. You can expect weeks or months of off-and-on-again mucus, alerting you that you will soon be ovulating. Of course, bleeding would be another signal that you need to begin charting.

It's not unusual for a woman's first ovulatory cycle after breast-feeding to have a luteal phase less than twelve days long, which suggests less than enough progesterone to sustain a pregnancy. (And you've probably heard of women who conceived before their first period returned: don't count on a short luteal phase for your first ovulatory cycle.)

If you want to postpone or avoid a new pregnancy while you're nursing and your fertility is ambiguous, you can observe the rules of Fertility Awareness presented below; you can use barrier methods (condoms or a diaphragm or cervical cap with spermicide); you can make love without genital-genital contact; or alternate between using various barrier methods and making love without intercourse. If you use a diaphragm or a cervical cap, it should be refitted after childbirth; also, be aware that the spermicide will interfere with your mucus readings. The CCL advocates for abstinence during potentially fertile days. I don't consider the Pill a viable option because all steroids pass through your breastmilk. The long-term effects of the Pill on nursing mothers and their babies have not been studied. Also, estrogen can decrease your milk supply. IUDs now commonly emit progestin and thereby can also disrupt normal hormonal functioning.

Again, it's the first few months of your baby's life that are key to establishing lactational amenorrhea. Allowing him or her continuous access to your breasts, including at night, can postpone your return to fertility *and* clear up confusing signals. With this style of nursing, mucus will typically become consistently dry—unambiguously infertile. Prolactin levels will be higher if you nurse, say, twenty to thirty times throughout the day and two to three times or more at night—rather than for a handful of extended feedings. In the early months of your baby's life, a little more nursing, perhaps at night, may stave off the signs that make you think you're returning to fertility, such as cervical mucus and breakthrough bleeding (bleeding that is not preceded by ovulation).

Taking a daily nap (nursing and actually lying down for about twenty minutes) with your baby may also help delay your return to fertility. When Sheila Kippley hears of an exclusively breast-feeding mother menstruating before her baby is six months old, she asks if they take a daily nap together; so far, the women she's queried do not. Based on anecdotal evidence, not being well rested might speed your return to fertility. Kippley and the Taylors also observe that once menstruation returns, you probably won't be able to guide your body back to unambiguous infertility. If your mucus returns before your baby is six months old, it's easier to reestablish dryness—and infertility—by increased nursing and perhaps a daily nap.

Donna Taylor explains, "The time to establish infertility is during your baby's first few weeks and months. Through frequent nursing and keeping your baby close, your body gets the message that it's nurturing a baby. It will show unambiguous dryness—unambiguous infertility. You'll be unable to conceive, and can enjoy lovemaking whenever you want." Taylor adds, "I've worked with hundreds of breast-feeding mothers, and they do most of the work that it takes to establish long-term infertility after childbirth. But because some are not aware that their baby's first twelve to eighteen months can be an infertile time, they don't get to reap the benefits of lovemaking without the chance of pregnancy."

Lovemaking While Breast-feeding

For many women, pregnancy and giving birth change the patterns of sexual desire. If you're breast-feeding, you've got sensuous, skin-to-skin contact happening frequently throughout the day. It may take a while for you to have enough energy for lovemaking. Some women, however, claim that sex while they're nursing is the best of their lives.

In either case, consider this a time for slow sex: twenty minutes won't be enough. Breast-feeding women are typically very dry vaginally, since elevated prolactin levels can decrease estrogen. Extra foreplay and/or lubrication (saliva is free and readily available) may be needed to enjoy intercourse. Also, the slightest movement from the baby can shift your focus from lovemaking and turn you off, so that the first steps to arousal have to begin again.

Even if sex is the furthest thought from your mind, keeping alert to your fertility signals will be much appreciated when your interest returns.

Night-Lighting's Effects on Fertility

As you'll see in chapter 10, night-lighting (sleeping exposed to or in the absence of light), can affect your whole body's functioning, including your fertility.

You can help delay your return to fertility by sleeping in complete darkness through the months you nurse and your mucus is dry. Once slippery mucus returns, introducing light can encourage a speedier return to more predictable ovulatory cycles: if your vaginal sensation or mucus was wet during the day, sleep that night with a lamp lit by a 40-watt bulb in your bedroom. Or keep a 75-watt bulb burning in the bathroom down the hall and keep the bathroom door open so that its light shaft comes to your bedroom—like bright moonlight. If your vaginal sensation and mucus were dry all day, sleep in darkness.

Sleeping with the light on four nights in a row (while mucus is wet), then returning to total darkness, can help trigger ovulation.

If you practice this regime and your temperature doesn't indicate that you've ovulated, then wait for your next slippery mucus buildup and again sleep with light on the nights you had wet vaginal sensation or mucus during the day.

Carolyn, forty-one, called me when she bled for the third time despite the fact that she was exclusively breast-feeding her eight-month-old twin sons. Her first period started 114 days postpartum; the second cycle was 88 days long; the next periods arrived 35, then 37, then 35 days later. At night, she nursed every two hours. With her first (now nine-year-old) child, whom she'd also breast-fed, she didn't menstruate until the girl was a year old. Given that she was nursing twice as much with the boys, why had her periods returned so quickly this time?

I asked about her night-lighting. Outside her bedroom window, neighbors flashed lights throughout the night for security purposes. When I explained that these flashing lights could affect her pineal gland and thereby her whole endocrine (hormonal) system, Carolyn wondered how they might affect her sons. Her husband blocked off their bedroom windows with dark cloth, and she immediately began to sleep better. The boys still woke frequently to nurse, which is typical of babies their age.

During the boys' first six weeks, Carolyn napped with them four or five times each week. After this initial period, she continued to nurse, returned to work (at home), and napped much less frequently. She felt extremely stressed during this time and tried smoking marijuana several times a week to help her relax. (Marijuana has high levels of estrogen; smoking it may also have contributed to Carolyn's return to menstrual cycles.) After several months, she stopped the pot, because she found herself more relaxed without it.

When the twins were eleven months old, Carolyn's family moved to a rural area with no night-lighting. While she didn't observe her fertility signals, she did note her periods. After moving to the country, her cycles stretched to forty-two and then forty-five days long. Before the boys were conceived, her cycles tended to be thirty-two days.

While it would have been interesting to see if Carolyn's cycles were ovulatory, what she did observe offers a wealth of information. As Sheila Kippley has suggested, once you menstruate, it may not be possible to shift back to dry, unambiguous infertility, including amenorrhea. The younger the baby, the easier it is to establish infertility.

Cloudy Skies Without Rain

Waiting for ovulatory cycles to return can be a maddening time, because the woman shows signals that her fertility is returning or about to return, when actually she's infertile. However, she *could* ovulate at any time. Donna Taylor says this is like having cloudy skies without rain. Either or both parents may be frustrated by a lack of intercourse and nervous about conceiving a new child before they're ready. Taylor suggests that giving your child the nursing that's asked for can also mean no crying or fighting—and allowing peace to reign.

A large part of the challenge of lovemaking while you're breast-feeding and approaching ovulation may come from our culture's assumption that having intercourse frequently, even daily, without becoming pregnant is normal. I liken this to expecting fresh apples in Boston in January. We have the technology. We can ship the apples in from South America, though that'll take a fair amount of fossil fuel; we can wax the fruit to make it shine—though waxing also seals in pesticide residues; and special packaging is required to keep the apples from being bruised until you buy them. Likewise, the Pill allows daily intercourse without becoming pregnant; if you're breast-feeding, it may dry up your milk. It will also alter your hormones, and that may affect your baby through your milk.

We might be more in sync with nature if we assume "seasons" of infrequent intercourse—such as while a woman is returning to fertility during or after breast-feeding; after coming off hormonal drugs; or while approaching menopause. When expectations about sex change, frustration levels can, too.

Once Cervical Fluid Returns

Once you feel wet vaginal sensations and/or observe cervical fluid, it means your fertility is returning—though it may be many months before you actually ovulate. Start charting your temperatures again when you see the cervical fluid. If your baby is less than six months old, nursing more frequently, including at night, may help dry up the mucus.

Note that a nursing woman's temperatures may be lower than normal, because her fats (fuel) are going to her breast milk. As you return to ovulatory cycles, temperatures typically will elevate.

Behaviors that commonly encourage ovulatory cycles to return include:

- Introducing solid foods to your baby's diet.
- Decreasing breast-feeding.
- Weaning.
- Your baby sucks a thumb or uses a pacifier.
- Exposure to light while sleeping.
- You are sick and nurse less often.
- Your child begins sleeping through the night.
- Your baby sleeps in his or her own bed.
- Going away for a night or two and leaving your baby with a sitter.

Once your mucus returns, you may feel eager to see a predictable, ovulatory pattern again. To encourage ovulation, sleep in complete darkness except for the days you see slippery mucus building; on these days, sleep with a little bit of light. You don't need to limit nursing.

The Rules for Preventing Pregnancy While Breast-feeding

Before ovulatory cycles resume, you're in an extended preovulatory phase. You can observe your vaginal sensation, mucus, and cervix changes to determine that you're about to ovulate. Your basal temperature can't give you much information until after you've ovulated, though you still need to chart it.

If you're charting for the first time while you're postpartum, that can be especially challenging, because it may take a while for you to determine the differences between tacky, creamy, and stretchy mucus. It may take a while to discern a firm cervix (which can feel like the tip of your nose) from a soft one (soft like your tongue). When in doubt, don't take chances.

- If you have one or two days of wet sensation or mucus and the next two days you're dry, consider yourself potentially fertile on the day(s) you've got a wet sensation and/or mucus. You'd be safe for intercourse the second evening you've been dry all day.
- If your mucus patch lasts three days, you're potentially fertile on the days your sensation is wet and/or you have mucus. Count four day(s) of dryness after your last day of wet sensation or mucus, and you're then safe to resume intercourse on the fourth evening.

The more Peak Days you have, the more likely it is that you're approaching ovulation. (Again, the Peak Day is the last day of wet mucus or wet vaginal sensation before drying up begins.)

If your cervix is soft, open, or high (indicating potential fertility) on a day that your CF and vaginal sensation indicate infertility, the cervix's signal overrides the signals from your mucus and vaginal sensation, and you should consider yourself potentially fertile.

Even if you know the basic rules for preventing pregnancy through charting, these breast-feeding rules can seem especially cumbersome. I didn't really get the rules myself until I saw Donna Taylor's charts of her fertility returning after her third child. I'll show them—but first, here are some telling stories.

When Donna and Bill's first child, Fran, was nine months old, Donna got the flu. Her mother offered to take the boy, including at night, so she could sleep. Donna hadn't menstruated as of that point. She also wasn't charting, so she doesn't know what her mucus was like at the time. Two weeks after she got sick, she menstruated. The Taylors' second child, Beth, was conceived within a few weeks of that first period and born nineteen months after Fran. "If I knew then what I know now," Donna says, "I'd have stayed in bed with the baby while I had the flu, and asked people to help by cooking dinner and cleaning the bathroom—rather than caring for Fran—although I'm very, very glad Beth's here!"

Donna's cervical fluid returned when Beth was fifteen months old; she ovulated when Beth was eighteen months. Her third child, Paul, was born three years after Beth.

"My mucus returned when Paul was only three months old," Donna says. "He was a dream baby, falling asleep at 8:30, then sleeping through the night. But I wanted to remain infertile for at least a year. To reestablish infertility, we decided that Bill would wake the baby at around 11:30 P.M., when he was ready to go to sleep, and put him next to me for an extra night nursing so I wouldn't have to get out of bed. (I usually went to bed a little earlier than Bill.) Paul would nurse a bit, and then we'd go back to sleep. At 4:30 A.M., he'd wake really hungry, then nurse off and on until 6:30. That extra feeding at 11:30 dried up the mucus almost immediately. It didn't return until Paul was eighteen months old. I didn't ovulate until he was two years old and still nursing some."

The Taylors did the night-lighting regime suggested above starting on December 8 (see figure 4.5), when Paul was twenty-two months, and Donna had slippery, stretchy mucus. Up to that time, they'd been sleeping in a moderately dark room; and then they bought room-darkening shades. On the first night of Donna's mucus patch (beginning on Day 23), they placed on the floor near their bed a lamp lit by a 40-watt bulb for four nights; they returned to sleeping in complete darkness on Day 27. The first time they tried this method for triggering ovulation, Donna ovulated.

Here are Donna's charts (see figures 4.2 to 4.5). They began when she was thirty-one and Paul eighteen months, and she noticed cervical fluid and wet vaginal sensation for the first time since he was three months old. Please note that Donna usually observed only her cervix's location and openness, not its texture. Also, even though she didn't bleed for the first few charts she filled up (with each chart lasting forty-two days), Donna considers the whole series (until she ovulated and menstruated) one cycle.

Note that all of Donna's temperatures in the chart beginning November 16 (figure 4.5) are 97.5 or higher, signaling that her fats are now going more to her

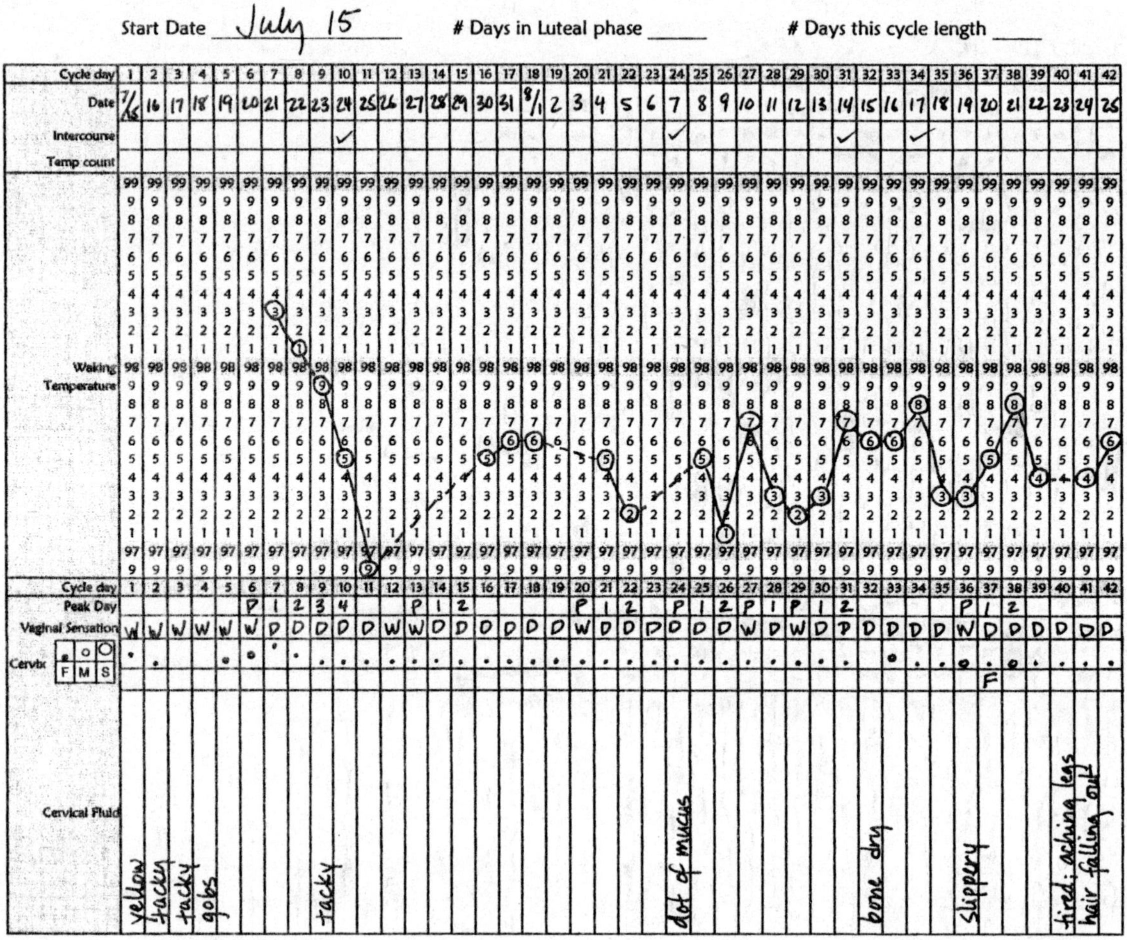

Start Date __July 15__   # Days in Luteal phase _____   # Days this cycle length _____

The chart shows cycle days 1–42 with dates beginning 7/16 through 8/26, recorded intercourse, waking temperature grid (97–99°F), peak day markings, vaginal sensation, cervix, and cervical fluid notations.

Cervical fluid notes (bottom of chart): yellow, tacky, tacky globs; tacky; dot of mucus; bone dry; slippery; tired: aching; less hair falling out

Figure 4.2.

Because of the "dot of mucus" on Day 24, intercourse was risky. Days 33 and 38 should be viewed as potentially fertile because of her slightly open cervix. Safe evenings were on Days 10, 11, 15–19, 22, 23, 26, 31, 32, 34, 35, and 38–42. Notice that Donna's temperatures were frequently lower than 97.5, which is typical of breast-feeding women, because her fats were going to her milk.

own system, rather than her breast milk. (Rising temperatures may also signal that ovulation is near.)

Donna also notes that her abdominal soreness on Days 9 and 10 (in figure 4.5), about two and a half weeks before she ovulated, is very common. "The feeling can be intense," she explains, "like strong cramps. A woman might think she's got the flu or a bad infection. But this is a common sensation when the body hasn't ovulated for a long while."

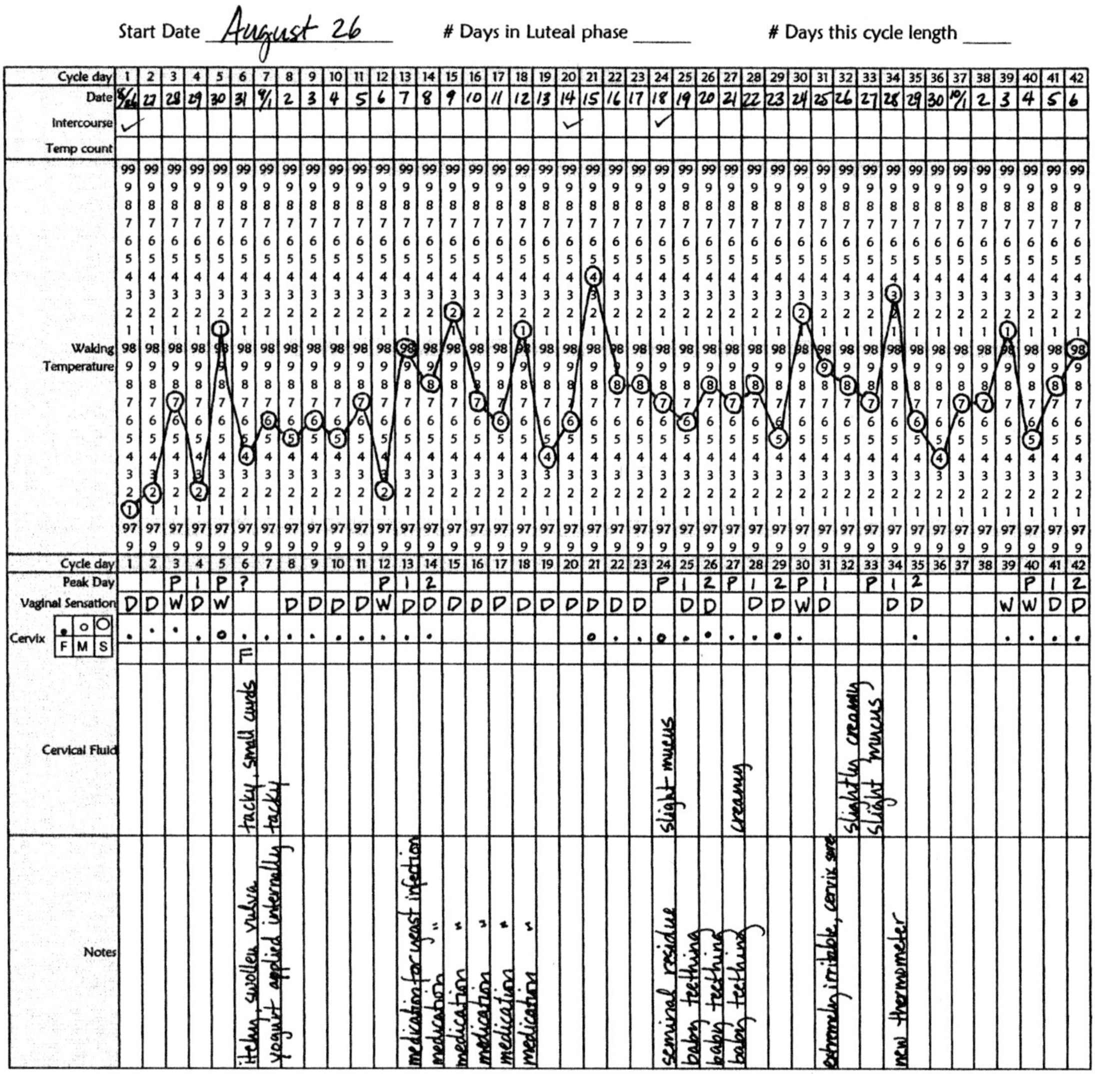

Start Date _August 26_   # Days in Luteal phase _____   # Days this cycle length _____

Figure 4.3.

Because Donna had slight mucus and a slightly open cervix, intercourse on Day 24 was risky. She was safe the evenings of Days 1, 2, 8–11, 19, 20, 22, 23, 26, and 35. Days 13–18 need to be seen as potentially fertile, because the yeast infection and medication could have obscured her reading. Because Days 36–38 were unobserved, they need to be considered potentially fertile.

Donna's next cycle was thirty-one days long; she was able to confirm ovulation by the evening of Day 23, with another eleven-day luteal phase.

When I remarked at the commitment it must have taken for her to observe and

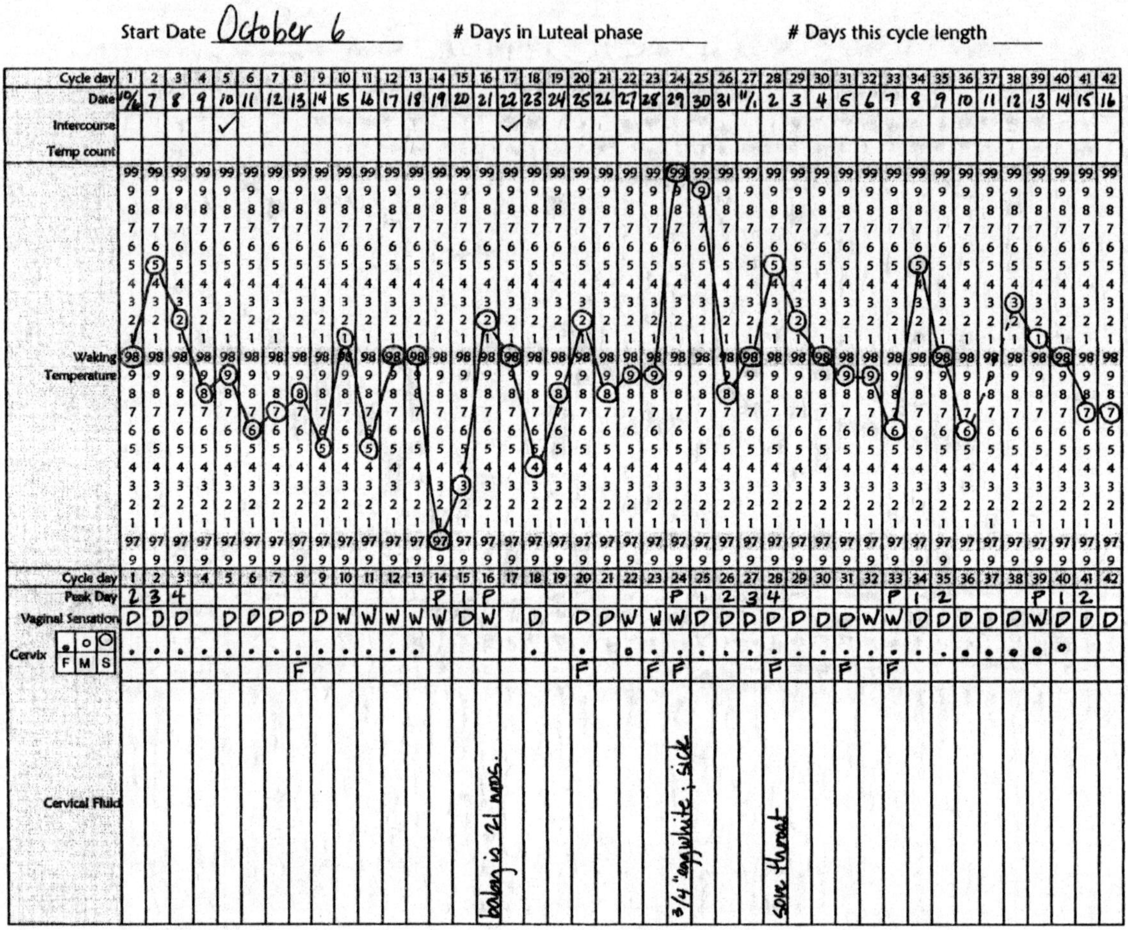

Start Date *October 6*   # Days in Luteal phase _____   # Days this cycle length _____

Cycle day	1	2	3	4	5	6	7	8	9	10	11	12	13	14	15	16	17	18	19	20	21	22	23	24	25	26	27	28	29	30	31	32	33	34	35	36	37	38	39	40	41	42
Date	10/6	7	8	9	10	11	12	13	14	15	16	17	18	19	20	21	22	23	24	25	26	27	28	29	30	31	11/1	2	3	4	5	6	7	8	9	10	11	12	13	14	15	16
Intercourse				✓													✓																									
Temp count																																										

Figure 4.4.

Paul turned twenty-one months on Day 16. Intercourse was safe on the evenings of Days 3–9. Because she didn't chart on Days 17 and 19, Days 17–20 were fuzzy—and therefore should be considered potentially fertile. She was safe again on the evenings of Days 21, 28–31, 35–37, 38, 41, and 42. With all of these mucus patches and the high cervix on Day 40, the couple expected that Donna would soon ovulate.

record her fertility signals while she had three children to care for, Donna said, "For me this was the path of least resistance. It let Bill and me enjoy lovemaking without becoming pregnant or harming Paul or me with harsh chemicals. It kept me in touch with my body. Bill charted my temperatures, so that made our method cooperative. One thing that does amaze me is that I'm an extrovert, and I like to be spontaneous. If charting were difficult, I'd be the first who couldn't do it."

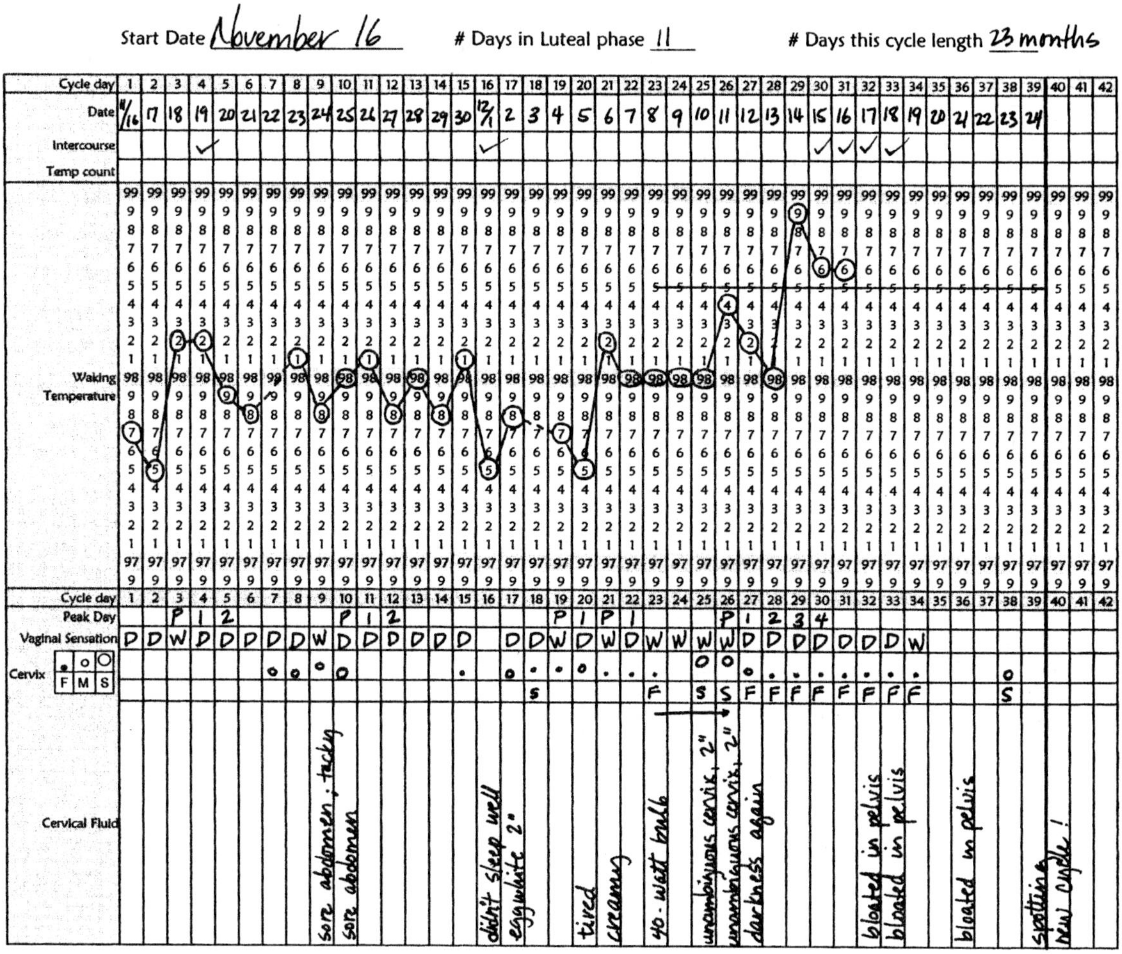

Start Date **November 16**   # Days in Luteal phase **11**   # Days this cycle length **23 months**

Cycle day	1	2	3	4	5	6	7	8	9	10	11	12	13	14	15	16	17	18	19	20	21	22	23	24	25	26	27	28	29	30	31	32	33	34	35	36	37	38	39	40	41	42
Date	11/16	17	18	19	20	21	22	23	24	25	26	27	28	29	30	12/1	2	3	4	5	6	7	8	9	10	11	12	13	14	15	16	17	18	19	20	21	22	23	24			
Intercourse			✓													✓													✓	✓	✓	✓										
Temp count																																										

Waking Temperature

Cycle day	1	2	3	4	5	6	7	8	9	10	11	12	13	14	15	16	17	18	19	20	21	22	23	24	25	26	27	28	29	30	31	32	33	34	35	36	37	38	39	40	41	42
Peak Day			P	1	2						P	1	2						P	1	P	1				P	1	2	3	4												
Vaginal Sensation	D	D	W	D	D	D	D	D	D	W	D	D	D	D	D		D	D	W	D	W	D	W	W	W	W	D	D	D	D	D	D	D	W								
Cervix (F M S)							•	•	•	•					•		•	•	•	•	•	•	•			•	•	•	•	•	•	•	•				•					

Cervix second row: ○ marks and S/F/S readings across days 19–30.

Cervical Fluid notes (handwritten, by day):
- Day 9: sore abdomen; tacky
- Day 10: sore abdomen
- Day 15: didn't sleep well; eggwhite 2"
- Day 19: tired; creamy
- Day 22: 40-watt bulb
- Day 28: unambiguous cervix, 2"
- Day 29: unambiguous cervix, 2"; darkness again
- Day 31: bloated in pelvis
- Day 32: bloated in pelvis
- Day 36: bloated in pelvis
- Day 39: spotting; new cycle!

Figure 4.5.

Paul (still nursing quite a bit, including at night) turned twenty-three months on Day 36 of this chart, in which Donna ovulated for the first time since he was conceived. Since she didn't chart her signals on Day 16, intercourse on that day was risky. By her CF and cervix readings, she was safe for intercourse on the evenings of Days 1, 2, 4–6, 12–15, and from the evening of Day 30 through to the end of the cycle. By her temperature, she couldn't confirm ovulation until the evening of Day 31. Donna thinks she ovulated around Days 27–28. The Taylors started a postovulatory party (!) on Day 30 (when, by the readings of her CF and vaginal sensation, she could consider herself infertile); they did not conceive as a result. Donna's luteal phase was eleven days long, almost sufficient for sustaining a pregnancy.

A SUMMARY OF FERTILITY AWARENESS RULES
WHILE BREAST-FEEDING

To Establish Unambiguous Infertility and Delay Your Return to Fertility

- Especially in the first few months, allow your baby continuous access to your breasts, including at night. During the day, you might nurse once or twice per hour or more. A feeding might last only thirty seconds. At night, you might nurse several times. Nursing can't be scheduled. It's not unusual for a baby to want another feeding fifteen minutes after the previous one. While your baby is teething or ill, it might seem like nursing lasts all night long or for an hour at a stretch. Other nights, your baby might sleep continuously for four or five hours.
- Keep your baby from thumbsucking or using a pacifier by pacifying at your breast.
- Keep your baby close to you in a sling, rather than use a stroller. When you go to the grocery store or on other errands, take your baby with you. A quick feeding before you shop can keep your baby quiet and satisfied until you arrive at a place where you can nurse again.
- Practice the family bed.
- Sleep in the absence of light. If you need light while you nurse at night, get a red bulb (the kind used in darkrooms) from a camera store.
- Take a daily nap (twenty minutes is fine) with your baby.

   With these behaviors, dry vaginal sensation, no mucus, no ovulation, and no bleeding will typically result. Once you've *established* unambiguous infertility, you may not need to nurse as frequently to maintain dryness and lactational amenorrhea.

To Encourage Ovulatory Cycles (Once Fertility Is About to Return)

- Nurse less frequently.
- When slippery mucus appears, sleep with a 40-watt bulb on in your room for three nights, then return to darkness. If you can't confirm ovulation (by your temperature), sleep with light when you observe mucus again.

The Rules for Preventing Pregnancy

- Establish unambiguous infertility and dry vaginal sensation.
- Once wet sensation and/or wet mucus return, begin charting them along with your temperature and cervix changes.

continued

- Look for the Peak Day—your last day of wet vaginal sensation or wet mucus before drying up begins.
- One or two days of wet sensation and wet mucus require two days of dry sensation and dry mucus to consider yourself infertile after 6 P.M. (your second dry day after your peak).
- Three days or more of wet sensation or wet mucus require four days of dry sensation and dry mucus to consider yourself infertile after 6 P.M. (the fourth dry day after your peak).
- If your cervix is soft, open, or high (indicating potential fertility) on a day that your CF and vaginal sensation indicate infertility, the cervix's signal overrides the signals from your mucus and vaginal sensation; and you should consider yourself potentially fertile.

If You Bottle-feed or Nurse Partially
- The older your baby is, the easier it is to establish ovulatory cycles.
- Expect that cycles may return when you introduce solids.
- Employing baby-sitters or going for long stretches without nursing can encourage ovulation.

Hannah, twenty-six. Our third child just turned eight months old. I'm nursing him exclusively (actually, he started drinking a little water when he was six months), and he still sleeps with us. My mucus just returned, so I figure I've got a few months or more of ambiguous fertility ahead. It's frustrating, sexually speaking. We don't want more kids. But Mark (my husband) hates condoms and doesn't want a vasectomy, I don't like spermicide, and we're both nervous that intercourse could lead to another pregnancy.

Recently it dawned on me that there are other ways to make love besides intercourse. We can take out massage oil. We can get to know each other slowly and learn other ways of being intimate. This is actually great for our marriage, because I can get fixated on my husband's frustration about what he's not getting, and make myself crazy. When we take time and communicate—instead of relying on a certain act to give us intimacy—I feel so much better about myself and our relationship.

I'm motivated to be really good at charting so I can pass it on to my daughter. She's only seven now, but I want to help her respect how her body works, learn to take care of herself, know what pleases her and how to make that known. I wish I'd started learning these things when I was younger.

Mark (Hannah's husband), twenty-six. *I'm an engineer, so I know that quick fixes have long-term consequences. Breast-feeding takes time, that's for sure; but infant formula simply can't provide what nature does. So I really appreciate that Hannah breast-feeds our kids, because they're healthier for it.*

Given that Hannah nurses and that we eat organic food as much as we can, it follows that we don't want to use chemicals for birth control. At first, I didn't believe that Fertility Awareness could be effective. Once we took a class and I learned the science of it, I felt confident. This actually improved our sex life—because before, whenever we made love, we'd be terrified afterward that we'd conceived again. That kind of squelched whatever pleasure we'd had.

Now that I know the method and understand what a woman's hormones and fertility signals do while she's breast-feeding, I'm not terrified about the situation. I can read Hannah's charts and help decide how we relate. I'm like most men, I suppose; I'd like intercourse every day. But this way, I feel secure about the long-term consequences of what we're doing. So even though we don't have intercourse every day, it's worth it.

Molly, twenty-eight. *I was twenty-six when Jake was born. He was a frequent nip and nurser; during the night, he usually nursed once or twice. At five months, he began drinking water; at six months, he began taking little bits of food.*

When Jake was five months old, I started bleeding and charting. My temperatures were low, and my mucus, when I remembered to chart it, was "globby." My cycles were about thirty-five days long, and anovulatory. I never established unambiguous infertility. I've wondered if I was just too stressed for my body to be dry and clearly infertile. We didn't have much money and had to move around a lot from relative to relative. To prevent pregnancy, I didn't want the Pill or an IUD or even a diaphragm—I didn't want to expose myself or my son to artificial hormones or chemicals.

During most of these months, I didn't want much sex. It was a very frustrating time for Ian (my husband) and me. We used condoms, but I never really felt comfortable making love.

Once I finally ovulated (when Jake was sixteen months) and could read my charts confidently, I realized that a big part of my not wanting sex was that I'd feared getting pregnant again. We took a Fertility Awareness class together around the time I started ovulating again (I'd learned how to chart from a book). The truth is that I didn't really know how to read my charts until I took the class—and Ian hadn't known that or basic anatomy. Once we could tell when I'm fertile and not fertile, the questions Is Ian attractive? *and* What's wrong with Molly? *went away.*

That first cycle I ovulated (I was still breast-feeding), my luteal phase was only nine days long—not long enough to sustain a pregnancy. But I finally had my fertility back—and my sex life.

Rebecca, thirty-one. *Despite my being a childbirth educator and a great advocate of breast-feeding, I didn't feel blissed, triumphant, or relaxed while I nursed either of my children. My daughter was very small at birth, and she nursed all the time. I mean 'round the clock. We moved twice in her first two months, eventually settling in a city where I knew no one except my husband. I was alone all day with our daughter, and finally, when she was four months old, I switched to bottle-feeding. I felt terribly sad that I hadn't found the key to making nursing work for us; but I also found myself feeling like a better mother once I gave her a bottle. She wasn't so clingy anymore.*

It was years before I identified my feelings as postpartum depression. I'm still sad I didn't find the right support and encouragement to keep nursing. Now, in my classes, I tell women that with breast-feeding, they have to discover their own rhythm.

Also, I've found it impossible to get consistent temperature readings when I have a child who doesn't sleep through the night. I can only rely on my mucus readings. For the last two months, our son (who's a little over a year old) will take only his father at night. This means I sleep much better—and I finally get a sensible BBT chart.

Jody McLaughlin, publisher of **The Compleat Mother,** *and mother of two grown daughters.* *When women go back to work and can't bring their baby, I like to tell them about Sacagawea, the sixteen-year-old Shoshone Indian whom Lewis and Clark hired in 1805. She served as an interpreter and helped guide them through the territories recently purchased by the United States from France. Through blizzards, bears, mosquitos, and tipped boats, Sacagawea helped Lewis and Clark; and she was still nursing her baby when their expedition ended two and a half years later. The baby was three months old when the journey began. Her husband accompanied her, and she didn't get pregnant on the trip.*

I consider Sacagawea the first federal employee who took her breast-fed baby to work.

Persist, not insist.

—AUTHOR UNKNOWN

Replace your ambition with curiosity.

—MARTIN KEOGH

Joyful fishing catches more than fish.

—CHARLES HOY

5. Enhancing Your Chances of Conceiving

WHEN I HEAR ABOUT A WOMAN WANTING to bear a child, I see her dancing with empty arms, open to receiving mysteries and gifts. She dances before her gods and goddesses, before her partner, her family, and community—and waits to see what she'll be offered. She can make wishes, but she can't control what comes to her. She can care for herself as well as possible. She can give thanks for what she receives.

I first thought of this image while reading Lewis Hyde's *The Gift: Imagination and the Erotic Life of Property,* a book about creativity in a market-oriented society.

Hyde explains that in medieval times, the village beggar with an empty bowl was considered the town's wealthiest member for being most open to receiving. I wondered if, while inviting biologic creativity, we can welcome the wealth of a woman with an empty womb.

When a couple has difficulty conceiving a child or sustaining a pregnancy, I may ask, *What are your questions?* For me, a question is like an empty bowl. The questions I carry, my hands cupped together and empty, affect what I receive. Some questions invite a yes or no or a maybe *(Will I be a mother?)*; some open us to technical information *(What can I do to strengthen my progesterone levels?)*; others move us to discover ourselves and our world more deeply *(What encourages my sense of family and belonging?).*

Questions are also like prayers. I've often defined prayer as what we give our attention to, and the way prayers are phrased can matter. For example, *We just want a healthy baby, in a year,* is dependent on a healthy baby's arrival. What if no baby arrives? What if the baby who arrives isn't healthy as you dream? Some prayers can open you to surprises: *We welcome the chance to include children in our family.*

"For fifteen years," a client once told me, "I gave myself the message, *'Don't get pregnant!'* I used all kinds of birth control, and I reminded myself, often, that I was not able to handle a baby. Then one day I changed my tune to *'Get Pregnant NOW!'* It's been eight months, and I'm still not pregnant. Apparently my body—and my mind—might need time to adjust to this new idea."

For many women and men, opening to conceive also heralds a fresh look at health, diet, pace, and spirituality. As naturopath and midwife Deborah Keller explains, "Healthy fertility emerges out of general health. When a couple decides they want to conceive, my focus turns toward strengthening their overall wellness."

Dagmar Ehling, a doctor of Oriental medicine, says, "When a woman seeks my help after having difficulty conceiving or sustaining a pregnancy, my best suggestion is for her to focus on restoring her health and appreciating her body as it is. Herbs and acupuncture can help. But it's just as important for her to be gentle and patient with herself—whether or not she becomes pregnant."

Through charting your fertility signals (perhaps for several months or more before you begin trying to conceive), you can see if aspects of your gynecological health might be strengthened. Charting can also tell you when to time intercourse to increase your chances of becoming pregnant.

Essentially, to use Fertility Awareness to help you conceive, you need the same

THE PRIVILEGE OF FERTILITY

One of the biggest reasons why hormonal imbalances are misunderstood is because modern medicine disregards the way the human body deals with its environment. Consider that the body's responses basically have not changed for 50,000 years. We still respond to our environment with the most primal of mechanisms: the "fight-or-flight" mechanism, the release of adrenaline and other stress hormones. The stress response, initiated in the hypothalamus and pituitary and regulated by the adrenal glands, is responsible for redirecting energy and resources away from the reproductive organs when we are under severe or chronic stress, directing it instead to the muscles and organs that are necessary for survival. This redirection is allowed to take place because, on the body's list of priorities, survival comes first and reproduction comes last.

The reproductive system is the only body system whose functions are biologically expendable. With this in mind, we see how the ability to reproduce becomes a privilege in the body, not a right.

—Michael Borkin, Naturopathic physician

information as you do to prevent pregnancy: how to determine that you're fertile and about to ovulate and how to confirm that you have ovulated. Now though, it's time to make love during your fertile phase.

Fertile Clues: *Cervical Fluid and Vaginal Sensation*

Cervical fluid and vaginal sensation provide the biggest clues to when you are fertile and about to ovulate. Remember that being fertile and ovulating are not the same: being fertile means you've got cervical fluid present that can keep sperm alive until you ovulate. After the menstrual period, once you observe CF (including tacky mucus) or a moist vaginal sensation, your follicular phase has begun: follicles are emitting estrogen, which in turn produces cervical fluid. Ovulation refers to the twelve to twenty-four hours your egg is alive in the fallopian tube.

Also, the Peak Day is the *last* day of fertile cervical fluid *or* moist vaginal sensation. Typically, you'll observe egg white on your Peak Day. The Peak Day is not the day of *most* mucus. It's your *last* day of slippery CF or moist sensation, and it signals that ovulation is about to take place. You won't be able to identify your Peak Day until the next day, when your CF and vaginal sensation have begun drying up. Typically, ovulation takes place plus or minus two days from the Peak Day.

Some women don't observe egg white. In that case, your last day of wet CF or wet sensation would be considered your Peak Day.

Sperm Counts and Timing

Once you know when you're about to ovulate, you can combine this information with awareness of your partner's sperm count and thereby time intercourse to optimize your chances of conceiving.

Typically, a woman has wet cervical fluid for two to four days each cycle; and usually it takes thirty-six hours for a man to replenish his sperm count after ejaculating. If your partner has a normal sperm count, you can have intercourse on each day that your mucus is wet before your Peak Day. If your partner's sperm count is low, have intercourse every other day that your mucus is wet. If his sperm count is especially low, make love every third day that you have wet mucus.

Whether your partner's sperm count is normal or low, try to have intercourse on the Peak Day as well, since the Peak Day usually occurs either on the day before you ovulate or the day you do. A recent study shows that the highest probability of conception occurs with intercourse one or two days before ovulation.[1] Since you can't identify your Peak Day until the next day, when drying up begins, you need to make decisions about timing intercourse based on past cycles' Peak Days. If, for several cycles, your Peak Day has been Day 17, you can time lovemaking accordingly. If it's fallen on Day 17 one cycle and Day 23 the next, make love every day or every other day (depending on your husband's sperm count) while your CF is wet.

Sperm counts are generally considered low when there are less than 50 million sperm per ejaculate; when less than 60 percent of the sperm have normal morphology (shape); or when less than 60 percent have normal motility (ability to move forward). If the man's sperm count is tested and found to be low, he should have it tested again within a few weeks, because an occasional low count might inaccurately reflect his normal count.

Hot tubbing, bicycling, wearing tight pants, spending the day cooking near a hot oven, smoking marijuana, environmental toxins, and age all can decrease sperm counts.

Here are two charts that show when to time intercourse to enhance your chances of conceiving:

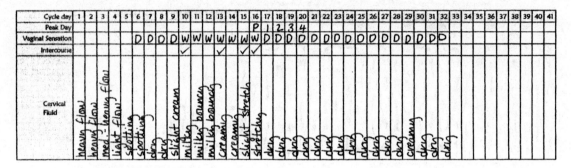

Figure 5.1.

The woman's peak was on Day 16. Her partner's sperm count is normal. Their best days to try began on Day 10 (because she had mucus and wet vaginal sensation). Their very best days to try were Days 15 and 16, when she had egg white.

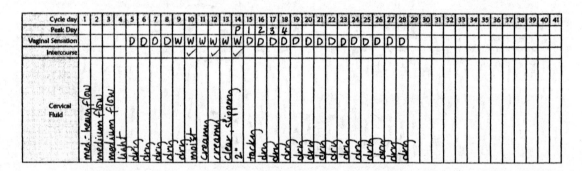

Figure 5.2.

The woman's peak was on Day 14. Her partner's sperm count is low. Their best days to try began on Day 10, when she had mucus and wet vaginal sensation; their very best days to try were Days 10, 12, and 14.

Split Peaks

Some women observe split peaks, whereby their mucus builds to a wet, slippery consistency then dries up—then becomes wetter again. The temperature doesn't shift (to confirm ovulation) along with the "false" peak.

If you experience a split peak while you are readying to conceive, you can take steps to normalize your cycle before you try. (You can read more about split peaks in chapter 3 on p. 49, in chapter 6 on p. 116, and in chapter 12 on p. 195.) You can also continue with intercourse every day or every other day (depending on your partner's sperm count) while your mucus is building up again. The days you've got egg white are ideal for trying.

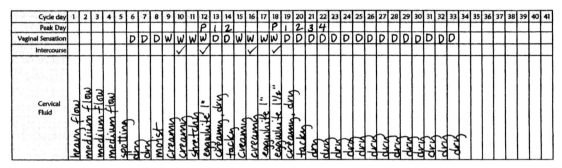

Figure 5.3.

The woman had a false peak on Day 12; her true peak was on Day 18. Her partner's sperm count is normal. Their best days to try began on Day 9 (because she had mucus and wet vaginal sensation). Their very best days to try were Days 11, 12, 17, and 18, when she had egg white.

If You Don't See Egg White

If your cervical fluid never gets very slippery, like egg white, you might try sleeping in the absence of light and making some changes in your diet (such as taking cod liver oil and eating organic butter). You can read more about these options in chapters 10 and 11.

The Basal Body Temperature

If you record your BBT every day, you can use it to confirm ovulation, to determine if you have sufficient progesterone levels to sustain a pregnancy, and to discover if you have become pregnant.

The postovulatory luteal phase (when progesterone is dominant) typically lasts twelve to sixteen days. At the end of this phase (in a nonpregnant woman), the corpus luteum dies, your temperature drops, and a new cycle begins with menstruation. If, before trying to conceive, you notice that your luteal phase consistently lasts less than twelve days, you may not have enough progesterone to sustain a pregnancy.

Also, if your temperature dips to or below your coverline after ovulation, you may not have enough progesterone to sustain a pregnancy. If you notice such patterns before trying to conceive, you can take steps to strengthen your cycle before you try. Part 2 describes these steps.

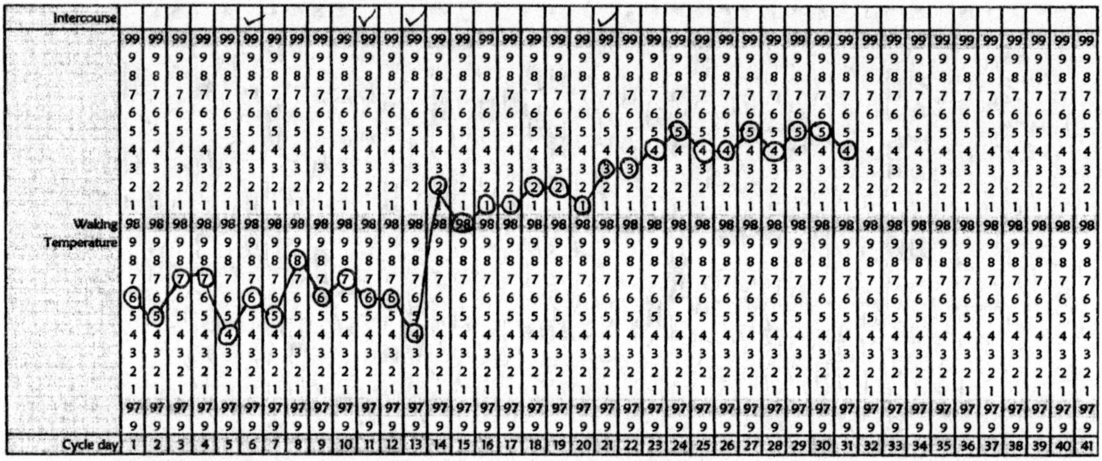

Figure 5.4.

Some women show a significant dip in their temperature on the day they ovulate. If you do, have intercourse on that day. For example, in figure 5.4, the woman's temperature dipped on Day 13, when she probably ovulated and then timed intercourse. (She could confirm pregnancy on Day 31.)

You can also have intercourse the morning of your temperature rise, even though you've probably already ovulated, because:

- If you release more than one egg at ovulation, you might still have one viable.
- In some cases, women don't release their egg until right after the rise.
- If ovulation occurred just before the rise, there's still a chance that the egg is alive.

Cervix Changes

Charting the cervix's changes can help women in special circumstances (such as breast-feeding and coming off the Pill) to gauge when ovulation is about to take place. Typically, the cervix softens and rises, and the os opens when you're fertile. Just before ovulation, it may become firm, lower in the vaginal canal, and the os may close. (The logic of this is that all sperm would be collected in the cervix before ovulation occurs; closing the os decreases the risk of an infection after conception has occurred.)

In figure 5.5, this breast-feeding woman found her cervix "unambiguously open" on Days 25 and 26. To conceive, she could time intercourse on those days.

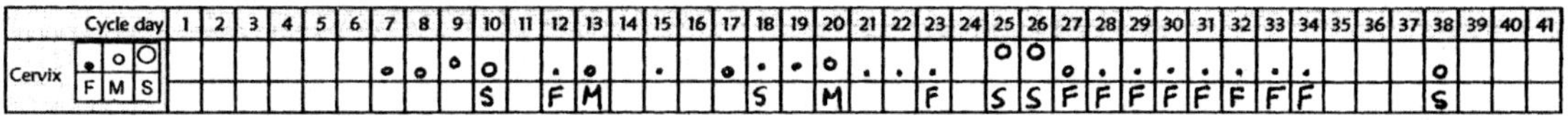

Cycle day	1	2	3	4	5	6	7	8	9	10	11	12	13	14	15	16	17	18	19	20	21	22	23	24	25	26	27	28	29	30	31	32	33	34	35	36	37	38	39	40	41
Cervix							•	•	•	O		•	•		•		•	•	•	O		•	•	•	O	O		•	•	•	•	•	•	•	•	•			O		
F M S										S		F	M				S		M			F			S	S	F	F	F	F	F	F	F	F				S		

Figure 5.5.

I know a lot of women who didn't conceive for several cycles because their timing was off. To conceive, you need to make love when you've got mucus! Figure 5.6 shows the chart of a couple who began trying to conceive on Day 13, several days into her follicular phase. The man's sperm count is low. They confirmed pregnancy (with eighteen temperatures above her coverline) on Day 35.

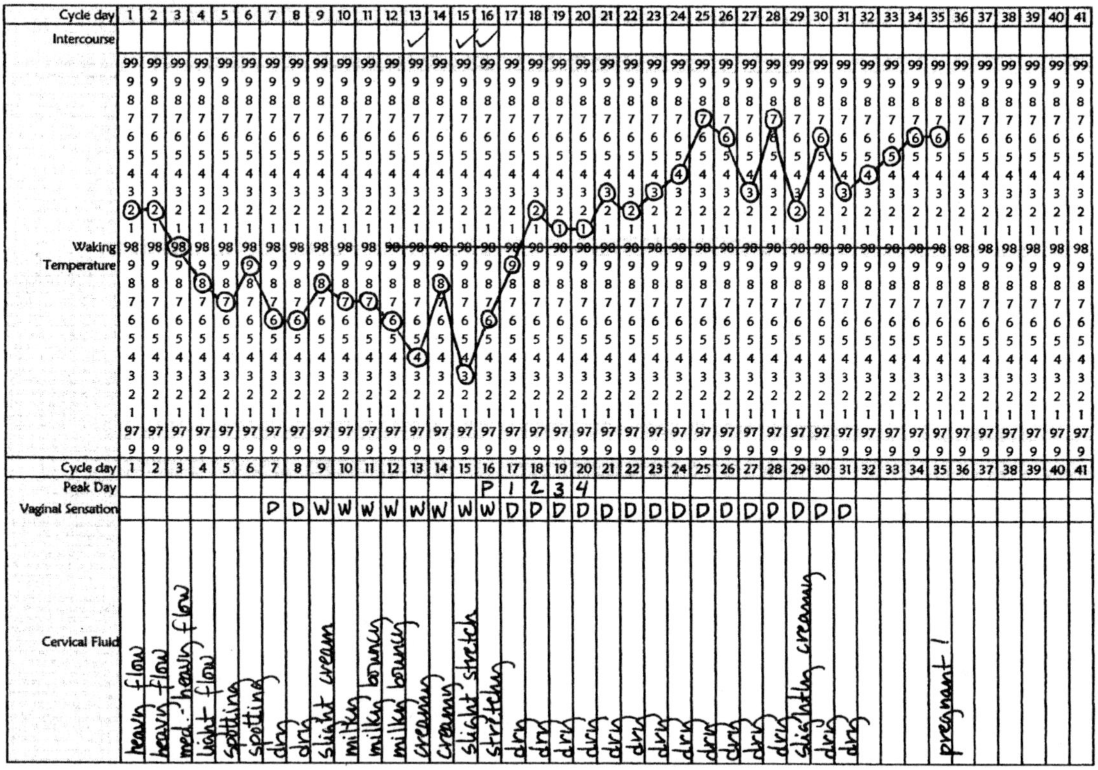

Figure 5.6.

Night-Lighting and Pregnancy

Sleeping in the absence of light, except for the few days around ovulation, has helped some women to conceive. (This is called Lunaception, and you can read more about it in chapter 10.) Once you do conceive, sleeping in complete darkness can help you maintain the pregnancy. This is so because sleeping with light can reduce your pineal gland's production of melatonin, which in turn can reduce production of progesterone, which is needed to sustain pregnancy.

How To Determine Whether You're Pregnant

If you have eighteen temperatures above your coverline and no period, then you're probably pregnant. (You can read how to draw a coverline in chapter 3.) You need eighteen high temps because the corpus luteum will not live longer than sixteen days unless you're pregnant; and it's possible that you don't conceive until a second egg is released at ovulation (which could be two days after the temperature rises). Add sixteen and two and you get eighteen days.

The rare exception to this rule is when a corpus luteum cyst is present. Also, women who take a fertility drug such as Clomid may have an extended luteal phase though they have not conceived.

The woman whose chart was shown in figure 5.4 could confirm that she was pregnant on Day 31, when she had eighteen temperatures above her coverline.

Calculating Your Due Date

Obstetricians usually predict your due date by subtracting three months from the first day of your last menstrual period and adding seven days. This system assumes you conceived during a textbook cycle, with ovulation (and conception) occurring on Day 14. With this system, if your last period started on January 1, your due date would be October 8.

To determine a due date that is probably more precise, you can calculate it based on information provided by your chart. Subtract seven days from the first day your temperature shifted into the luteal phase, then add nine months. For example, if your last period started on January 1 but you didn't ovulate and show a temperature shift until January 25, your due date—based on when you ovulated and conceived, not when your last period began—would be October 18.

A recent issue of *Family Foundations,* the Couple to Couple League's bimonthly journal, featured a story about a woman whose insurance company declined to cover her pregnancy and birth—until she mailed them her chart and the CCL explained that she didn't ovulate (or conceive) until she was in fact covered by their policy!

Defining Infertility

I use the term *infertile* very cautiously. I've seen many people jump to call themselves infertile when they're simply not conceiving within their planned time frame. A study presented by Dr. David Dunson at the 2001 European Society of Human Reproduction and Embryology found that most healthy couples who don't conceive after a year of trying will conceive during the second year. The new research shows that even couples in their late thirties have a 91 percent chance of becoming pregnant naturally within two years.

When pregnancy doesn't occur despite healthy charts, healthy sperm counts, and right timing, I'm reminded of our inability to control nature, including our fertility. We can spend so much time waiting to conceive and waiting to know if we're pregnant, and then pregnancy is a long wait, and giving birth can be, too. The dictionary says that *wait* means "to remain or be in readiness; to serve the needs of, be in attendance on." Its Indo-European root is *weg,* which means "to be strong, be lively."

I'm also intrigued by the common experience of couples conceiving a healthy child after they've adopted another, or otherwise "given up" their chances of becoming pregnant. Is there a mechanism that constricts people from becoming pregnant? Is there a way to soften or open that mechanism?

The mysteries and gifts of fertility cannot be possessed: to circulate and sustain their aliveness, they must be given away. "In the spiritual world," Lewis Hyde writes, "new life comes to those who give up."

Katherine, thirty-five. After much discussion about whether or not we're really ready for a baby, my husband and I recently started making love without barriers. I knew I was ready, but despite his assurances, I still doubted that he was. Then I noticed that even though he can't read my chart, he's become very interested in lovemaking when I'm fertile. This feels like a yes from him, at an unconscious level. It convinced me that he really is as ready as he says he is.

Brenda, thirty-two. In the first cycle we started trying to conceive, I got a bladder infection just before I ovulated. I told my husband, "I don't care if it hurts when we make love—I want a baby!" As soon as I heard myself say this, I thought, "Is this how I want to invite a child into our lives?"

In fact, it isn't. I've still got some irritation with my bladder, and I'm starting to think it's helping me slow down, get to know myself while I open to a baby (which I've never done before), and let go the idea that I can control my body or when I get pregnant.

Phoebe, thirty-eight. I miscarried pretty quickly after we started trying to get pregnant three years ago and haven't conceived again. By my charts, it looks like I've got low progesterone. I've tried herbs, therapy, acupuncture, and naturally compounded progesterone to remedy the situation—all, so far, to no avail.

Recently, I imagined myself ten years into the future, still without a child. I sensed I could accept my life like that—in ten years. But I'm not accepting of my life now. This is what hurts so much. Since realizing this, inch by inch I've turned my focus from trying to get my charts just so to simply trusting and accepting myself, even when my body's not giving me what I want.

Rachel, twenty-seven. When I didn't conceive in nearly a year, I went to a rabbi and asked his opinion about fertility drugs. This rabbi said, "Sure you can take the drugs. But first: Do you eat breakfast? If not, try eating breakfast every day for a few months before you try the drugs."

I had indeed been skipping breakfast. Once I started eating it, I got pregnant in three months.

Sandi, fifty-eight. Many years after our son was born and we were on our way to divorce, my husband told me that he had deeply resented having "sex on command" when I was fertile. He felt controlled and bossed around by me and my chart. He didn't feel ready for parenthood but went ahead because I wanted it so much. For our marriage, this was a recipe for disaster.

Bernice, fifty-three. The first time I got pregnant, I was forty-two. I miscarried at six weeks. I'd begun charting several months before the miscarriage because I started having hot flashes and I'd missed a period. Frankly, because of my age, I hadn't thought I could get pregnant. After the miscarriage, I brought my charts to the doctor's office. He could tell from my charts (which had returned to a healthy ovulatory pattern) that I was fine and that I didn't need a D&C. Then he asked if I'd like a fertility workup.

I asked him if it's more difficult to get pregnant or keep pregnant. He said that at my age, getting pregnant is harder. Well, I'd just done that. So I declined the fertility workup. I decided I didn't want Clomid, either, after I did a little research and read that it can increase a woman's risk of ovarian cancer. My mother died of ovarian cancer.

We conceived our daughter within a few months after the miscarriage. She's nine years old now—and delightful!

WRITING GAMES

- Ask your grandparents if there are family tales of miscarriages, stillbirths, abortions, adopted babies, and/or infertility that would help you understand your family constellation and your place in it more fully. Just live with these questions for a while and see what answers come to you (kind of like living with an empty bowl). If your relatives are still alive, and you feel comfortable, ask them!

- If the ones who could answer your questions are dead, get a blank notebook and a few great pens, unplug your phone, or go to a quiet hiking trail, and invite your ancestors to tell you their stories. If you think you're just making stuff up as you write, that's probably the case; and that's fine. Let the stories come out as you would with a dream. You can also live with them as you would with a dream.

- If you've been trying to conceive for a while, ask your ancestors what's blocking you. Ask them what you need to carry a health pregnancy to term. If the stories you get feel true to you, or if they linger with you and give you stuff to ponder, great. If not, not to worry. Keep your hands soft around your empty bowl. What you need will come to you.

- Imagine a good friend of yours wants a baby. She hasn't conceived in a year, or maybe she's had several miscarriages. She's heartbroken, and her partner and her friends can't comfort her. What advice would you give her? Write this down—and consider it your best medicine.

Some Other Tips

Residual semen can interfere with your CF observations. In order to get a more accurate reading, do Kegel exercises (see p. 22) a few hours after sex. By that time, the sperm with potential to fertilize an egg will have had plenty of time to travel into the cervix.

If you need lubrication, note that saliva can impede sperm; so can K-Y Jelly. Try Kegeling slowly for a few minutes each day to increase arousal fluid.

In the day or days before you try to conceive, enjoy sexual cuddling that doesn't involve ejaculation (to build up sperm). After you make love to conceive (and your partner has ejaculated), focus on your connection with each other.

If you are considering conceiving with a donor's sperm, the Sperm Bank of California is the first such organization to provide donor-identifying information to offspring who are eighteen or older. They have also pioneered a family contact program, which allows families that use the same donor to conceive their children to be put in contact. The Sperm Bank of California, 2115 Milvia St., 2nd Flr., Berkeley, CA 94704; www.thespermbankofca.org; 510-841-1858.

A SUMMARY OF WAYS TO OPTIMIZE CHANCES OF CONCEIVING

1. Have intercourse on your Peak Day—the *last* day of egg white or wet vaginal sensation. If you don't observe egg white, your Peak Day is still the *last* day of the wettest cervical fluid you have.

2. If the man's sperm count is normal, have intercourse each day you have fertile cervical fluid. If his sperm count is low, have intercourse every other day that you have fertile CF. In either case, try to have intercourse on your Peak Day, through to and including the first morning of your rise in temperature.

2

Fertility Awareness and Gynecological Health

*More than any other tool or system, Fertility Awareness gives
a woman avenues to connecting with her own body and
to knowing the vital signs her menstrual cycle offers,
as well as a vocabulary for communicating effectively
with her health care provider.*

—JUSTINA TROTT, MD
President, American College of
Women's Health Physicians

6. Gauging Gynecological Health by Fertility Signals

WHEN YOU KNOW HOW TO READ FERTILITY
charts to prevent or achieve pregnancy, learning how to interpret them for basic
gynecological health is an easy next step. Charts provide a way to observe the rise
and fall of your hormone levels. They can tell you whether you're ovulating and
how to predict when your period will come; they can indicate your progesterone
levels, if you've miscarried, and whether you're at risk for thyroid problems or
ovarian cysts. Moreover, when you observe your fertility signals, you know what's
normal for *you;* if you observe changes in your cervical fluid or temperature that
are abnormal to your patterns, you can opt for diagnostic tests in a timely manner.

Indeed, once you learn the basics about reading your body, you become a more active player in your own health care.

Looking for Patterns

Several theories presented in this chapter come from traditional Chinese medicine. The Chinese have observed the relationship between geological patterns and human health for thousands of years: Oriental medicine stems from the idea that life arises from the endless interplay of the opposing forces of yin and yang, heaven and earth, masculine and feminine, heating and cooling, moistening and drying, active and passive, light and dark, contracting and relaxing. Diagnosis of a person's health includes looking at the tongue (for color, shape, and coating) and feeling the pulse at the wrists (for qualities of yin, yang, heat, cold, dampness, dryness, excess, and deficiency). A practitioner determines a person's "pattern of disharmony," which can then be addressed with acupuncture and herbs.

In the mid-sixties, when some Chinese doctors began using a woman's waking temperature (BBT) to confirm ovulation, they found it could also be used to gauge other aspects of gynecological health. Bob Flaws, an American doctor of Oriental medicine (DOM), has translated Chinese studies that gauge gynecological health by the BBT and brought them to the West. For example, the Chinese found that transitions taking more than three days between the follicular and luteal phases might indicate yang deficiency. In Western terms, this can translate to progesterone deficiency. The Chinese term *excess yin* can mean excess estrogen in Western terms.

Before describing what a healthy fertility chart looks like, I'll say that I rarely meet women who consistently have "textbook" charts; and most women's cycles differ from one month to the next.

The menstrual cycle and its hormones are parts of a woman's whole complex body—part of her whole complex life—and she is part of a much wider ecosystem. As the Chinese have observed, we all participate in dynamic, ongoing cycles of heating and cooling and moistening and drying. A woman isn't her diagnosis; she's a whole person with an energetic makeup. Our body parts and their functions are all interrelated, and related to our environment. And so much of what affects us—like love, for example—isn't measurable.

Hormones (messengers that travel through the blood from one organ to another) are delicate players in a body's overall wellness. We've learned a lot about them in the last fifty years. And still, much about hormones is mysterious and hard to track down. Like emotions, like weather, they change from day to day. Their levels can even fluctuate within a few hours.

This is one reason to advocate for using fertility charts to gauge gynecological health: they allow you to observe your cycles over time, at no cost. In gathering information about your menstrual cycle, charting your fertility signals is an excellent first step.

When reading your charts to gauge gynecological health, look for patterns. One strange cycle might be just that—a strange cycle. Keep in mind that the situations presented here are not unusual. Indeed, this chapter shows the most common problems. If your charts indicate a problem or two, you're not alone. Then, there are remedies for all of these situations. If you think you've got a problem, chapters 8 through 12 describe options for addressing specific situations. You can also use the introductory information presented here to help you raise questions with your health-care provider. The Resources section of this book can lead you to more information.

Also, please note that this chapter only explains how to use charts to help diagnose your cycles. I've separated these sections about gauging and strengthening gynecological health because recognizing a problem is one step; choosing a remedy is another. The problems described here likely developed slowly, over time. Remedying them can also take time.

That said, let me remind you of a few key vocabulary terms:

- The *follicular phase* is the phase before ovulation, when follicles (sacs containing eggs) are emitting *estrogen*. Estrogen stimulates production of cervical fluid, cools your body temperature, encourages interest in sex, and begins building your uterine lining with blood in preparation for a possible pregnancy.
- The *luteal phase* comes after ovulation; it ends when the new cycle begins, at menstruation. The luteal phase is dominated by *progesterone*—which dries your mucus, warms your temperature, and continues preparing your uterine lining for pregnancy.

A typical healthy fertility chart shows:

- A steady, red, clot-free bloodflow during the menstrual cycle's first three to five days.

- Dry vaginal sensation and no mucus for a few days after the period.
- Cervical fluid building up from a tacky or creamy texture, "peaking" at a slippery, egg white–like texture just before ovulation, then transitioning to dryer CF after ovulation.
- Lower temperatures before ovulation and higher ones (at least two tenths of a degree higher) after ovulation.
- The temperature shift indicating ovulation takes three days or less.
- The temperature shift from the luteal (postovulatory) phase to the new cycle takes three days or less.
- A twelve- to sixteen-day luteal phase.
- The luteal phase temperatures stay above the coverline.

In figure 6.1, Sara turned thirty-nine. She never took the Pill and has never conceived, nor tried to. Through her temperature, she shows a slight progesterone deficiency, because her transition from the follicular to the luteal phase takes four days (Days 15 through 18). But basically she's got a healthy cycle: lower temperatures before ovulation and sustained higher temperatures after ovulation. She probably ovulated on Day 16 or 17. Her Peak Day of cervical fluid and her temperature shift line up exactly: each signal confirms ovulation by 6 P.M. on Day 20.

Using Charts to Predict When You'll Menstruate

Once you've charted several cycles, know how to confirm that you've ovulated, and are able to determine the length of your luteal phases, you can predict when your period will come—even if the number of days in your preovulatory phase varies from cycle to cycle. If you get cramps with your period, or otherwise like to take it easy when you menstruate, you can use your charts to schedule accordingly.

Remember the corpus luteum, the sac that emits progesterone during your luteal phase (after ovulation) and typically lives twelve to sixteen days? When it dies, your temperature drops and menstruation usually begins within a day or two. Typically, the length of the luteal phase (from ovulation until menstruation) is predictable.

For example, in figure 6.1, Sara had a fourteen-day luteal phase—as she usually does. Once she's got three temperatures above her coverline and can confirm ovu-

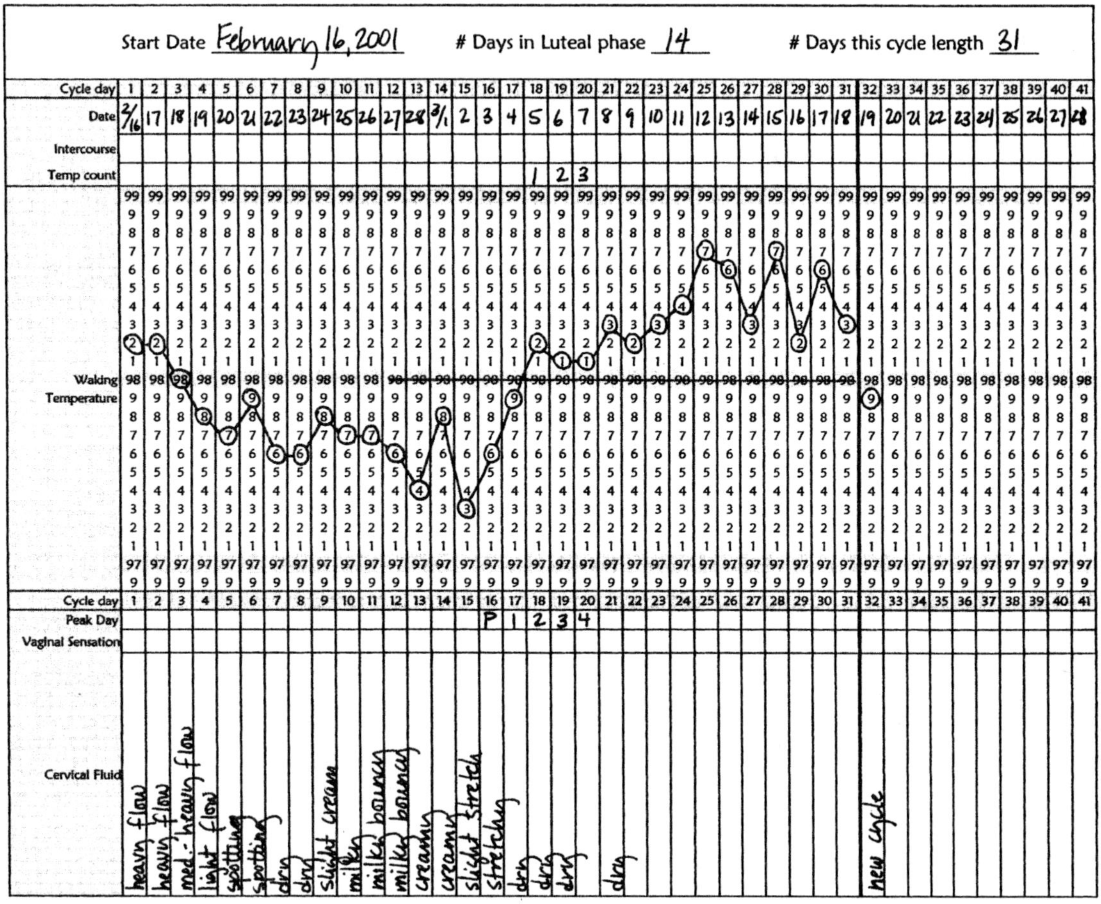

Start Date **February 16, 2001**   # Days in Luteal phase **14**   # Days this cycle length **31**

Figure 6.1. A healthy chart.

lation (on Day 20/March 7), Sara can count eleven more days (for a fourteen-day luteal phase) and predict she'll start menstruating on March 19.

The preovulatory phase—the follicular phase—tends to be less predictable. For example, you might ovulate on Day 12 in one cycle and Day 18 in the next. In either case, the postovulatory, luteal phase is usually more predictable; and it won't last longer than sixteen days unless you're pregnant.

The rare exception to this rule is when a corpus luteum cyst is present. In this situation, which might happen once in a woman's lifetime, the corpus luteum doesn't dissolve after its normal twelve- to sixteen-day life span; and, though you're not pregnant, your temperature may remain high. Around the time your period is expected, you might have mild pain and spotting. Usually, a corpus luteum cyst will dissolve on its own. If your temperature remains high for more than eighteen days, your pregnancy test is negative, and you haven't menstruated, a bimanual exam and an ultrasound can determine if you've got a corpus luteum cyst.

Here's another example of a healthy chart. In figure 6.2, Helen, thirty-four, has a very crisp temperature shift between Days 17 and 18, indicating probable ovulation on Day 17. Her cervical fluid peaks on Day 15. By her CF, she can consider herself infertile at 6 P.M. on Day 19. By her temperature, she can't confirm ovulation until 6 P.M. on Day 20. To prevent pregnancy, she'd wait to have intercourse until after 6 P.M. on Day 20. This slight difference between when the two signals confirm ovulation indicates no health problem.

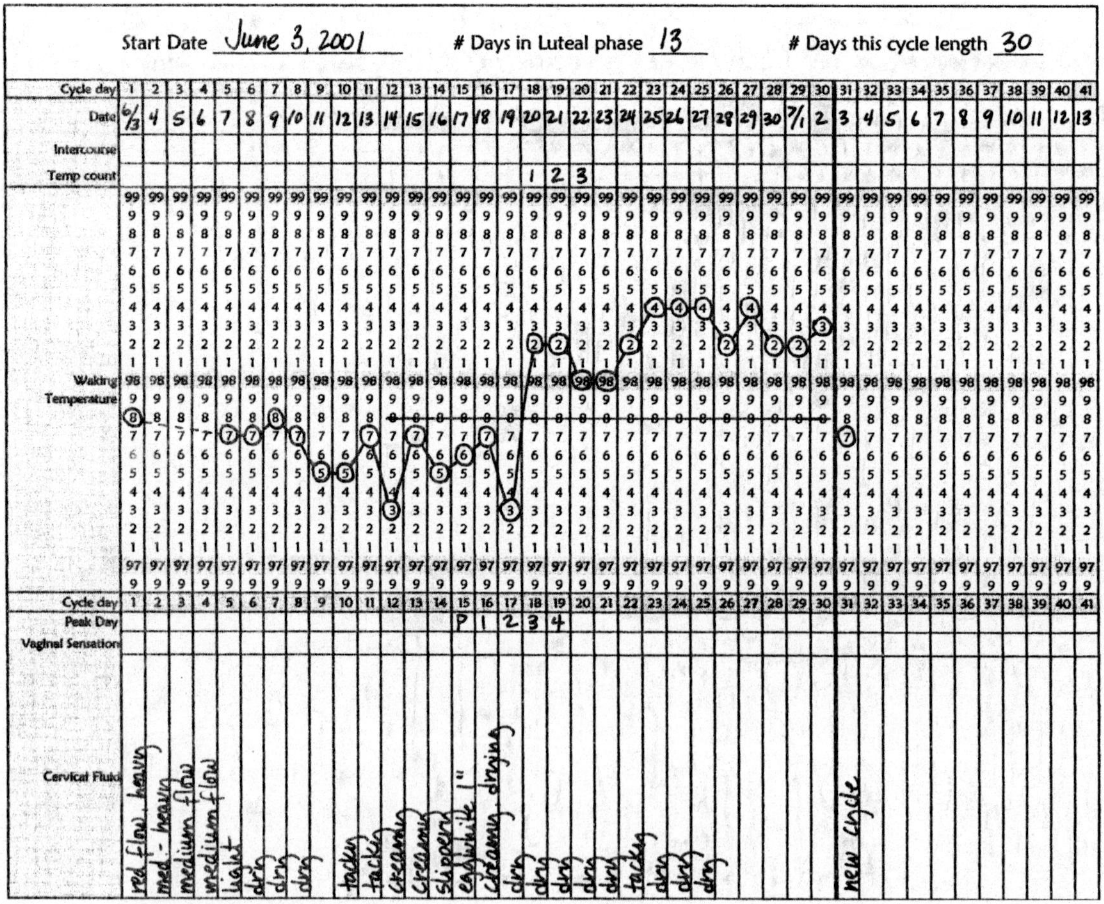

Start Date June 3, 2001   # Days in Luteal phase 13   # Days this cycle length 30

Figure 6.2. A healthy chart.

Helen's luteal phase is almost always thirteen days long. Beginning with her third temperature above her coverline on Day 20/June 22, she can count ten more temps (for a total of thirteen, the typical length of her luteal phase), and predict that she'll begin menstruating on July 3.

Anovulation

Anovulation means not ovulating. It's common among teenagers, women who are on or coming off the Pill, and overweight and underweight women. Weaknesses in the pituitary or thyroid gland can lead to anovulation. It's also common (and perfectly healthy) among breast-feeding women and those who have recently stopped nursing, since prolactin levels tend to be high while a woman is breast-feeding, and this hormone suppresses ovulation. Women who are approaching menopause also tend to have anovulatory cycles. *And,* it's possible for women in each of the above situations to ovulate and carry a healthy pregnancy to term.

Anovulation can also mean that you're pregnant.

Amenorrhea is the absence of menstrual bleeding. An eighteen-year-old woman who has never menstruated has primary amenorrhea; if your menses have stopped for at least three months, you have secondary amenorrhea.

Many people are surprised to learn that it's possible to have an apparent period without ovulating. Called *breakthrough bleeding*, this occurs when estrogen has caused enough endometrial growth for bleeding to appear normally. However, ovulation does not occur, and there isn't enough progesterone to sustain your uterine lining. Since it does not follow ovulation, breakthrough bleeding is not true menstruation.

With anovulation, hormone levels may be strong enough to build the uterine lining, while FSH (follicle-stimulating hormone) and LH (luteinizing hormone) may not be strong enough to cause ovulation.

The easiest way to tell whether you're ovulating is by your temperature. If you don't see a *sustained* shift (with temperatures staying high for at least three days after a rise of two tenths of a degree), you're probably not ovulating.

If you don't show a shift in temperature and you think you are ovulating (perhaps you show a clear buildup of cervical fluid followed by dryer mucus, you have midcycle pain around your Peak Day, and/or menstruation follows about fourteen days after your mucous peak), talk with your doctor to find out if you're among a very small group of women who ovulate without a temperature shift. An ultra-sound might be used to determine whether you're ovulating.

Ovulation requires FSH, estrogen, LH, and progesterone to work in concert with hormones secreted by well-functioning thyroid and adrenal glands. If you're not ovulating, you might have low levels of one or several of these hormones (which is common among premenopausal women).

Ovulation also requires a healthy ratio of weight to height and fat to muscle. Fatty tissue is necessary, for example, for estrogen to be produced and stored properly. Women who are underweight or extremely thin may not ovulate because their hypothalamus gland may not properly stimulate their pituitary gland to secrete FSH and LH—which are both necessary for ovulation. Nutritionist Marilyn Shannon suggests that women of "supposedly ideal weight" who have unexplained anovulation may benefit from gaining three to five pounds in order to encourage ovulation.

Being overweight can also inhibit ovulation, because too much body fat can create elevated estrogen levels. Elevated estrogen can "confuse" the pituitary gland, so that FSH levels remain low, and an ovulatory follicle does not develop. Also, an overweight woman may have increased insulin, which can interfere with follicular development.

See figure 6.3. Gabrielle began menstruating at eleven, and took the Pill for two months when she was fifteen. She was twenty in this chart. She's 5'4", 115 pounds, muscular, and healthy. Sometimes she bled monthly, sometimes every two or three months, sometimes every four or five months. After a year of charting, she had six ovulatory charts.

There's a myth that one day's rise in temperature means that the woman has ovulated. But each time Gabrielle's temperature rises here, it goes back down: she doesn't have a *sustained* rise. There's no place to put a coverline. Some people might think that Gabrielle ovulated between Days 20 and 21. But she has only four (not six) low temperatures before her rise. This is anovulation.

Because her temperatures are frequently below 97.5, Gabrielle may also have a thyroid problem. (See "Thyroid Disorders" on p. 108.)

As for mucus in anovulatory cycles, typically, it's unchanging—either dry, creamy, watery, or some combination of these. Gabrielle's egg white on Day 15—a false peak—could be related to elevated estrogen levels.

I recently spoke with a twenty-six-year-old woman who's been charting for a year. She bleeds monthly, although she hasn't ovulated for six cycles. After a yearly

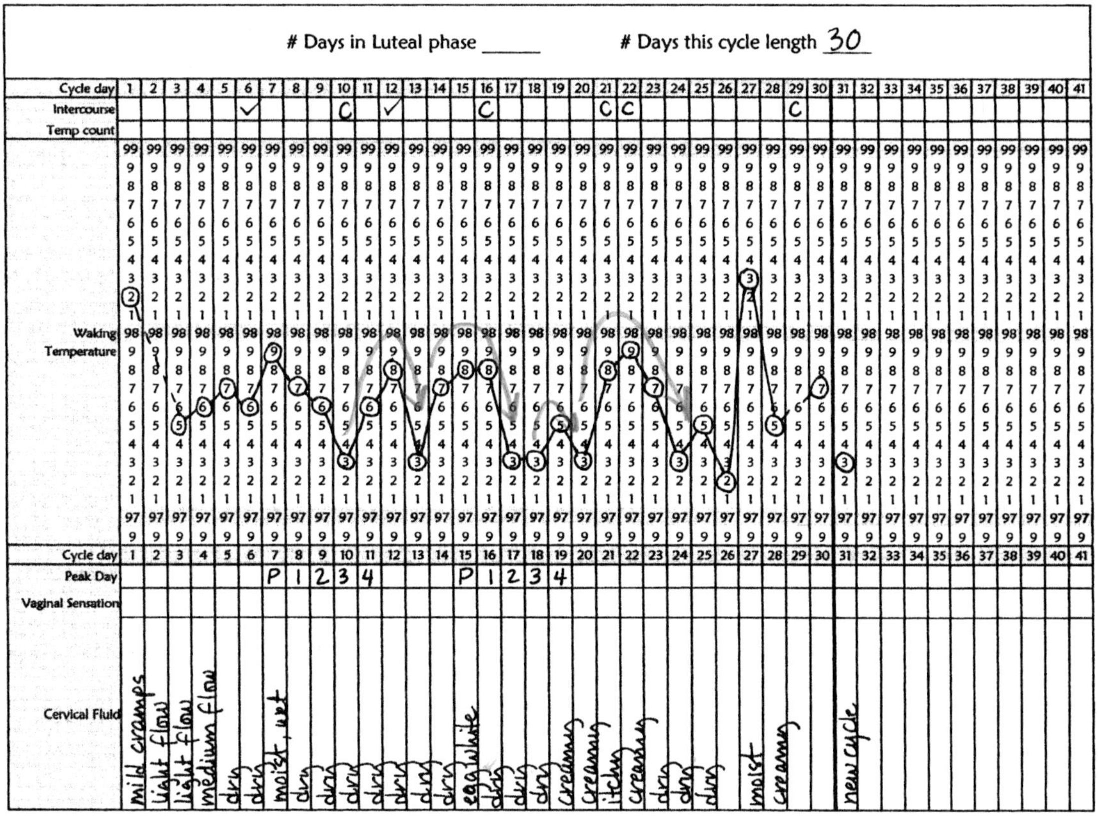

 # Days in Luteal phase _____   **# Days this cycle length _30_**

Cycle day	1	2	3	4	5	6	7	8	9	10	11	12	13	14	15	16	17	18	19	20	21	22	23	24	25	26	27	28	29	30	31	32	33	34	35	36	37	38	39	40	41
Intercourse						✓				C		✓				C					C	C						C													
Temp count																																									

(Waking Temperature grid, cycle days 1–41)

Cycle day	1	2	3	4	5	6	7	8	9	10	11	12	13	14	15	16	17	18	19	20	21	22	23	24	25	26	27	28	29	30	31	32	33	34	35	36	37	38	39	40	41
Peak Day											P	1	2	3	4		P	1	2	3	4																				
Vaginal Sensation																																									
Cervical Fluid	mild cramps	light flow	light flow	medium flow	dry	dry	moist wet	dry	dry	dry	dry	dry	egg white	dry	dry	creamy	creamy	itchy	creamy	dry	dry	moist creamy					new cycle														

Figure 6.3. An anovulatory chart.

checkup, including a pap smear, blood pressure test, etc., her doctor declared that "everything's in order." She wondered about this: Doesn't anovulation signify some kind of problem?

About a third of the women who've taken my classes in their twenties and thirties are not ovulating regularly. What might cause anovulation? Stress, a thyroid disorder, an eating disorder, a diet high in fast foods and weak in nutrient-dense foods, exposure to urban lighting, exposure to environmental toxins, coming off hormonal medication? All of these possibilities need to be considered.

Beth Kennard, MD, reproductive endocrinologist. *A woman who doesn't ovulate regularly has an increased risk of polycystic ovarian syndrome, diabetes, heart disease, stroke, and endometrial (uterine) cancer. Some nonpharmaceutical remedies (including diet modification and exercise) may be worth trying to encourage regular ovulation. If she doesn't ovulate for six months or more, the woman should see a health-care provider for a general checkup. If she's unable to achieve semiregular ovulation, I tend to recommend either the Pill or progesterone supplements to reduce her risk of uterine cancer.*

*✳ **Bev, thirty-two.** I've been charting for two years. I usually ovulate on Day 12, then have a fourteen-day luteal phase. This cycle, it's Day 23, and I still haven't ovulated. Nothing unusual has happened in the last month, and my diet hasn't changed, either. Not knowing what's going on makes me feel a little crazy! Today, another charter told me, "It's within our power to be aware of our menstrual cycles and to support them; it's not within our power to understand them completely or to control them."*

Just for today, this is what I needed to hear.

Thyroid Disorders

The thyroid gland's primary function is to produce thyroid hormones, which affect metabolism and overall energy levels. The thyroid regulates the body's use of fuel. According to the late Broda Barnes, MD, author of *Hypothyroidism: The Unsuspected Illness*, "Too little thyroid hormone (in hypothyroidism) causes your motor to run sluggishly. . . . Too much thyroid hormone, in hyperthyroidism, makes your motor race."

The October 2000 issue of the *National Women's Health Report* says that "approximately one woman in eight will develop thyroid disease in her lifetime." Symptoms of a sluggish thyroid (*hypothyroidism*) can include low temperatures, low energy, cold hands and feet, swollen feet, slow speech, heart palpitations, hair loss, dry or itchy skin, difficulty concentrating, muscle achiness, shortness of breath, nervousness, constipation, depression, lack of sexual energy, persistent vaginal infections, excessive and/or painful menstruation, and anovulation and/or low progesterone levels. Because these symptoms develop gradually and can also signal stress, hypothyroidism is often unsuspected and misdiagnosed.

Hyperthyroidism is less common. Symptoms can include high temperatures, weight loss, bulging eyes, a fast or irregular heart rate, heat intolerance and increased perspiration, trembling, insomnia, decreased menstrual flow, and infertility.

Men's thyroid disorders can be expressed in conditions like high blood pressure, low sex drive, bulging eyes, rapid heart rate, insomnia, and impotency.

Strange as it may sound, it's not unusual for people to have symptoms of both hypothyroidism and hyperthyroidism. For example, a woman may have cold hands and feet and dry skin (symptoms of hypothyroidism) and difficulty maintaining weight (a typical hyperthyroid symptom). Or, her weight might fluctuate rapidly, without a change in eating habits—which can also be a symptom of thyroid problems.

According to Dr. Barnes, "Production of thyroid hormone can make or break a person's health." Around 1940, he developed the Barnes Basal Temperature Test: he tested the basal (waking) temperature of hundreds of students at the University of Denver and learned that it provided a highly accurate indicator of hypothyroidism—more accurate than a blood test. Dr. Barnes's studies still hold true, and women who chart their basal temperature as a fertility signal can also read it for thyroid problems.

If a woman's waking temperatures are below 97.5, she may have thyroid problems; men indicate hypothyroidism when their waking temperatures are below 97.8. However, it's not unusual for people with low basal temperatures and other symptoms of hypothyroidism to show "normal" levels of thyroid-stimulating hormone (TSH) when their blood is tested. According to Mary Shomon, author of *Living Well with Hypothyroidism* and herself a hypothyroid patient, this is likely because the range for normal TSH levels is very broad. If your temperatures are below 97.5 and you have some of the other symptoms listed above, find a practitioner who's aware of the discrepancies in blood tests for thyroid disorders and knowledgeable about treating them.

In *Solved: The Riddle of Illness,* Dr. Stephen Langer lists numerous causes of thyroid problems, including the Pill, hormone replacement therapy, sulfa drugs, antidiabetic agents, fluoridated water, aspirin, cigarette smoke, alcohol, and soy products. Vegetables grown in depleted soil have lower mineral content at the dining table; this, too, can affect the thyroid.

Dagmar Ehling, a doctor of Oriental medicine and the author of *The Chinese Herbalist's Handbook,* says, "According to traditional Chinese medicine theory, low temperatures may indicate cold kidneys (kidney yang deficiency) and, subsequently, poor circulation. Women with these indications may have difficulty becoming pregnant, because an embryo may not want to implant into what the Chinese call a cold uterus. I rarely see women get pregnant when they have temps in the 96s. One of my goals is to raise their temperatures above 97.5 during the follicular phase."

Prolactinemia (elevated prolactin levels that occur while a woman is not breast-feeding and which in turn inhibits ovulation) can be caused by hypothyroidism. Addressing the thyroid problem can clear the prolactinemia. Thyroid disorders can also be exacerbated while pregnant or postpartum, and they are common among menopausal women.

A blank chart for women with temperatures below 97 degrees can be found in the appendix and on www.gardenoffertility.com.

Stephanie, age thirty (see figure 6.4), has low energy, a sleep disorder, and unexplained weight gain. A year before she learned Fertility Awareness, she tested negative (through a blood test) for hypothyroidism. Once she began charting, her low temperatures suggested to her that, despite the negative blood test, she needs to continue investigating hypothyroidism. Her mother has been on thyroid medication since Stephanie was born.

While her temperatures were very low here (with all of her preovulatory temps well below 97.5), Stephanie's cervical fluid had a clear transition toward dryer mucus around ovulation, and her ovulation was crisp (between Days 18 and 19). Her postovulatory phase was a healthy fourteen days.

I've rarely seen women with charts like Stephanie's carry healthy pregnancies to term; I've also seen such women have great difficulty becoming pregnant, or with increased hypothyroid symptoms once their baby is born. I've known women (and doctors) who think nothing of their having low waking temperatures and cold hands and feet (even in warm climates) for years. At menopause, their hypothyroid symptoms may increase. Knowing how to read your fertility charts for a thyroid problem allows you to address it early.

Erica, thirty-seven. I started charting right after I went off the Pill, and we started trying to conceive about three months later. When I brought my charts to my doctor for a preconception exam, I pointed out that I had a lot of temperatures below 97.5, chronic, low-grade depression, and plenty of relatives with a variety of thyroid problems. My doctor said, "Don't worry. You're probably fine. Just enjoy getting pregnant."

Six months went by with no pregnancy. I went back to my doctor and said, "I need to know what's going on here. I still think these low temperatures mean something."

This time, she felt my thyroid and found it was enlarged. A blood test showed low TSH (thyroid-stimulating hormone) levels, indicating hyperthyroidism. A second blood test (which an endocrinologist administered) showed high TSH levels and Hashimoto's disease, a form

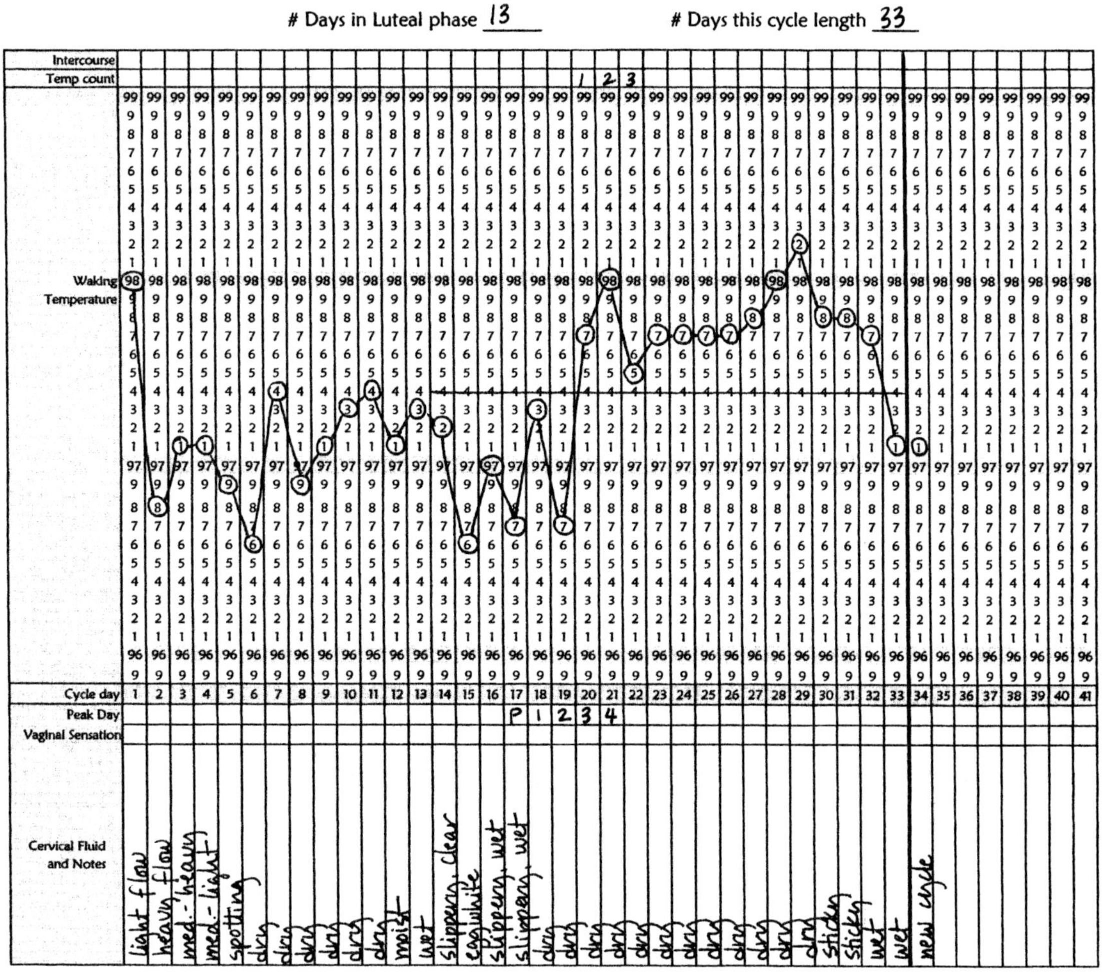

Days in Luteal phase _13_   # Days this cycle length _33_

Intercourse																																									
Temp count																			1	2	3																				

Cycle day: 1 2 3 4 5 6 7 8 9 10 11 12 13 14 15 16 17 18 19 20 21 22 23 24 25 26 27 28 29 30 31 32 33 34 35 36 37 38 39 40 41

Peak Day: P 1 2 3 4

Cervical Fluid and Notes: light flow / heavy flow / med.-heavy / med.-light / spotting / dry / dry / dry / dry / moist / wet / slippery clear / eggwhite / slippery, wet / slippery, wet / dry / dry / dry / dry / dry / dry / dry / dry / sticky / sticky / wet / wet / new cycle

Figure 6.4. A chart indicating possible hypothyroidism.

of hypothyroidism. Apparently TSH levels can fluctuate. I've also learned that antithyroid antibodies can be a factor in preventing implantation and that I'm a candidate for this problem, too.

Finally, I can address my infertility—and my overall health—at their roots. I'm reading about hypothyroidism, the kinds of alternative and pharmaceutical options available, and I'm starting to make changes. I'm learning that doctors can't know everything and that I run into trouble when I think they should. It's my charts that got me here and gave me the courage to take responsibility for my own health care.

Low Progesterone Levels

If estrogen is like yin (feminine, dark, moist, cooling), progesterone is like yang (masculine, light, dry, warming). Like yin and yang, estrogen and progesterone are in perpetual relationship to each other.

Women who don't have sufficient progesterone often have PMS (premenstrual syndrome), dysmenorrhea (painful periods), and menopause problems. Low progesterone can exacerbate low libido. Progesterone also contributes to bone building, efficient fat building, normalizing of blood sugar, and more. Other women may experience drowsiness, depression, and PMS as a result of elevated progesterone.

Low progesterone levels (also called *luteal phase deficiency,* or *LPD*), can also indicate a propensity for miscarriage, since progesterone is needed to sustain a pregnancy. When you hear progesterone, think "pro-gestation." Progesterone helps make your uterine lining spongy in preparation for implantation of the embryo; it creates the dry mucus that covers your cervix so that the uterus remains closed off and sterile during pregnancy; and it keeps you (and your uterus) at a slightly elevated temperature, which is what a fetus likes in the womb. Throughout pregnancy, progesterone levels (produced by the placenta after the first trimester) remain high.

The following signals might indicate low progesterone levels:

- The temperature zigzags up and down around ovulation.
- The luteal phase lasts eleven days or less.
- The transition from the follicular to the luteal phase takes more than three days.
- The transition from the luteal to the follicular phase takes more than three days.
- Temperatures dip onto or below the coverline during the luteal phase.

See figure 6.5. At the time of this chart, Cathy was in her third cycle off the Pill. She probably ovulated between Days 18 and 19. This cycle shows low progesterone levels because her luteal phase is only eleven days long, and two of her temperatures fall onto her coverline.

Common stuff like soy products, mercury amalgams, and birth control pills can disrupt hormones, increase estrogen levels—and in turn decrease progesterone. Eating healthy fats, giving your body plenty of rest, and carrying a healthy preg-

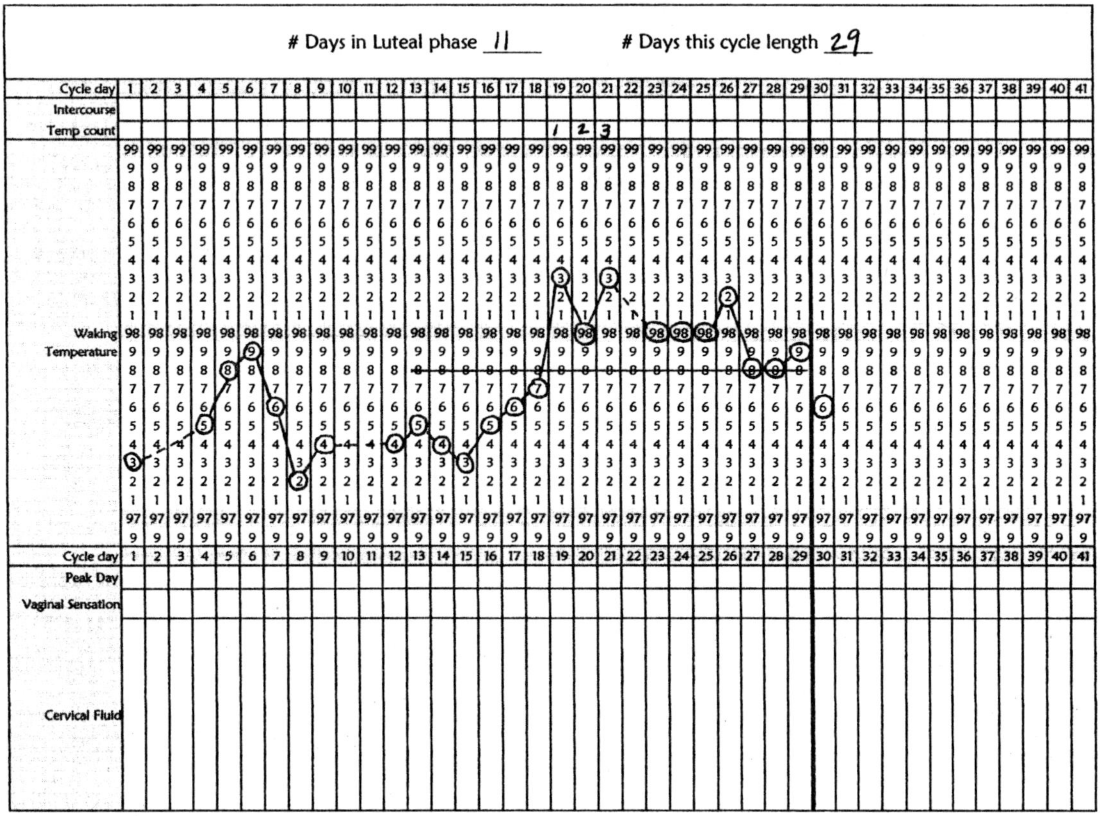

Days in Luteal phase _11_   # Days this cycle length _29_

(Fertility charting grid — Cycle days 1–41, with Intercourse, Temp count, Waking Temperature, Peak Day, Vaginal Sensation, and Cervical Fluid rows. Temp count marks 1, 2, 3 at cycle days 19, 20, 21.)

Figure 6.5. A chart indicating low progesterone levels.

nancy to term are a few of the things that can strengthen progesterone. (You can read more in chapters 10 through 12.)

Progesterone Deficiency and Hypothyroidism

It's not unusual for a woman's chart to show progesterone deficiency *and* a thyroid problem. Barbara, for example (see figure 6.6 on page 114), who's never been on the Pill, was twenty-three in this cycle. She took six days (Days 18–23) to shift from the follicular to the luteal phase and three days from the luteal phase to her new cycle. Her last three temperatures dip below the coverline or fall onto it. The long shifts and the dips all indicate progesterone deficiency.

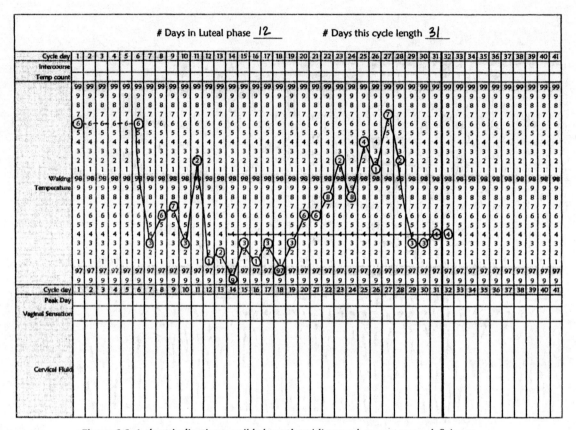

Figure 6.6. A chart indicating possible hypothyroidism and progesterone deficiency.

By her temperature rise on Day 20 and the coverline at 97.4 degrees, it looks like she probably ovulated on Day 19. Because of her gradual shift (stair stepping) between the follicular and the luteal phases—and because she didn't chart her mucus—it's difficult to confirm when she ovulated. Barbara's thirteen temperatures below 97.5 signal that she may also have hypothyroidism.

Elizabeth's chart (see figure 6.7) also indicates hypothyroidism (because fifteen of her temperatures fall below 97.5) and low progesterone levels (because her luteal phase is only ten days long)—even while her crisp temperature shift indicates ovulation. She probably ovulated on Day 21. Her coverline is at 97.2. Day 21 was her Peak Day. She entered her postovulatory, infertile phase on Day 24. Elizabeth was twenty-five during this cycle.

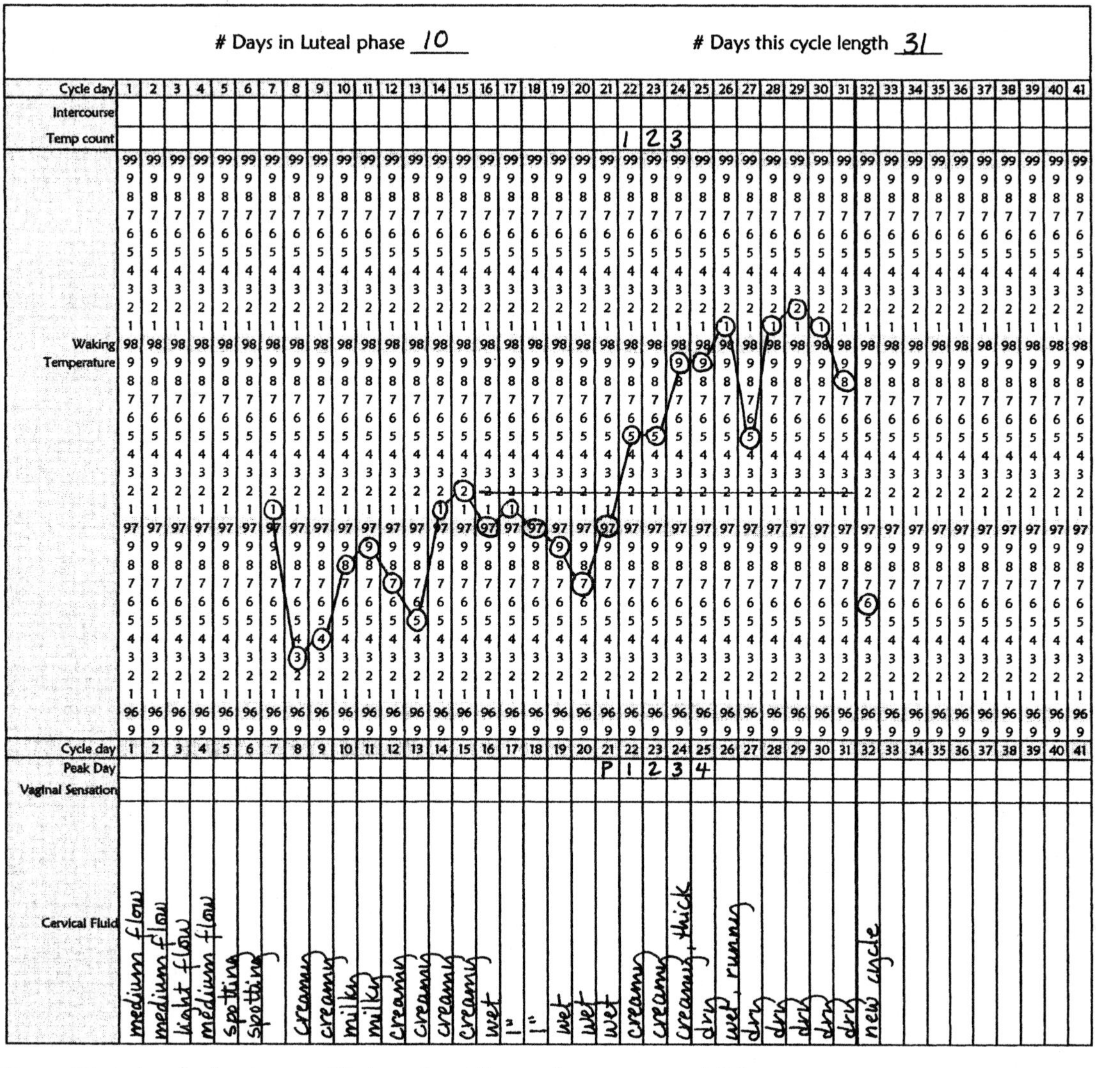

Days in Luteal phase _10_   # Days this cycle length _31_

Cycle day: 1 2 3 4 5 6 7 8 9 10 11 12 13 14 15 16 17 18 19 20 21 22 23 24 25 26 27 28 29 30 31 32 33 34 35 36 37 38 39 40 41

Intercourse

Temp count: 1 2 3

Waking Temperature

Cycle day: 1 2 3 4 5 6 7 8 9 10 11 12 13 14 15 16 17 18 19 20 21 22 23 24 25 26 27 28 29 30 31 32 33 34 35 36 37 38 39 40 41

Peak Day: P 1 2 3 4

Vaginal Sensation

Cervical Fluid: medium flow, medium flow, light flow, medium flow, spotting, spotting, creamy, creamy, milky, milky, creamy, creamy, creamy, wet, 1", 1", wet, wet, wet, creamy, creamy, creamy thick, dry, wet, runny, dry, dry, dry, dry, new cycle

Figure 6.7. A chart indicating possible hypothyroidism and progesterone deficiency.

Ovarian Cysts and Polycystic Ovarian Syndrome

Anovulation or long cycles (and infrequent ovulation) typically signal elevated estrogen levels; they can also indicate that a woman's at risk for ovarian cysts or *polycystic ovarian syndrome* (PCOS).

An *ovarian cyst* is a partially developed follicle that doesn't release an egg at ovulation—and it doesn't dissolve, either. While most ovarian cysts do resolve on their own, they can cause pain or discomfort in the lower abdomen, pain during intercourse, and unexplained abdominal swelling. A fluid-holding cyst can also rupture and cause severe abdominal pain and bleeding. A cyst can be detected through a bimanual pelvic exam or ultrasound.

When a woman's ovary is covered with a tough, shiny, white cover and shows (through ultrasound) many cysts just under the ovary's surface, she's considered to have PCOS. Follicles are readying to burst, but not quite doing so. Rather than dissolving (as they typically do after healthy ovulation), they form cysts at the ovary's surface that produce testosterone.

The syndrome's most common signs are anovulation or infrequent ovulation, hirsutism (excess hair), and obesity—though not all PCOS patients are overweight. Women with PCOS may also experience high blood pressure, insulin resistance (when your cells resist the insulin necessary for metabolizing glucose), and abnormalities in lipid (blood fat) levels.

Indeed, the syndrome has a broad spectrum of complex symptoms. About 20 to 30 percent of women of childbearing age have polycystic-appearing ovaries.

Fertility Awareness can help you detect if you're a candidate for ovarian cysts or PCOS. If you've got cycles lasting two months each or longer, or if you get a cycle with a false peak more than once a year, you may have a propensity for ovarian cysts or PCOS. A false peak means your cervical fluid builds up to a wet texture, you transition to dryer CF—but you can't confirm ovulation with your temperature. Wet cervical fluid and/or wet vaginal sensations reappear with another buildup of mucus. You may have several "false peaks" of mucus without ovulation before you can actually confirm ovulation by your temperature. Or you might have frequent anovulatory cycles with breakthrough bleeding.

Rosie, twenty-seven. Because I've got facial hair and acne, my grandmother is diabetic, and I usually ovulate only every two or three months, I'm probably a candidate for polycystic ovarian syndrome. Just the possibility of this scares me. I feel out of control with my body, which, through Fertility Awareness, I'm just beginning to understand. I'm learning that my body isn't perfect. That doesn't feel good right now.

At my next checkup, I've decided to talk with my doctor about PCOS. Meanwhile, I'm still charting. Before I charted, I knew I had long cycles, but I never kept track of them. And even though it might take me sixty days or more to ovulate, I love seeing that there is something working here!

Miscarriage

About one third of all pregnancies end in miscarriage, often before the women even know they're pregnant. By charting your fertility signals, you can know whether you're pregnant, and whether you've miscarried rather than had a "late period."

If you haven't had a menstrual period and you're expecting it, either your ovulation was delayed, you haven't ovulated yet, or you're pregnant. The postovulatory (luteal) phase won't last longer than sixteen days unless you're pregnant or you have a corpus luteum cyst.

Charlene, thirty-seven, was able to confirm pregnancy on Day 31, since she had eighteen temperatures above her coverline (see figure 6.8). (Eighteen postovulatory temperatures are required to confirm pregnancy since it's possible to release

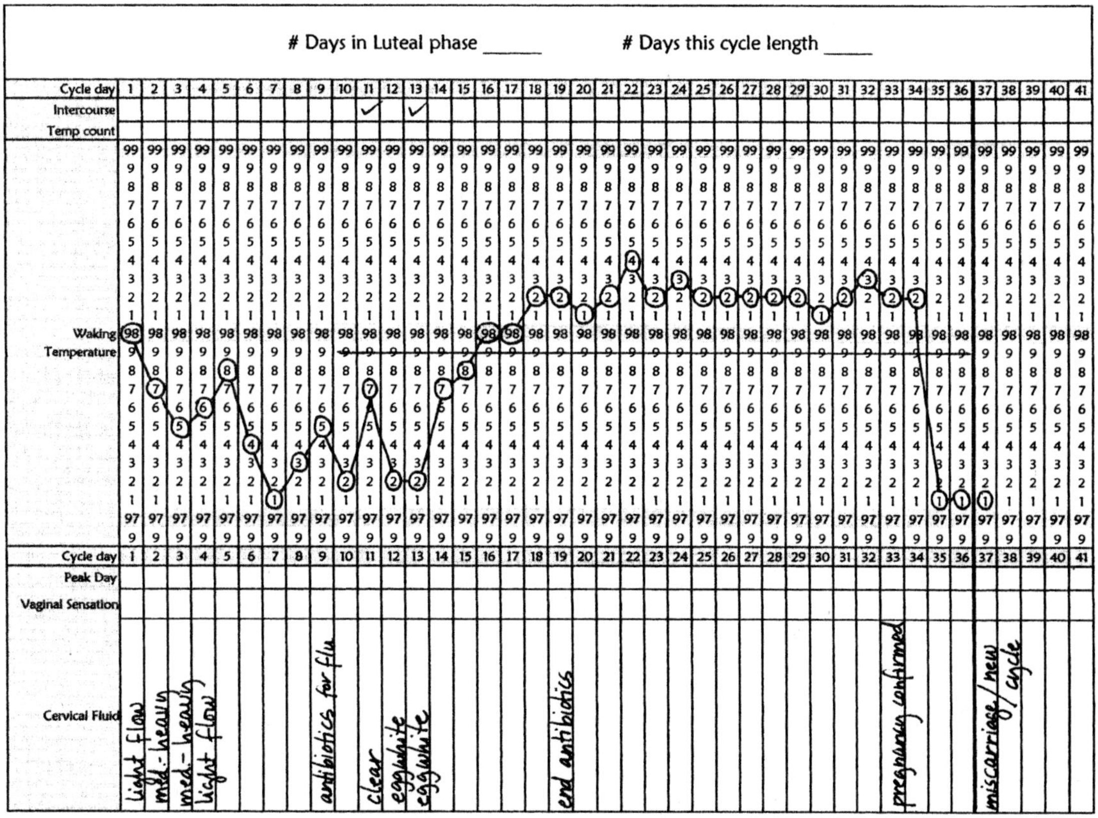

 # Days in Luteal phase _____   **# Days this cycle length** _____

Cycle day	1	2	3	4	5	6	7	8	9	10	11	12	13	14	15	16	17	18	19	20	21	22	23	24	25	26	27	28	29	30	31	32	33	34	35	36	37	38	39	40	41
Intercourse											✓		✓																												
Temp count																																									

(Waking Temperature grid and Cervical Fluid annotations as shown in figure.)

Cervical Fluid annotations: light flow, mid–heavy, med–heavy, light flow; antibiotics for flu; clear; eggwhite; eggwhite; end antibiotics; pregnancy confirmed; miscarriage/new cycle

Figure 6.8. A chart showing pregnancy and miscarriage.

two eggs at ovulation, to conceive with the second egg [which might not be released until two days after the temperature rise], and the corpus luteum doesn't live longer than sixteen days unless you're pregnant.)

On Day 29, Charlene took a home pregnancy test, which also confirmed her pregnancy. Her temperature dips on Days 35 and 36 signaled low progesterone levels. She miscarried on what would have been Day 37, twenty-three days after she ovulated.

Charlene and her husband were heartbroken. They had been trying to conceive for a year. The grief of a lost pregnancy, whether intended or unintended, and including one at such an early stage as Charlene's, is often kept private in our culture; and yet miscarriage can be so painful. (Please read chapter 9 for ways to honor yourself and what you've lost.)

Discovering that you've miscarried (whether or not your pregnancy was intended) lets you know that you've ovulated and conceived, which can be encouraging. With this information, if you want to bear a child, you can focus on ways to sustain a pregnancy. Often this means strengthening overall health and progesterone levels—although many other factors besides low progesterone can contribute to miscarriage. (Remedies for low progesterone can be found in chapters 10 through 12.)

Cervical Fluid and Gauging GYN Health

While this chapter focuses on how the waking temperature can be used to gauge gynecological health, cervical fluid can also provide signals. In *Teaching the Billings Ovulation Method* (based on mucus changes and vaginal sensation), Drs. Evelyn and John Billings describe a woman in her early thirties who had one child. After several years of observing cycles with a clear Peak Day followed two weeks later by menstruation, she had a cycle with several days of abundant, slippery mucus *after* her Peak Day. The woman decided that the unusual pattern warranted a Pap smear—which she was due for. Her cervix was found to be cancerous, and treatment was provided.

Vaginal Infections

If you're familiar with your cervical fluid patterns, it'll probably be easier for you to notice when your mucus isn't normal and when you may have an infection. Sexually transmitted infections like chlamydia or gonorrhea can produce unusual, thick secretions. Not all sexually transmitted infections have observable symptoms; some take a week or two or longer to present symptoms. If your mucus doesn't change throughout your cycle, or if it has a greenish tint or a foul odor, you may have a vaginal infection.

If you think there's even the slightest possibility that you or your partner have a sexually transmitted infection, get medical attention as soon as you can. Don't have sex until you and all your current partners have been tested, treated, and cured. (For more information about STIs, please check out my website, www.gardenoffertility.com, and the resources listed in this book on page 256.)

A vaginal infection such as yeast can be caused by diet (perhaps too much sugar, too much alcohol, insulin resistance, diabetes, or immunodeficiency); it can create an itchy, cottage cheese–like discharge.

Also, please note: the cervical fluid of women who are on the Pill typically does not change unless the Pill isn't working. Women who are coming off the Pill may not show a change in their mucus for several cycles or more, or they might cycle normally right away.

Other Reasons to Chart

An open os, lubricated by cervical fluid, can make Pap smears less painful. Try to schedule Paps when your os is open and your vaginal sensations are wet.

If you have decided to use a diaphragm or a cervical cap, try to schedule your fitting during your fertile phase. The shape and texture of the cervix change throughout the cycle, and to prevent pregnancy you want it to fit when you're fertile!

Breast lumps are least affected by hormones at the end of your period. You can use your charts to remind yourself to do a breast self-exam on your period's last day. If you find lumps at that time, you can opt for further evaluation.

Studies show that for women who are still cycling, surgery outcomes are greatest when estrogen levels are high (in the days before ovulation)—*except* for breast surgery. In that case, outcomes are best when surgery is performed during the period's first two days or after ovulation, when estrogen levels are low.

Indeed, we've only begun to tap into the applications of Fertility Awareness. When women chart their fertility signals, they often raise excellent questions about their gynecological health and about environmental factors that might influence it; they often give more attention to their diet and lifestyle.

So many women are thrilled when they see that they have ovulated through data they have gathered themselves. When we understand through charting that our progesterone levels are low, and that this may contribute to menstrual cramps and/or affect our ability to sustain a pregnancy, many of us commit more easily to making dietary and lifestyle changes that could improve our health. Indeed, I've been inspired by women who chart, by their curiosity, their great questions, their commitment to their own wellness, and their respect for their bodies.

I have also seen men take a stronger interest in their partner's health as well as the environmental and lifestyle factors that might contribute to their own well-being when Fertility Awareness is practiced.

All of these factors give more reason to chart!

We are so curiously made that one atom put in the wrong
place in one original structure will often make
us unhappy for life.

—WILLIAM GODWIN
(1756–1836)

Whatever befalls the earth befalls the (children) of the earth.
Man did not weave the web of life; he is merely a strand in it.
Whatever he does to the web, he does to himself.

—CHIEF SEATTLE

7. Common Products That Can Be Hazardous to Reproductive Health

FOR MANY WOMEN, LEARNING FERTILITY Awareness dovetails with becoming aware of the way common products can affect health. Say you begin (or stop) taking a medication for headaches. Over time, on your chart, you may notice if your cervical fluid or temperatures are affected. You might question how common products like tampons (which need to be purchased and discarded month after month) affect the health of the earth.

Most of the food, cleaning products, and medicines available today are prepared far from our local communities. We usually have no contact with the manufacturers of our butter or the remedy we buy for a vaginal infection. We may not know an item's ingredients or how it is made. We may be attracted to a product because it's advertised as "natural," though the true meaning of this word has become pretty fuzzy.

I vote for the Precautionary Principle. Developed by scientists, farmers, and breast cancer action groups, the Precautionary Principle advocates not waiting for absolute proof of a given product's dangers, but rather not using a substance or product when there's a reasonable suspicion of its dangers.[1] Perhaps because they've been around for a while, perhaps because (on their own) they may not cause immediately noticeable adverse reactions, many products are assumed to be safe. However, used alone, repeatedly or in combination, items such as the Pill, fertility drugs, bras, fragrances, mercury amalgam fillings, phthalates (plastics), tampons, disposable diapers, and many other products can be hazardous to reproductive health.

Groundbreaking books like *Silent Spring* by Rachel Carson and *Our Stolen Future* by Theo Colborn, Dianne Dumanoski, and John Peterson Myers show how commonly used chemicals can have a deadly effect on wildlife and can also be traced to birth defects and reproductive failures.

While this chapter presents (in alphabetical order) only a few products that can harm reproductive health, it's hard to swallow. It's not unusual for people who learn this information in my classes to blurt out, "This is all stuff we use!" Digest the information slowly. Do your own research. Choose products that feel right for you.

Assisted Reproductive Technology

In *The Elusive Embryo: How Women and Men Approach New Reproductive Technologies*, anthropologist Gay Becker describes couples who pursue their desire for a child "until emotional and financial resources are exhausted." She observes that with the proliferation of assisted reproductive technologies, "the emphasis has shifted from diagnosing and correcting abnormal physiology to achieving a pregnancy in the fastest and most direct manner possible, regardless of the cost or invasiveness. This approach aggressively augments the natural reproductive cycle, or bypasses it altogether, and aims for results regardless of the underlying infertility diagnosis."

If you are considering using reproductive technology to help you conceive, please, first research its potential hazards—to yourself and to your potential offspring.

Clomiphene citrate, also known as Clomid, a common drug prescribed when a woman has difficulty conceiving, hyperstimulates one aspect of the reproductive system—which then requires the rest of the system (which was perhaps out of sync before the drug was administered) to grasp for health and wholeness in response to being overstimulated. It works by binding itself to estrogen receptors in the brain so that naturally occurring estrogen cannot be detected by the body. Clomid tricks the body into producing more and more follicle-stimulating hormone, causing more follicles to grow than they normally would. In turn, more estrogen is produced by the follicles, and more eggs are matured. Typically, a woman taking this drug produces double or triple the amount of estrogen (and releases more eggs at ovulation) per cycle compared to pretreatment cycles. In *Our Stolen Future,* the pivotal work about how chemicals threaten our ability to reproduce, Theo Colburn and her coauthors report that "numerous studies have linked estrogens, even those occurring in the body, to cancer, suggesting that the greater a woman's lifetime exposure, the greater the risk."

According to a package insert about Clomid (available from any pharmacist by request) from Merrell Pharmaceuticals, Inc., one of the drug's manufacturers, "The majority of patients who are going to ovulate will do so after the first course of therapy. If ovulation does not occur after three courses of therapy, further treatment with clomiphene citrate tablets USP is not recommended. . . . If menses does not occur after an ovulatory response, the patient should be re-evaluated. Long-term cyclic therapy is not recommended beyond a total of about six cycles." Merrell Pharmaceuticals also recommends that the first dose of Clomid be 50 mg.

Unfortunately, I have heard from women who have taken Clomid for as many as twelve cycles and from others who took the drug at double or even triple the dosage recommended by pharmaceutical companies in their first treatment. (A colleague worked with a woman who took Clomid for forty-three cycles.)

Educate yourself as much as you can before using reproductive technology. Judith Steinberg Turiel's *Beyond Second Opinions: Making Choices About Fertility Treatment* (University of California Press, 1998) explains that fertility drugs are commonly given before (or perhaps without) diagnosing a couple's particular infertility problems; she describes the hazards of various treatments in accessible terms. Studies show that high-tech treatments like Clomid and in vitro fertilization increase a woman's risk of ovarian cancer (with increased risk if she never conceives)[2,3] and her offspring's risk of birth defects.[4,5,6] Also, Clomid can dry up cervical fluid, so that sperm cannot easily reach mature egg(s).[7]

Leah Morton, MD. *Some women want to be pregnant immediately once they start trying. I see this desire as part of a wider idea in our culture that we can and should be able to control our lives. Already, technology can be used to help us control lovemaking, pregnancy prevention, conception, and labor and delivery. But really, technological controls have nothing to do with fertility, with the mystery of life or the joy, darkness, and awe that we experience.*

I've never prescribed Clomid. It's been established that even one cycle on Clomid potentially puts a woman at risk of ovarian cancer. Double-blind controlled studies haven't been done, which I find questionable. But already there are many articles about the hazards of reproductive technologies. Women should be informed about the risks.

If a couple is having difficulty conceiving or sustaining a pregnancy, my first concern is whether they're eating food that's not genetically modified, that is organic, whole, and low glycemic (this means with little or no refined sugars or starches). Improving one's diet is one of the hardest things to do in our culture. But slowing down enough to reflect on one's emotional and spiritual life is conducive to fertility. It also makes for healthier parenting!

Bras

According to Sydney Ross Singer and Soma Grismaijer, who conducted the study, "Bras and Breast Cancer," women who choose a bra for its appearance and ignore the soreness and swelling it causes have twice the rate of breast cancer of those who do not.

From 1991 to 1993, Singer, a medical anthropologist, and Grismaijer interviewed four thousand women from five large American cities and found that 75 percent of the women who kept their bras on at night while they slept contracted breast cancer; so did one out of seven women who wore a bra more than twelve hours a day. Women who don't wear a bra have 1 chance in 168 of being diagnosed with breast cancer—the same as men.

Toxins that accumulate in breast tissue are usually flushed by lymphatic fluid into large clusters of lymph nodes, which nestle in your armpits and upper chest. In their book, *Dressed to Kill: The Link Between Breast Cancer and Bras,* the researchers write, "Because lymphatic vessels are very thin, they are extremely sensitive to pressure and are easily compressed." Chronic minimal pressure on the breasts can cause lymph valves and vessels to close. Fifteen or twenty years of bra-constricted lymph drainage can result in cancer.

Singer and Grismaijer were also struck by the low incidence of breast cancer in poor nations, which are typically doused with pesticides—but women from these countries likely don't wear tight bras. Japanese, Fijian, and Maori women who do wear bras have rates of breast cancer similar to women in North America and Europe.

The researchers caution: don't sleep in your bra. If you must wear one, choose a loose-fitting cotton bra and wear it for the shortest time possible. Make sure you can slip two fingers under the shoulder straps and side panels. Take it off when you're home. Each time you remove your bra, massage your breasts gently to encourage lymphatic health.

Fertility Awareness can help prevent breast cancer: your chart can remind you to check your breasts after your period, around Day 7 of each cycle. Hormonally, this is the best time to check.

Depo-Provera

Depo-Provera is an injectable, hormonal method of preventing pregnancy that requires a shot every three months. Even one shot before a woman is twenty-one can result in bone loss. Adolescent women who use Depo may be more likely to suffer fractures when they reach menopause than those who never take the injections.[8, 9]

Women who take Depo-Provera shots for two years or more before they're twenty-five have an almost triple risk of breast cancer.[10]

Sophie, twenty-seven. I recently began a nursing job that required me to get a measles immunization shot. Because measles is a live vaccine, it's known to cause birth defects in fetuses that are exposed to it. So it's crucial that women not become pregnant during the first three months following the shot, while the vaccine is still alive. Most physicians recommend that their patients take "risk-free" birth control such as the Pill during this time. I was actually offered Depo-Provera. It was a great moment for me, because I realized how much I trust Fertility Awareness. After a year and a half of charting, I know when I'm fertile, I know the method is effective, and I don't need the "insurance" of hormonal drugs.

Disposable Plastic Diapers

During a boy's first six months, he normally has testosterone levels nearly equal to those of a mature man. According to a recent study, the scrotal temperature of baby boys who wear plastic disposables is significantly higher than that of boys who wear cloth diapers.[11] Researchers are now studying to see if there's a link between the use of plastic disposables during this crucial phase of boys' development and the increase in male infertility, retarded or stunted sexual development at puberty, and testicular cancer.

Furthermore, chemicals that absorb babies' urine (including sodium polyacrylate crystals, which are associated with the development of toxic shock syndrome through tampons;[12] and nonylphenl ethoxylate, which mimics estrogen[13]), may enter the body through broken skin in the area covered by the diaper.[14]

Cloth diapers are also better for the environment: about 4 percent of our landfills are now filled with plastic disposables, which can take hundreds of years to de-

compose. Cloth diapers, which can be used over and over, decomp_e
months.

Mothering Magazine's January 2003 issue includes an excellent dis_e
politics of diapers.

Mercury

Mercury can be ingested or inhaled by:

- Eating deep-water, bottom-dwelling fish like tuna, swordfish, and shark.
- Vaccines and other drugs that contain mercury-based preservatives such as thimerosal.
- Dental work.

According to dentist Hal Huggins, DDS, and Thomas Levy, MD, authors of *Uninformed Consent: The Hidden Dangers in Dental Care,* exposure to mercury (which is commonly used in dentistry) can create incurable disorders, including multiple sclerosis, lupus, leukemia, chronic fatigue syndrome, Parkinson's, mental disorders, breast cancer, infertility, and birth defects.[15] Avoiding mercury in dentistry and fish can help prevent these disorders.

The ovaries and the testicles can accumulate mercury. According to Dr. Huggins, "When the (fertilized) human egg is exposed to mercury, it sometimes loses its ability to become implanted in the wall of the uterus." Further, some men's low sperm counts can be attribted to mercury toxicity.[16]

During pregnancy, do not consume fish high in mercury (such as tuna, shark, sea bass, and swordfish), avoid drugs that contain thimerosal, and do not have mercury amalgams newly applied or removed. Mercury passes easily through the placenta; ingesting it or inhaling mercury vapor could harm your growing baby's nervous system. Dentists in Austria, Germany, and Sweden are not allowed to give pregnant women mercury amalgams. If dental work is necessary, insist on non-mercury fillings.

Phthalates

Phthalates (pronounced thalates) are industrial chemicals that are used as solvents or to soften plastic in numerous consumer products. Millions of tons are produced worldwide each year. Phthalates can be absorbed through the skin, inhaled as fumes, ingested when they leach into food wrapped in some brands of cling wrap, or when children bite or suck on plastic toys; they can be inadvertently but directly administered to patients while they receive medication from an IV bag made from polyvinyl chloride (PVC). Phthalates are especially recognizable by their smell: new (vinyl) car seats and shower curtains, for example, have the unmistakable smell of phthalates.

The Centers for Disease Control and Prevention (CDC) has found that while all Americans have been exposed to phthalates, women of childbearing age show evidence of the highest levels of exposure, perhaps because they typically use more cosmetics than other groups. Phthalates are commonly used as a solvent in cosmetics and as a softener in PVC plastic products, including sex toys, car dashboards, wallpaper, flooring, and raincoats. To date, the FDA has not required manufacturers to label products that contain phthalates.

In 2002, Health Care Without Harm (HCWH), a research and action group working to make health care more environmentally responsible and sustainable, released "Not Too Pretty," a report that outlines the harmful effects of exposure to phthalates in popular fragrances, hairsprays, and deodorants. HCWH's researchers found phthalates in most of the popular beauty products they tested. The report suggests that women ages twenty to forty would most likely be more exposed to phthalates than other Americans because this group purchases more cosmetics and other personal-care products.[17]

Meanwhile, a new peer-reviewed study suggests that diethyl phthalate (DEP), a chemical commonly used in fragrances and other grooming products (such as deodorant and shampoo) damages the DNA of sperm in adult men.[18] Dr. Ted Schettler, science director of the Science and Environmental Health Network, explains: "The last thing you want is DNA damage to sperm, which can lead to infertility and may also be linked to miscarriages and birth defects, and cancer and infertility in offspring." The male reproductive tract, as it develops, appears to be the most vulnerable body system exposed to phthalates (although effects on the liver, kidneys, lungs, and blood clotting are also of concern).

While manufacturers of phthalates continue to argue that there is little evidence that people can be harmed by phthalates, Health Care Without Harm refers to several hundred animal studies, which show that phthalates cross the placenta, contaminate breast milk, and cause reproductive damage—particularly in male offspring. Scientists have agreed that these studies can be used to predict human health effects.[19]

Solutions

- Store leftovers in glass or stainless-steel containers.
- If you must microwave, use oven-proof glass or ceramics with an oven-proof glass lid or plate.
- Read the labels of bottles and other products in plastic containers. Choose #1 (PETE) or #2(HDPE) whenever plastics can't be avoided; these are the most commonly recycled plastics. Avoid plastics labeled #3 or V (PVC), #6(polystyrene), and #7(polycarbonate), which leach toxic chemicals. Labels or numbers can be found on the bottom of the bottle.
- Bring your own mug to work and your own bowl to the salad bar.
- Check out Health Care Without Harm's websites, including www.nottoopretty. org (which lists products that don't contain phthalates) and www.noharm.org (which has info about phthalates in medical devices).
- Avoid perfumes and colognes.
- Read nail polish labels. Nail polish manufacturers are required to indicate if their product includes phthalates.
- If you have a favorite brand of some type of cosmetic, phone the manufacturer and ask if it contains phthalates.
- Choose nonvinyl products such as cloth car seats and shower curtains.
- To release harmful fumes from new cars, keep car windows open on warm days.

The Pill

Oral contraceptives are made from artificial steroids that mimic the effects of estrogen and progesterone. The Pill works by:

- Suppressing the release of follicle-stimulating hormone (FSH) and luteinizing hormone (LH), thereby preventing ovulation.

- Stimulating the cells in the cervix's crypts to produce thick cervical mucus, thereby preventing sperm survival and ability to swim to a ripe egg in the fallopian tube in the event that ovulation does occur.
- Disrupting the ability of the cilia (that line the fallopian tube) to move a fertilized egg toward the uterus in the event that conception does occur.
- Preventing buildup of the uterine lining and thereby inhibiting implantation of a fertilized egg in the event that conception occurs.[20]

It's worth noting that the mini-Pill, or progestin-only pill, may not supress ovulation or conception from occurring.[21, 22]

In *The Breast Cancer Prevention Program,* Sam Epstein, MD, writes, "[M]ore than twenty well-controlled studies have demonstrated the clear risk of premenopausal breast cancer with the use of oral contraceptives. These estimates indicate that a young woman who uses oral contraceptives has up to ten times the risk for developing breast cancer as does a non-user, particularly if she uses the Pill during her teens or early twenties; if she uses the Pill for two years or more; if she uses the Pill before her first full-term pregnancy; if she has a family history of breast cancer." Thus, a woman who takes the Pill for two years before she's twenty-five, and before she's had a pregnancy to term, increases her risk of breast cancer up to ten times.

A study conducted by the World Health Organization found that women who carry HPV (human papillomavirus) and who have taken the Pill for five to nine years are nearly three times more likely than non-Pill users to develop cervical cancer.[23] (HPV affects one third of all women in their twenties.) Women with HPV who've taken the Pill for more than ten years are four times more likely than non-users to develop the disease.

Women who have a history of migraine headaches and who take combined oral contraceptives (COCs) are two to four times more likely to have a stroke than women who have migraines and don't take the Pill.[24]

Women who use low-dose oral contraceptive pills have a twofold increased risk of a fatal heart attack compared to non-users.[25]

Women who take oral contraceptives and smoke have a twelvefold increase in fatal heart attacks and a threefold increase in fatal brain hemorrhage.[26]

Women who use the Pill after the age of forty-five have a 144 percent greater risk of developing breast cancer than women who have never used it.[27]

Because of blocked hormone production, women who take the Pill have decreased sensitivity to smell. In turn, this may decrease their sex drives.[28]

In *Solved: The Riddle of Illness,* Dr. Stephen Langer writes that "the Pill, an effective birth control method, can cause severe bodily damage in hypothyroidism."

Dagmar Ehling explains that, "in its listing of the side effects of oral contraceptives, the *Physician's Desk Reference* includes increased blood clotting, uterine bleeding, and carcinoma of the breast and endometrium. In Oriental medicine, these conditions could be categorized as Blood Stasis, a kind of 'pattern of disharmony.' Blood Stasis describes sluggish blood circulation, which might manifest as blood clotting, varicose veins, tumors, nodules, or cysts. While acupuncture and herbs can address these conditions, from an Oriental perspective, the longer a woman stays on the Pill, the more she increases her risk for these kinds of problems."

If you have taken the Pill and feel it has thrown your cycles out of sync, please read about the options presented in chapters 10 through 12.

Leah Morton, MD. While many women who ask for the Pill have a strong sense of responsibility and a simple intention to control the possibility of an unwanted pregnancy, I'm very wary of prescribing it.

First, I'm pained to see women thinking we need to be sexually available all the time, without being mindful of our true desires. Being on the Pill essentially shuts down the reproductive system—and shuts down a woman's awareness of herself as a fertile being. Young women need education about how their bodies work, and to experience a sense of authority about their desires and who they are. In my experience, the Pill discourages such explorations.

Second, the Pill can lead to a significantly increased risk of breast cancer. I once heard Dr. John Lee compare a breast to a tree: the branches are like ducts, and the leaves are like glands. (For an illustration of a breast's anatomy, see page 65.) In the same way that branches don't grow out of leaves, ducts don't grow out of glands. While they're rapidly growing, ducts are more susceptible to cancer-causing estrogens, radiation, and/or environmental toxins. Glands, in contrast, are more resistant to toxic damage. Once the glands are established, there's more protection against breast cancer, since they block further development of the ducts. With a complete pregnancy, a woman's breast goes through a maturation process. A complete pregnancy exposes her to high doses of progesterone, and thereby establishes glandular development.

If a young woman (whose ducts are still developing) takes the Pill, which contains progestin (a synthetic hormone) and estrogen, it encourages further development of her ducts. The bottom line here is that progestins and strong estrogens are toxic to the breast.

The Pill can also increase a woman's tendency to depression; and it can suppress the immune system by depleting B-vitamins, thyroid hormones, and other essential nutrients.

Third, the Pill is frequently prescribed "to regulate" a woman's cycle—when she is prone to painful menstruation, for example, or ovarian cysts, even acne. But the drug merely suppresses the symptoms that indicate a root problem. It does nothing to discern or heal the real problem.

There are so many things we don't understand. First and foremost, to be healthy, we need to respect nature and our bodies. Exposing women's bodies to high doses of unnatural hormones moves us away from nature's evolutionary design.

Claire, twenty-five. *I got really depressed on the Pill, which I took to be a clue that it was harming my body. I'm an active Green Party member. Practicing Fertility Awareness meets my philosophy of taking action toward creating a clean environment, with the first environment being my own body.*

Norah, fifty-two. *My daughter and her boyfriend live in different cities and are able to see each other only one weekend a month. When I learned that she's on the Pill, I told her about its potential risks—and about Fertility Awareness. She told me she's not willing to risk giving up a few days of intercourse with her boyfriend. It pains me that sex is more important to her than her long-term health, but then I took the Pill when I was younger (and the doses were much stronger). Since I let her know my opinion, I figure my job is to support her, whatever she chooses.*

Progesterone Creams and Gels

Progesterone creams and gels are available over the counter and by prescription from compounding pharmacies in the form of lozenges and troches. Women may use progesterone supplements to relieve premenstrual tension, menstrual cramps, endometriosis, and premenopausal symptoms and to help sustain a pregnancy.

According to Dr. Elias Ilyia, medical director of Diagnos-Techs, a lab in Kent, Washington, that evaluates hormone levels from saliva, "Over 95 percent of women who apply progesterone creams or gels are overdosing on them. They show progesterone levels that would be normal for a pregnant woman at twenty-four or twenty-five weeks gestation." Dr. Ilyia's observations are based on saliva tests of more than 20,000 women who applied these creams or gels. Overdosing can take anywhere from seven to thirty days and may be associated with symptoms such as anovulation, water retention, increased weight, breast engorgement, and mild-to-moderate depression. The return to acceptable levels of progesterone may vary from thirty to two hundred days.[29]

If you're thinking about taking a variety of progesterone, consider how long you intend to use it and how you will determine if you've "overdosed" on it.

Dr. Ilyia suggests that progesterone applied under the tongue (available with a prescription in troches or sublingual drops from compounding pharmacists) is safer and more effective. Other options for strengthening progesterone levels are described in chapters 11 and 12.

Ginny, thirty. I was recently diagnosed with endometriosis and prescribed a transdermal progesterone cream to inhibit my estrogenic activity and keep the endometriosis from growing further. I apply it Days 5 through 19 of my cycle and usually begin bleeding around Day 27.

Within a month of using the cream, I stopped getting any slippery (fertile) mucus; and I've now had six cycles without a temperature shift. Apparently, I've stopped ovulating. But I'm continuing with the cream, because it's the only thing so far that's given me relief, and otherwise I'm unable to perform daily functions.

Tampons

Most tampons are made from rayon (for absorbency) and cotton; most are bleached. Dioxin, a chemical produced in the bleaching process, can be toxic to the immune and reproductive systems. Dioxin is potentially cancer-causing, and it's been linked to endometriosis. The Environmental Protection Agency reports that there is no acceptable level of exposure to dioxin, given that exposure to it is cumulative, and the chemical disintegrates slowly. The real danger with dioxin comes from repeated contact.

In a lifetime, a woman may use 8,000 tampons.

Because it's very absorbent, rayon contributes to the danger of a woman being exposed to dioxin through tampon use; when rayon fibers remain in the vagina after the menstrual period (as they commonly do), so, too, does dioxin.

The alternatives are to use tampons made from unbleached, organic cotton; sanitary napkins; reusable silk sponges; washable organic cotton pads; and The Keeper, a reusable menstrual cup made out of gum rubber.

Natracare (303-320-1510; www.natracare.com) and Organic Essentials (800-765-6491; www.organicessentials.com) make unbleached feminine hygiene products. Lunapads (888-590-2299; www.lunapads.com) and Glad Rags (800-799-4523; www.gladrags.com) make washable pads.

Furthermore, 6.5 billion tampons (and their sometimes plastic applicators) end up in landfills or sewer systems each year. Organic cotton tampons are significantly less harmful to the environment, especially if there's no applicator, or if the applicator is also biodegradable.

The Precautionary Principle

As I completed this chapter, colleagues suggested I include information about other things that can be hazardous to reproductive health: alcohol, antibacterial soaps, aspirin, chlorine, marijuana, microwaved food, nicotine, sodium laurel sulfate—the list grew on and on. Indeed, this chapter is merely an introduction. More books and research about all of these subjects are sorely needed. Meanwhile, refer to the resources listed in the appendix to learn more. Research a product before you choose to make use of it. And remember the Precautionary Principle!

We thought we had given away to doctors and
ability to heal. But here it was, still in our poss
ours after all, we were more than we had tho

—ÁLVAR NÚÑEZ CABEZA DE VA
to the king of Spain, early sixteenth ce

The wife and mother is, so to
the natural physician of the family.

—ANNA FISCHER-DUECKELMANN, MD
The Wife as the Family Physician (1908)

When
more c
plete
yo

Throughout time, women have taught
each other about the body's basic functions and shared the remedies they've discovered for easing menstruation, pregnancy, childbirth, and menopause. They've
observed their menstrual cycles in relation to the phases of the moon.

Fertility Awareness affirms these traditions. Once you know how your reproductive system works, chart your fertility signals, and begin questioning how stress,
relaxation, and different foods affect your cycles, you're on the road to strengthening your health.

you observe your fertility signals, you may notice your general health closely as well. You may find that some foods and medicinal remedies de-health. With ongoing charting, you may also notice the impact of nourishing urself.

Human beings need healthy food, clean water, proper light, sufficient rest, and love. Throughout history, most of our attention has gone into acquiring these things for ourselves and our families. In the last one hundred years or so, while processed foods, night-lights, and other new technologies have seemingly made life easier, we may have lost some traditions for maintaining health. Still, we can learn the nourishing, regenerative skills that our ancestors knew by puberty: how to feed ourselves and our children, how to pace ourselves, how to help our bodies heal when we're sick.

Over and over again, I hear from friends, clients, and colleagues that health is best restored and built by eating well and resting regularly. This chapter and chapters 10 through 12 present the strongest self-nourishing information and techniques I've learned. My book introduces this material, but it's not meant to be comprehensive. Because each person is unique and changing, I usually offer general rather than specific remedies. What's best for you may not suit your sister. What eases menstrual cramps in your twenties (for example) might not work in your thirties or forties.

If you feel the need for remedies, educate yourself as well as you can about your options. Read, follow your nose, take classes. Give yourself the attention and research you want from the health-care provider of your dreams. When you feel the need for a practitioner's support, look for one who takes the time to hear your observations and concerns, and work with him or her to create a treatment plan that feels right for you.

The Six Steps of Healing

In the late 1970s, after studying scientific medicine, herbalism, various diets, homeopathy, and more, herbalist and author Susun Weed became increasingly confused—in regard to healing—about what to do *first*. Once she phrased her question, she realized the reply: *First, do no harm.*

Weed began to group healing techniques and remedies based on the likelihood of a technique or remedy harming or even killing her. In her first book, *Wise*

Woman Herbal for the Childbearing Year, she described the Wise Woman Tradition's Six Steps of Healing and outlined a way to increase health and decrease harm.

Susun has continued to write about the Six Steps of Healing in her newer books, including *New Menopausal Years the Wise Woman Way: Alternative Approaches for Women 30–90.* The Six Steps dovetail beautifully with Fertility Awareness. They help you connect with your body's wisdom and healing mechanisms. They encourage you to address problems at their root, rather than mask them, and to strengthen your relationship to yourself.

Here are the Six Steps of Healing, applied in the context of menstrual cramps:

Step 0. Do Nothing

Weed describes this as "a vital, invisible step." She explains: "This is not 'Don't do anything.' You must actively do no-thing." Essentially, step 0 is about taking time for yourself. If, for example, you've got menstrual cramps, unplug your phone and your TV and go to sleep. If your cramps worsen or are acute, go to step 1.

Meditation and sleeping in complete darkness are also included in this step. (You can read more about sleeping in darkness in chapter 10.)

Step 1. Collect Information

Charting your fertility signals is one excellent way to collect information. Writing down your questions and observations (e.g., does drinking more or less coffee affect my menstrual cramps?) is another. Talking with friends and health-care practitioners, reading books, and searching the Internet are also part of step 1.

Step 2. Engage the Energy

Notice what emotions come up around menstruation. Attend to your dreams. Write out a conversation between your period and you. Find out what it wants. Find out what you want from your period.

When bleeding begins, take a bath and relax. To ease cramps, try a homeopathic remedy. Pick one remedy from step 2 and set a time limit for working with it. Weed says it's vital to set time limits for every step. If your cramps worsen or are very acute, try another step 2 remedy, or go on to step 3.

Step 2 can also mean giving thanks for your life, for the food and water that sustain you, for your parents and grandparents who gave you life, for your woman-hood and fertility. Give thanks for your interest in your own wellness. A spirit of thankfulness—or the lack of it—can make or break your day.

Step 3. Nourish and Tonify

Feed yourself well. Replace processed, sugary, fast foods and drinks with freshly made, nutrient-rich meals.

Prepare herbal infusions (which you can learn about from books, a naturopath, or an herbalist) to give yourself high levels of minerals and vitamins; nourish and tonify your uterus so that it doesn't cramp. Keep your body and mind toned with regular physical activity. Take a yoga class. Grow some of your own food. Go for a walk.

If your cramps worsen or are not relieved within your time limit, add another step 3, or go on to step 4.

Step 4. Sedate and Stimulate

Acupuncture, chiropractic, Swedish massage, and most herbal tinctures fall into this category. Weed cautions that "there is always risk of developing dependence on step 4 remedies. Be aware of the frequency, dosage, and duration of your treatments—and your time limits."

If your cramps worsen or are not relieved within your time limit, add another step 4, or go on to step 5a or 5b.

Step 5a. Use Supplements

In this step, Weed includes all concentrated, extracted, and synthesized substances—including cod liver oil, vitamin and mineral supplements, standardized herbal tinctures, and all herbs in capsules. (Supplements can be made from foods grown with pesticides and include concentrations of pesticides.)

Step 5b. Use Drugs

Over-the-counter and prescription drugs as well as all hormonal medications (including progesterone creams) are included in this step.

Step 6. Break and Enter

Besides surgery, Weed includes psychotropic drugs, "fear-inspiring language," shots, and diagnostic tests such as laparoscopy as part of step 6. "If all other steps fail and you are a woman with severe menstrual cramps," she says, "a hysterectomy is a reasonable choice."

Susun further explains, "When you do nothing, collect information, engage the energy, and nourish and tonify (steps 0–3), then functioning and joy increase: you build health. True healing takes place in these early steps. Whether your problem is chronic or acute, steps 0–3 (along with realistic expectations of the time healing takes) are worthy of your attention.

"Although the impulse in our culture is to jump to step 4 or 5, each step up increases the possibility of severe side effects. While healing can and does take place with the aid of drugs and surgery, once you get to step 5, you can damage or destroy health. Drugs might get rid of menstrual cramps, but they don't address the cause or nourish your body. Drugs mask symptoms. Even common over-the-counter drugs like aspirin can injure health. In the Wise Woman Tradition, symptoms are not enemies to be destroyed but cherished messengers who encourage us to take good care of ourselves."

In the following women's stories, Susun Weed notes which steps the women took and offers further insights in plain type.

Natalie, thirty-two. *I took the Pill* (step 5b) *for six months when I was twenty. I became an emotional roller coaster; I felt like a different person. As soon as I went off it* (step 0), *I swore I'd never go back on again. To prevent pregnancy, we used condoms* (still step 5 if the condoms include nonoxynol-9; step 0 if they're untreated).

Then about a year ago, my acne got out of control. I saw a TV commercial that said the Pill can clear acne. I felt desperate, so I went to my doctor. She promised that a low dose of the Pill wouldn't hurt me; she said it would also take away my menstrual cramps, which had been getting stronger. So I went back on it (step 5b).

Within a few months, my skin cleared up about 85 percent. When I bled, my cramps were really faint. But by the sixth month on the Pill, I'd totally lost my sex drive. I mean totally. And each month I became more and more depressed and withdrawn—similar to how I'd been when I took the Pill at twenty.

I took my last pill and started learning Fertility Awareness (step 1) on the same day. For the first three months, I didn't ovulate, my menstrual cramps were so painful I had to leave work, and my skin got messed up again.

But learning how my body works had opened my eyes. I stuck with the charting (step 1). I started looking at the roots of my depression (step 2), which actually stopped as soon as I went off the Pill. I stopped drinking caffeine in the week before I menstruate (step 4—not step 3, since she drinks caffeine in the rest of her cycle), *started taking crampbark, magnesium, kelp, and evening primrose oil in pill form (step 5a). I'd like to make my own teas, but given my schedule, the pills are more practical.*

Once I started ovulating again, about three months after I went off the Pill, I could tell exactly when to expect my period. I scheduled myself for acupuncture on the day my period arrived (step 4). The acupuncturist was thrilled with all the information I was able to give her about my menstrual cycles. With her help and the other stuff I do, about 90 percent of my cramps have been alleviated.

As for my skin, I still wanted a quick fix, so I got an antibiotic facial cream from a dermatologist (step 5b); but it just clogged my pores and made things worse. I searched around (step 1) and found some herbal-based skin-care products that are a lot more friendly to my skin, though it's not perfect at the moment.

I'm not using Fertility Awareness to avoid pregnancy—yet. We've gone back to condoms. It's been six months since I learned FA, and I've used the charts to help me get in touch with myself. I learned the rules for preventing pregnancy, but I don't think I know them well enough to use them. I figure that's my next step.

Susun comments: "When Natalie first went off the Pill, she jumped from step 5 to 0. Going back from step 4 to 3, then 2, then 1, step by step as she came off the Pill could have helped her make an easier transition.

"Before jumping back to the Pill the second time, steps 2, 3, and 4 could have been tried to help her prevent or ease her cramps and acne.

"Natalie got a lot of benefit from working steps 1 and 4 when she came off the Pill the second time. Adding steps 3, 2, and 0 could remove the remaining 10 percent of her menstrual pain, and perhaps decrease her need of acupuncture."

Liz, thirty-nine. *My periods returned when my daughter was just over a year old, and then we tried conceiving again. My OB said to try for six months on our own (step 0). So, I did that, and I also decreased nursing (step 4).*

After five months, I figured I had an infertility problem. I didn't know about Fertility Awareness at the time. I didn't know that it's common for a woman not to ovulate—even though she may bleed—while breast-feeding or in the months after weaning. I didn't know you need progesterone to sustain a pregnancy, or that low levels of progesterone aren't uncommon after breast-feeding.

I called a reproductive endocrinologist (RE) (step 1). She said I absolutely needed to stop nursing, so I did. My daughter was then eighteen months old. The RE gave me a Clomid Challenge Test (step 5b) to test my FSH level, which in fact was high—13.1. (FSH levels typically increase as women age, showing that the ovaries are requiring more of this hormone in order to mature a viable egg for ovulation. Most doctors say that if your FSH level is higher than 10, you don't have much chance of getting pregnant.) As a result of taking the Clomid, I got what I call my $1,500 ovarian cyst. Then, the doctor said I had a 3 percent chance of conceiving. "Even if your FSH level goes down," she told me, "because it's been 13.1, you don't have much chance of getting pregnant." (Step 6, using fear-inspiring language.)

I felt devastated. She was an expert. But I didn't want to believe her (step 0).

I took a Fertility Awareness class (step 1) and learned some basic facts about breast-feeding and fertility. I began charting my fertility signals. I felt scattered—I had what seems now a ridiculous sense of urgency, probably because I believed the RE's prognosis. I consulted a nutritionist and an acupuncturist (step 1), and I got a prescription for injectable gonadotropins from my RE (step 6). I remember feeling I didn't have time to breathe.

*The supplements the nutritionist suggested (step 5a) didn't feel right for me (step 1—*Liz is collecting intuitive information here). *I took a few days worth of the injectables (step 6) and became nearly psychotic. So I stopped the shots and made a commitment (step 2) to acupuncture once a week (step 4) and Chinese herbs, which my acupuncturist prepared for me in a powder (step 5a). I also searched the Internet (step 1) and found a chat site for women with high FSH levels. I got a lot of support there (step 2).*

I conceived within two months. The cycle I conceived, my FSH level was 7, determined by a test that didn't require Clomid. A new RE gave me progesterone suppositories (step 5b), which I took during the first trimester. Our second daughter is six months old now.

I practically want to scream to other women: "Be careful about putting all your stock in 'experts.' Be careful about calling yourself infertile, and telling yourself you have a problem. You do have time to breathe!"

Susun comments: "Setting reasonable time limits—neither rushing things nor hanging back when action is required—is very important when using the steps.

When Liz called herself infertile after five months of trying, I think she was rushing. Most midwives I know suggest waiting for twelve to twenty-four months before deciding you have a problem. Liz's OB suggested six months, but she began identifying herself as infertile after only five months.

"By jumping from step 0 to 5b (the Clomid challenge test), Liz did some damage to her health. Researching Clomid before she took it (step 1) might have forestalled her use of it.

"Using steps 1 and 2 strengthened Liz's health and improved her chances of conceiving. Step 3 would have been helpful as well."

With the Six Steps of Healing in mind, I present introductory information about what different kinds of health-care providers can offer, followed by natural remedies for strengthening your gynecological health.

And ever has it been that love knows not its own
depth until the hour of separation.

—KAHIL GIBRAN

9. Healing Childbearing Losses

I AM CONTINUALLY AWED BY THE UNIQUE-
ness and the universality of every fertility story I've heard, including the stories of childbearing losses. I've known women who feel that their experience with birth control was a kind of loss—when it weakened their overall health or reproductive system, or made them infertile. I've been deeply touched by women and men whose grief and confusion feel unresolved, even decades after sexual abuse, a miscarriage, an abortion, a stillbirth, traumatic delivery, infertility, or releasing a child to adoption. I've known people who are strongly affected by their parents' childbearing losses as well as those of their grandparents or siblings. So many of these

experiences are not discussed; so many are invisible to others, even those close to us. And yet everyone in a family is touched by them. While understanding your reproductive anatomy and learning to chart are often healing, many people report that their pain still has no place to go.

I've also heard as many healing stories as I have ones about loss.

The dictionary defines *fertile* as—among other things—"rich in material needed to sustain growth." The Indo-European root of *fertile* is *bher*, which means "to carry" or "to bear children." "Burden," "suffer," and "offer" all have the same root. These words remind me of a friend's report of delivering her first child. "Giving birth is no bed of roses," she said, "unless you take all the thorns into account. It's not a Hallmark card; it's not a pillow of clouds. It's slimy and bloody and messy. It hurts like hell. I felt like I was dying. My midwife said, when a woman gets to that place close to death, she knows birth is near."

Sexual Abuse and Fertility

Discovering your fertility can also enhance awareness of how your sexuality was awakened. For many people, the experience was abusive and painful. For many, the desire to heal forms a strand that weaves with desire for a child, the decision not to bear children, or the inability to conceive—and creates a thick braid with the daily ritual of observing fertility signals.

Carl Jung once wrote, "The gods no longer rule from Mount Olympus, but from the solar plexus." Indeed, when women begin to observe their fertility signals, grief and anger about sexual abuse or childbearing losses may rise to the surface. To understand this juxtaposition, I've often turned to the relationships between the Greek gods Demeter, Persephone, and Hades. Our civilization's core fertility myth, the story is also about sexual abuse. In the myth, Demeter and Persephone (mother and daughter) live inseparably until the younger woman reaches childbearing age. Then, Hades rapes Persephone and brings her to the Underworld, where her focus turns inward. Eventually, the mother and daughter establish a cycle of being apart and reuniting. (See "The Myth of Demeter, Persephone, and Hades" on p. 145.) Their relationship is like the seasons, which are fruitful in the summer and fall and dormant in the winter.

Essentially, this myth is about a mother passing on the mysteries and joys of fertility to her daughter. And it's about every person's relationship to Hades, the most feared and mysterious of all the Greek gods, perhaps because he ruled the world of the dead.

Where's the healing in this myth? Consider that mythic characters are symbols of contradictory thoughts and feelings about peace and healing, symbols of our own raw nature. Descending to Hades (after sexual abuse, losing a baby, losing a dream) takes a person on a soul search through raw emotion and the unknown. Persephone's abduction brings her from the security of her mother's world, wherein her thoughts about life may have been unexamined. In the Underworld, alone with her pain and questioning her assumptions, she has only her own truth to rely on. Rising from Hades (as Persephone does each spring) symbolizes a woman freeing herself from concepts that no longer serve her—including naive ideas about how life should be. Now she knows the depths of life and her own self. She can be more accepting of life as it is—and thereby more at peace.

If you are a survivor of sexual abuse, you are not alone; and healing is possible. I highly recommend *The Courage to Heal: A Guide for Women Survivors of Child Sexual Abuse* by Ellen Bass and Laura Davis. Many people find support at twelve-step programs such as Survivors of Incest Anonymous. For a listing of local chapters, send three dollars and a SASE to SIA, PO Box 190, Benson, MD 21018; 410-893-3322; visit www.siawso.org. For a technique that helps you make peace with your own thinking, see The Work of Byron Katie, described on page 154.

THE MYTH OF DEMETER, PERSEPHONE, AND HADES

Demeter was the goddess of fertility, some say of agriculture. She also ruled over the Eleusian mysteries, sacred women's rites whose goals were regeneration and forgiveness of sins.[1] In most versions of the myth, she had only one child, a daughter. She called her daughter Kore, which has been translated to mean "the daughter" and "the inner soul of Mother Earth." The Roman version of her name was Ceres. The words *corn*, *kernel*, *core*, *carnal*, and *cardiac* are all rooted in her name.

Demeter and her daughter are often considered to be different aspects of the same goddess. They adored each other. Kore was very beautiful and had a mysterious quality about her that revealed a rich inner life. She knew the beauty of flowers and fruit, and also the brevity of this beauty. To keep her daughter close as long as possible, Demeter guarded Kore from men to a point of being possessive.

continued

Hades, one of Demeter's brothers and King of the Underworld, was especially attracted to Kore. Hades was god of the depths, god of the invisibles, and known for being narcissistic. He knew the location of all gems and precious metals in the earth. One day when Demeter's back was turned, Hades raped Kore and brought her to the Underworld to be his bride. In Hades, her name changed to Persephone.

Perhaps because of her focus on her interior, emotional life, Persephone was considered Queen of the Underworld even before Hades abducted her.

Demeter became distraught to the point of insanity when she realized that Hades had abducted her daughter. Demeter was powerless over Persephone's return. Through her depression, she withheld rain and refused to let anything grow on earth, even though people starved. She disguised herself as an old woman without relations and refused to be comforted.

Zeus, chief of the gods, sent his siblings to Demeter to persuade her to let the earth bear fruit again. She wouldn't hear any of them. She wanted only to see her daughter. Finally Zeus decided that Hades must give way. Hades agreed and let Persephone go— but first he offered her a pomegranate, a fruit that symbolizes fertility. She ate six of the red, juicy seeds.

While Demeter and Persephone rejoiced in their reunion, Hecate (a midwife who traveled between worlds) reported that Persephone had eaten in Hades. Anyone who eats in Hades is not allowed to leave. Demeter became distraught again. Zeus then arranged a deal: Persephone would spend half the year with Demeter and half in Hades.

In agricultural terms, Persephone is with Demeter during summer's warmth and the autumn's harvest; she's with Hades during the cold, dormant winter. The myth shows that fruitfulness and barrenness are both included in the cycles of fertility.

Julie, twenty-five. I decided I was a woman when I turned fourteen, and I wanted a ritual to mark it. I told an older man that I wanted to lose my virginity with him. I lied and told him I was sixteen. I also promised myself that I would always respect the young woman I was then. The man gave me what I wanted. But over the years, I felt abused by him. Even though I asked him to do what he did, because I was a child, he shouldn't have done it. He should have protected me and said no.

It took me a while to see that because of my promise to myself, my anger seemed to turn toward the man. Really, though, I was angry with myself. I still am angry; I still don't feel at peace with myself.

Learning Fertility Awareness three years ago also initiated me into womanhood—in a way I renew with each charted cycle. I wonder if I'd known I didn't need sex to be a woman, if I'd learned FA when I was fourteen, if I would have chosen a different entry into adulthood.

Sonia, forty-one. When I was twenty-five, my fiancé punched a hole through a wall. I felt shattered. Though I sensed that our troubles would intensify if we stayed together, it took me several months to leave him—partly because after fighting, we would make love very tenderly. By the time I left, I could see my contributions to our violent dance. I made a pact with God: until I'm ready for a relationship that isn't violent, I'd rather be alone.

I sort of studied myself, my relationships with my father (who molested me) and mother (from whom I felt very distant), and the violence in their marriage. Nine to five, I was blessed with very satisfying work. On weekends, I went to twelve-step meetings and leaned against the trunks of a lot of large trees. I took dance classes that helped me enjoy my body. I considered my menstrual periods personal holidays. They didn't come predictably, and during especially long cycles I felt grateful to celibacy for sparing me from wondering whether I was pregnant each month.

A few years went by. A man I wouldn't sleep with asked if I intended to become a saint. The truth was, I ached to be held. There were days when I felt absolutely out of my mind. As for family, I didn't feel able to relate sanely with a partner or with children. Seven long years of celibacy went by.

I met my husband when I was thirty-four. We took a class in Fertility Awareness shortly after we got together—we've used the method to avoid pregnancy. Sometimes I wonder if there's something wrong with me that I haven't wanted children. But from my very first chart, FA has shown me that I can try to conceive each cycle—or not. For whatever reason, I haven't felt moved to try. I have trusted my instincts and seen that understanding my menstrual cycles gives me (and my husband) a way to cherish my body.

Miscarriage

A miscarriage is a death without a public face. Losing a baby affects a woman physically, emotionally, and spiritually, often in solitude. Often, the reason for miscarrying isn't known. That miscarriage is a common experience doesn't lessen its intensity or pain.

Claudia Panuthos and Cathy Romeo, co-directors of a childbirth counseling center in Boston in the early 1980s, wrote a lovely book, *Ended Beginnings: Healing Childbearing Losses*, which offers help for creating a place to grieve and heal. The book includes a meditation for encouraging spiritual resolution after miscarriage, which they've generously permitted me to reprint here, along with their introductory and concluding comments, and the story of a couple who found this meditation healing.

If you're moved to try, this meditation can be used for situations besides miscarriage—perhaps for your grandmother's stillborn baby, a child your mother released to adoption before you were born, or an abortion your daughter had.

A Meditation for Encouraging Spiritual Resolution After Miscarriage

Whether one believes in afterlife, reincarnation, or something else, the following meditation/visualization is offered as an opportunity for parents to create a safe, supportive space for "visiting" and grieving with another soul. It is a daydream that may become or resolve a night dream. This exercise can be applied to any loss. It may be used as a means of connecting with lost children. It may also serve as a means of honoring lost dreams. As a way of reaching peace with whatever you have lost, we invite you to meet what is gone here, in the safe haven of a visualization you create. You may first want to read this exercise through and then do it with closed eyes.

Find a place where you can be quiet and undisturbed. You may want to play a favorite piece of music that you find particularly peaceful. Follow a relaxation process that works well for you, or simply breathe slowly and rhythmically, allowing yourself to let go of tension, pain, or anxiety through your breath. The oxygen in your breath reaches every cell in your body without your even having to think about it; you might pretend that your breath can bring peace to every part of your body as well.

When your body and mind are more peaceful and calm, allow yourself to drift off to some place in the world that you feel would support a meeting once again between you and your child. You may have visited this place many times, or perhaps you've never been there before. Take your time and locate yourself in a place that will truly honor this meeting—a beach, a forest, a meadow, a special room. You are creating a sanctuary, a haven of perfect peace, acceptance, and understanding. Your sanctuary is a place that no one can violate and where no one can interfere. Breathe evenly. Remember that all is safe here; all is understood. Blame and cruelty cannot exist here, for unconditional love reigns. No performance ratings; only complete acceptance. Lean into those feelings now; let them fill you and heal you. Breathe.

Now imagine that you are surrounding this place with complete protection. Perhaps you may envision the protection in the form of white healing light, or perhaps you will choose guardian angels or spirits who may already seem to be protecting your child. Breathe.

When you feel ready, look off into the distance and see your child in some physical form. (Or you might choose to envision your lost dream, somehow manifested in physical form.) This is a meeting beyond the body; it is a meeting of love and of the essence of each person. You may see your son or daughter as an infant or as a young child. Allow your loved one to take any age or appearance that feels right. Follow the vision intuitively, not intellectually. Whatever physical image you envision, remember that it is a meeting of one essence with another. Allow the image to come closer, close enough so that you are able to communicate with one another. Breathe.

If you feel tears, welcome them—for tears are the rivers of life that cleanse the heart and soul. They are signs of sorrow but also of love.

Please give your child the power to communicate in a way that you will be sure to understand. The essence of one's soul may communicate regardless of whether he or she has language. Take some moments to be fully with each other, experiencing each other's deepest capacities for love and understanding. Breathe.

Ask your child if there is anything she needs from you in order to be at peace. Allow all the time you need for an answer. If you do feel some need in your child, take the time now to provide for her. Remember that in this space everything is possible, and all wishes may be granted. Breathe. If there is anything further you need to learn, share, or say, allow it to be freely communicated. Take all the time you need.

You might then choose to offer a gift to your child, a gift that represents your eternal love. Then ask your child for a gift as well—an essence gift. An essence gift is a present that symbolizes some deeper meaning. Open your heart to receive this gift, even though you may not understand it fully.

Take the gift into your possession—keep it always as a sign of the permanent and indestructible bond between you and your child. Stand together in your sanctuary and see a star (or any other symbol of peace) above your heads, gently raining down peace, healing, and love on the two of you.

Now it is time to begin to slowly leave this place. Before you do, bless your child. As you bless her, the star above both of you melts into two stars—one will follow each of you wherever you go. Allow your child to drift away just as she appeared, remembering that you may visit with her at any time on this plane.

Bring with you the gift you received. See that gift as a symbol and draw from it new strength and healing. Make a commitment to find for yourself some actual, physical manifestation of what you've received. It need not be an exact replica but a symbol that feels right—trust yourself to know when you have found it.

Over the past several years, we have been using this meditation/visualization with grieving parents. We have no technological or scientific explanation that can adequately describe its effects. Parents consistently report a greater sense of peace. Some have shared stories that can only be explained in a spiritual context. Here is such a story:

Nina's answer. Nina's twin sons were delivered prematurely at six and a half months. They were stillborn, and Nina's grief shaped her life for many months. She willingly agreed to the visualization exercise, searching for some connection with the sons she had lost. She asked her boys to join her on a beach. They appeared, in her visualization, as young children. They each clutched a shell and held it throughout her mental imagery. Nina envisioned playing with her boys, fully feeling their presence, and then she asked them for gifts that she could keep with her as ever-present reminders of their love for and connection with each other. Nina told us later that she thought the boys would give her the shells they held, but to her surprise, they didn't. Instead, one gave her a flower, and the other a piece of driftwood. Nina cried and smiled and felt closer to her sons than she ever had before. "I couldn't believe," she says, "how it all worked! I didn't consciously think any of it, it just unfolded before me like a movie. It was one of the most beautiful experiences of my life." When asked to find some manifestation or symbol, on the physical plane, of her sons' gifts, Nina smilingly replied that she didn't even need to do that. She thought she might, anyway, but she knew that the flower and the driftwood were forever ensconced in her heart.

Nina was so delighted with her newfound pathway to her sons that she couldn't wait to share it with her husband. However, rather than just telling him about it, she asked him to experience the visualization himself. She did not share her experience but instead guided him through the relaxation until he, too, chose a sanctuary—also a beach—and then asked the boys to be with him. Nina could barely speak when he told her, through his tears, that they each gave him a shell.

Abortion

I believe that fertility is a privilege and a mystery and that the choice to continue or terminate a pregnancy belongs to each woman. Like choosing to act on sexual desires, like choosing a method for preventing pregnancy or trying to conceive, the way you respond to an unintended pregnancy encompasses emotional, physical, spiritual, and political terrain.

Half of the pregnancies that occur in the United States are unintended. Often, on learning that she's conceived unintentionally, a woman panics; at the same time, she may be awed that her body is actually fertile. When the question of an unexpected pregnancy is real and palpable, it's like being at the edge of a cliff. Each woman answers for herself how life will move forward with grace and respect. Every woman is different; every situation is unique. In those days of deciding whether to continue with or terminate her pregnancy, may every woman be heard as deeply as she needs. Whatever she chooses, may she have continued support from within herself and her community.

Facing the possibility of an unintended pregnancy can seem like a match of wills between you, your partner (if he or she is present), and the force of life itself. You may feel like you're in something beyond your control. You may feel unable to move forward, unable to carry the pregnancy or care for a child at this time, unable to continue relating with the father, unable to say yes or no to the mystery unfolding inside you.

Charting and being aware of the possibility of conception move each person who practices Fertility Awareness closer to the intricate web of life, death, and fertility. A woman faces those mysteries again when she conceives unintentionally.

A choice to abort can lead to a renewed commitment to life. And, after an abortion, you may feel deep grief—either immediately or many years afterward. I've known many women who, in their attempt to conceive a much-wanted child, feel fresh grief about an abortion they experienced years earlier.

If you feel unresolved about an abortion, however many years ago it was, consider your thoughts juicy messengers inviting you to make peace with yourself and your choices. You can still give yourself time and space to heal. You might experiment with the meditation suggested for those who've miscarried. Bert Hellinger, a German therapist and author, suggests doing something special to acknowledge the one you aborted, like planting a tree.

Leslie, thirty-eight. *Starting from when I was fifteen, sex was where I looked for love. I didn't know my body, didn't feel connected to it, and as a result I had several unplanned pregnancies. I've read that it's common for young women who were adopted, as I was, to have multiple unintended pregnancies (and abortions) at an early age. After all these years, I can see the pattern: my mother conceived me, gave birth to me, and said no to me. Essentially, I did the same with the ones I conceived.*

I take responsibility for my choices. Just recognizing the pattern helps me accept myself, and understand why I've resisted becoming pregnant with my husband.

Once I started charting, I began to appreciate the power of fertility—my fertility—and integrate it with awareness of myself. Recently, Jason and I finally felt confident in our ability to read my chart. We made love without a condom for the first time in six years of marriage. It felt like a great opening, like trust between ourselves and nature. Like honoring the sacredness of sex.

Jeff, forty-eight. *When Robin (my first wife) and I got together, she told me she didn't think she was fertile. I just said, "Oh. Okay." Within two months, she was pregnant. We were so new to each other, we didn't think we were ready for a baby. Without talking much about it, she had an abortion. About a year later, we did feel ready, and we had two great kids.*

By the time our oldest was seven, Robin and I had become strangers to each other. We divorced amicably, with shared custody of our children.

Lily (my second wife) practices Fertility Awareness. While she taught me the method, I faced the possibility of a pregnancy with her. I don't want another child. I also might not be able to say no if one showed up and surprised us. Just thinking this, I felt grief for aborting that first child. I'd never felt it before.

I wouldn't change what Robin and I did—I can't change it. And, there are still things about the abortion I haven't explored. I still don't know Robin's experience of it. I wrestle with this, and also realize we did the best we could with what we knew at the time. I'm still pro-choice. And I'm glad for Fertility Awareness in my life, for helping me complete one part of a circle I didn't even know was still open.

Lynn, forty-seven. *I didn't keep great charts after Sam was born. I'd been charting for fifteen years, and I guess I felt overconfident about knowing when I'm fertile. I was shocked to become pregnant again, when Sam was two.*

Perhaps it happened because part of me wanted another child. I adored raising Sam and longed to experience more of that pure love that a small child gives. But Jason (my husband) was certain he wanted only one child. Jason is keenly aware of how much energy it takes to raise children, and he believes in dedicating his energy to the wider society rather than nurturing a large family. I love this visionary part of him. It's one of the reasons I married him. When a friend suggested I just have the baby and let Jason deal with it, I knew I couldn't. I decided to abort the baby.

For several years afterward, I agonized about whether to have another child. I felt like the life force was knocking on my door incessantly. Around the time Sam turned seven, the knocking stopped; since then I've felt mostly at peace with our small family. I've come to appreciate that having one child allows me to give him my undivided attention, while my friends struggle to give each of their kids enough. Jason and I have created a unique nonprofit organization that affects some of the changes we care about—something we probably wouldn't have had time for if our family were larger. Ten years later, I see that the abortion affirmed my acceptance of Jason, his passions and limitations, and our life together.

It breaks my heart that time and money are spent fighting for and against legal abortion. I wish those resources were poured into something we all agree on: learning more about how our bodies (and minds) work, so unintended pregnancies can be prevented.

Traumatic Birth

I first heard the following story by Johana Moore nearly ten years ago and continue to share it with people in a variety of situations.

Prayers for David. I went into labor when I was about twenty-nine weeks pregnant. This birth came on the heels of several miscarriages; my first son was then five years old.

There had been no exceptional activity that day other than being unusually upset with my husband. No time to even think of that. As I lay in labor at the hospital, the doctor said he preferred doing C-sections for preemies, but my child was too far in the birth canal and would have to be delivered vaginally.

I dilated quickly and was rushed to the delivery room. My doctor saw the cord across the baby's blue head. "There's no time for a spinal," he told me. "I'll have to remove the child with high forceps—immediately."

The pain was enormous—so enormous that I froze with the thought, I can't contain this anguish.

Then the pain was over, and there was a tiny, blue, crying body that a dozen people were nervously handling: David. He was placed in a space suit and handheld all the way to the nearest neonatal unit, an hour away.

My body, achy as it was, was deeply relieved—as though I couldn't have contained my son's body another second. I had to work very hard not to feel guilty about how great I felt after the birth.

My mentor at the time was Hugh Prather. As soon as it was practically possible, I spoke with him. "Pray that David knows that you love him," Hugh said. "Tell him over and over again that you love him if he goes or if he stays. Don't pray for him to live, because if he doesn't, you'll feel unsuccessful. If he lives and isn't happy, you'll blame yourself. But do tell him, over and over, how very much you love him."

The next seventy-two hours were critical. Being male and only two pounds, twelve ounces, David had a fifty-fifty chance of survival at best.

I'd planned a home birth, and now my baby was in a completely "unnatural" setting. I learned quickly that God is in everything. In every being caring for my beloved child, in the technology, in the drugs, in the very structure of the hospital that housed his body when I no longer could. To love this child meant to love and embrace everything in his world. It meant to love myself whether or not he lived. The event brought me completely to a here-and-now reality. I cannot imagine a greater gift.

My prayers from David's tender beginning continue to give me the freedom to love and be loved by my son. He is thirteen now, with limitations and challenges (some of them remnants of his prematurity and divorced parents) I know he can handle. Still, guilt can take hold of me for a few, fleeting moments. Then I remember this is Love's child and Love is taking care of him.

Infertility

A woman recently told me, "Knowing fertility doesn't mean you know infertility." She explained that infertility includes questioning your worth as a woman and a human being; it leads to doubting your relationship with your partner, and every health-care and career choice you've made. It's about feeling jealousy, selfishness, hunger, and shame. It's about thinking that only holding your own baby in your arms will give you peace.

One of the best tools I can recommend for clarifying that you're with your thoughts and you're separate from them, that they don't define who you are—is The Work of Byron Katie. The Work offers a way to make peace with your thinking about a situation, including infertility and other childbearing losses, whether or not the situation changes.

Reading fiction about childbearing losses can be wonderfully healing. May I recommend:

- Gretchen Moran Laskas, *The Midwife's Tale,* Dial, 2003. When Elizabeth Whitely comes of age in the early 1900s, the last of a long line of midwives, she learns what her foremothers did with babies who weren't welcome and she struggles with her own infertility.
- Katie Singer, *The Wholeness of a Broken Heart,* Riverhead, 1999. Just after Hannah Fried leaves home, she makes a casual comment that offends her mother, who then refuses to speak with her daughter for ten years. For insight and solace, Hannah turns to her ancestors, including a miscarried child, who dedicated their lives to the next generation's freedom.
- Jane Smiley, *A Thousand Acres,* Knopf, 1991. A beautifully told story of three women, their family farm, and their complex, incestuous relationships with their father. One sister dies of cancer, another repeatedly miscarries her babies—possibly because their water is contaminated by pesticides. The youngest distances herself from the others in order to leave home.
- Mark Spragg, *The Fruit of Stone,* Riverhead, 2002. A riveting novel about a rancher who finds himself without children at forty.
- Diane McKinney Whetstone, *Tumbling,* Morrow, 1996. When babies mysteriously appear on Noon and Herbie's doorsteps, they take them in. While raising the girls, Noon finds comfort in church; Herbie finds it with a jazz singer named Ethel—until Noon fights to preserve her South Philadelphia neighborhood and to know her own passion.

In 1986, after forty-three years of thinking her life should be different than it was, Byron Katie realized that without a story about how life is supposed to be, she was left with a sense of peace. By giving up "what should be," she experienced the peace of "what is."

How does this relate to Fertility Awareness? Probably every woman has thought things like, *My body should have normal menstrual cycles,* or *I won't be motivated to chart my cycles until I have a decent partner,* or *My doctor should take the time to teach me about my medication.* Many an infertile woman has thought things like, *Only a baby can give me the love I need,* or *A loving God would give me a healthy baby.*

Byron Katie has developed a simple process of inquiry that helps you honestly reexamine the "shoulds" that you have believed. She suggests you write down your judgment of another person or a thing, ask four questions about this thought, including *Is it true? How do you react when you think this thought?*, and *Who would you be without the thought?* After inquiring, you "turn around" your statement. For example, *My doctor should take the time to teach me about my medication* becomes **I** *should take the time to teach myself about my medication. Until I can embrace my own baby, I can't know peace* becomes *Until I can embrace myself, I can't know peace.*

By welcoming our arguments with reality and exposing them to the clear light of investigation, the mind wakes up to its innocent mistake and lets go of its losing battle with reality. The result is peace.

Like Fertility Awareness, I consider The Work a basic life skill. To experience it for yourself, check out www.TheWork.org (where you can download a free worksheet); or read *Loving What Is,* which Byron Katie coauthored with Stephen Mitchell.

RESOLVE, a national organization with over fifty local chapters, offers support, education, and advocacy for those experiencing infertility. For more information, see the Resources section at the back of this book.

Smita, forty-two. Because of my career and because my first husband didn't want children, I didn't start trying to conceive until I was a month shy of forty-one. At first, when Paul (my second husband) and I started trying, we just enjoyed each other. A few months later, when I still wasn't pregnant, I began taking my temperature. It was nice to see the curves each month, but even when we enthusiastically checked the box for sex on key days, I still didn't get pregnant. Each cycle's rhythm of hope then letdown began to break my heart. I put away my thermometer and my charts. I had figured out the days I was fertile each month, and the charting only made me more obsessed.

I've been to all sorts of healers and doctors. I've been told to give up hope and to hold on to it. I got a prescription for progesterone, but when I read the warnings accompanying the pills, I put these in my drawer, too. I like to be friendly with my body, and these pills just don't seem friendly. The high-tech alternatives are even scarier.

Disappointment is such a hard emotion to live with. I've also struggled with bitterness, and my lack of generosity when other women seem to become pregnant so effortlessly. Lately, when my period arrives and heartbreak immobilizes me, I try to disengage from my own self-pity by sending prayers to the other women in the world who face this same disappointment. I know there is a big sisterhood of women who are caught in this net of pain.

I don't want frantic grief over being childless to undermine my life. I have so much to be grateful for each day. I want to be happy, to accept what life has brought me, and choose my next steps from a tranquil place.

A Wilderness of Fertility

Eliza, fifty-six. *I didn't marry until I was thirty-nine. I took a course in Natural Family Planning before my wedding, and then a year passed without my becoming pregnant. An OB/GYN put me on the Pill for several months—he figured this would clear up what he thought was endometriosis. When I stopped taking the Pill, I still didn't get pregnant.*

I prayed and asked others to offer prayers on my behalf. I thought if I just had strong faith, maybe I would conceive. I suggested to my husband that we adopt, but he wasn't interested in pursuing that. Mother's Day was one of the hardest times each year.

By this time, I had taught school for sixteen years. Slowly, I realized I wasn't going to have my own children. One evening, I was at Mass. During the liturgy it seemed God told me, "Motherhood is an infinite mystery. Even if you had twenty children you would not grasp the fullness of this mystery." It's hard to communicate this now in words—but I felt a sense of affirmation: I was not denied fertility. It was just not to be physically manifested in a child of my own. If having ten children did not exhaust this mystery, then zero children did not disqualify my participation in it, either.

Invisible rhythms underlie most of what we assume to be constant in
ourselves and the world around us. Life is in continual flux, but the
change is not chaotic. The rhythmic nature of earth life is perhaps
its most usual yet overlooked property. Each day, as earth turns
on its axis, we experience the alternation of light and darkness. The
moon's revolution, too, pulls our atmosphere into a cycle of change.
Night follows day. Seasons change. The tides ebb and flow. These
various rhythms are also seen in animals and man. We, too,
change, growing sleepy at night and restlessly active by day.
We, too, exhibit the rhythmic undulations of our planet.

—GAY GAER LUCE
Biological Rhythms in Human and Animal Physiology

10. Night-Lighting and Reproductive Health

MANY OF US HAVE HEARD THE STORY THAT before the introduction of street lamps and other forms of modern lighting, women ovulated when the moon was full, and bled while it was new. We've heard that factory-farmed chickens are exposed to light twenty-four hours a day to increase their egg production. These tales are based on the fact that exposure to light influences circadian rhythms and our hormonal systems, including the menstrual cycle. (*Circadian* comes from the Latin word *circa,* which means "approximate," and *dian,* which means "day.")

The earth's primary rhythm comes from rotating on its axis every twenty-four hours, bringing sunrise and sunset, the daily pattern of light and darkness. Seasonal patterns of light and darkness are determined by the earth's revolving around the sun every 365.25 days. And the moon waxes and wanes as it revolves around the earth every 29.5 days (the length of a typical menstrual cycle), offering a great variety of visible light.

Light from the sun and moon and artificial light affect circadian rhythm, which keeps humans, plants, and animals in sync with the earth's twenty-four hour rotation.

Our circadian system is regulated by the *pineal gland,* which is located in the brain. The pineal gland directs your body's rhythmic activities—including sleep, appetite, and the onset of puberty—through its production of *melatonin.* This hormone is primarily secreted at night, and it requires darkness to be produced. Bright light suppresses melatonin secretion.[1]

The *hypothalamus gland,* also located in the brain, is richly supplied with melatonin receptors. This gland regulates your body's overall homeostasis, including things like blood pressure, emotions, temperature, and the endocrine (hormonal) system. Hormones secreted by the hypothalamus stimulate the anterior pituitary gland to secrete its hormones; and these, in turn, stimulate the thyroid gland, the adrenals, and the ovaries to secrete yet other hormones. The ovaries (and the testicles) are also thought to contain melatonin receptors.[2] You can see how melatonin production—and thereby sleeping in darkness or with light—can affect your whole body's functioning, including your menstrual cycle: if the hypothalamus doesn't receive sufficient melatonin, its ability to regulate your hormonal system could be impaired.

Lunaception

In the late 1960s, writer Louise Lacey realized that being on the Pill took her body away from its natural rhythm. She went off it and subsequently had very irregular cycles. She began reading about circadian rhythm as well as the sexual cycles of some primates, which suggested peaks of sexual activity relating to the lunar cycle. Lacey wondered if the moon's cycles relate to human reproduction and, if so, how? She wondered if artificial lights interrupt the moon's effect.

A newspaper article that reported the effects of night-light on the menstrual cycle then caught her attention. John Rock (the OB/GYN whose experiments with giving infertile women synthesized progesterone led to the creation of the Pill) and physicist E. M. Dewan found that women's menstrual cycles became regular by sleeping in complete darkness Days 1 through 13, sleeping with a 100-watt bulb burning all night (under a lampshade in the bedroom) Days 14 through 17, and then returning to sleeping in complete darkness until the new period began.[3]

Thrilled by the possibility that she could return to healthy cycles, Lacey tried variations on the above experiment, beginning in 1971. She also began to chart her temperature. She found that sleeping in complete darkness except for three nights each cycle (when she slept with a 40-watt bulb under a lampshade *or* with a 75-watt bulb beaming a shaft of light from a nearby bathroom, essentially mimicking full-moon light) triggered ovulation. She called the technique "Lunaception" and found that it could be used to direct her fertility—and that of her women friends. By avoiding intercourse on the days they slept with light, Louise Lacey and twenty-seven of her friends developed regular, healthy menstrual cycles and used Lunaception to avoid pregnancy effectively until menopause.[4]

Sleeping in the Absence of Light to Strengthen Gynecological Health

After reading about Louise Lacey's work, the Couple to Couple League (CCL), which has taught Natural Family Planning since 1971, conducted a study to see if sleeping in darkness except for three nights midcycle could help women with very short or very long cycles develop a more normal cycle length. Indeed, 92 percent of the women in the CCL's study experienced at least some reduction in cycle irregularity.[5]

Joy DeFelice, a registered nurse and director of the Natural Family Planning Program at Sacred Heart Medical Center in Spokane, Washington, also read an article by Louise Lacey about her findings. In 1976, DeFelice and her NFP students began studying the effects of night-lighting on the menstrual cycle. Unlike Louise Lacey and the CCL (whose groups found that darkness-only regimens did not work), most of Joy DeFelice's students have found they seldom require sleeping with any light at all in order to normalize their hormonal patterns. DeFelice instructs her students to sleep in complete darkness for three to six months before deciding to introduce light for a few days each cycle.[6]

According to research conducted by the Couple to Couple League and Joy De-Felice, eliminating light while sleeping helps women create healthy menstrual cycles in a variety of situations:

- Women with anovulatory cycles have become ovulatory.
- Women with unclear mucus readings develop discernible, healthy mucus buildup.
- Ovulation occurs in sync with fertile mucus buildup.
- Cycles that had been very short (twenty-six days or less) or very long (thirty-five days or more) become twenty-seven to thirty-one days long.
- FSH levels become healthy.
- Spotting at various times during the cycle is significantly reduced.
- Progesterone levels are strengthened.
- Women with a history of miscarriage(s) are able to sustain pregnancy.
- During breast-feeding, an infertile mucus pattern is easily established.
- During weaning or bottle-feeding, sleeping in darkness (and then introducing light during a slippery mucous patch) can help trigger a return to ovulatory cycles.
- Premenopausal women develop a more discernible mucus pattern; and the intensity of their premenopausal symptoms—including hot flashes, sleeplessness, and mood changes—is reduced.

So what does sleeping in total darkness mean? Fifteen minutes after turning out the lights, you can't see objects in the room, including your own hands. Exposure to the moon and stars (from a skylight or another window) probably provides too much light.

To sleep in the absence of light:

- Cover your bedroom windows with room-darkening blinds or curtains backed by light-blocking fabric. Customized blinds can be ordered from local and online companies that do window treatments. Light-blocking fabric can be sewn on to the backs of existing curtains for about seven dollars per yard.
- As a temporary measure, cardboard can block out a fair amount of light.
- Cracks of light from under your door can be covered with a towel. Cracks around the edges of your windows can be covered with aluminum foil.
- Cover the light from your digital clock.

If you live in a warm climate, tightly woven red cloth can block out light and allow fresh air. If you need light in the middle of the night (in the bathroom or while nursing), use as dim a light as possible; perhaps purchase a red bulb (like those used in a photographer's darkroom) from a camera store. When traveling, a scarf (folded several times) or a mask can be placed over your eyes while you sleep.

Practicing Lunaception

In the twenty-first century, sleeping in the absence of light usually takes time and attention. Eliminate sources of light from your bedroom gradually: cover your window one night and the crack under your door the next. While it may take several months, a healthier hormonal sequence should result. It's up to you, of course, to try Lunaception (wherein you'd introduce light for three nights midcycle) or to sleep only in darkness, as Joy DeFelice's students have found to be most effective.

If you choose Lunaception, there are several variations to try:

- To support healthy, ovulatory cycles, begin your cycle by sleeping in the absence of light. Then, after you observe two consecutive days of slippery cervical fluid or wet vaginal sensation, on the night of the second day allow full moonlight, a lamp lit by a 40-watt bulb in your room, or a 75-watt bulb beaming toward your room from another nearby room. Sleep with the light for three nights and then return to sleeping in darkness.

- If you are not ovulating and haven't bled for a month or longer, first sleep in the absence of light for twelve days. Then introduce light in your room (as described above) for the next three nights. Then return to sleeping in darkness for two weeks. Continue with this technique to encourage healthy ovulatory cycles.

- If you want to ovulate later than usual in your cycle, first sleep in the absence of light up to and including the day you normally ovulate. Introduce light on the next night, and sleep with it on for three nights. Then sleep in the absence of light until your next period begins. For example, if you normally ovulate on Day 10, and want to ovulate on Day 14, in your first cycle with Lunaception, sleep in darkness Days 1 through 10; introduce light Days 11 through 13; then return to darkness. If this helps you to ovulate one day later, then in the next cycle introduce light Days 12 through 14. The idea is to shift your ovulation gradually.

- If you want to ovulate earlier in your cycle, first sleep in the absence of light until the day before you normally ovulate. Sleep with light for three nights, then return to sleeping in darkness. For example, if you normally ovulate on Day 20, in your first cycle, sleep in darkness Days 1 through 18; introduce light Days 19 through 21; then return to darkness. If this helps you to ovulate one day earlier, then the next cycle, introduce light Days 18 through 20. Again, the idea is to shift your ovulation gradually.

The darkness and the light should feel right to you. You may also find that you (and your whole family) sleep better in complete darkness. Male fertility may also be enhanced by sleeping without light. More research about sleeping in the absence of light would be most welcome!

Emma, twenty-nine. I went on the Pill when I was seventeen to regulate my cycles because they were so long and far apart. By the time I was eighteen (and still on the Pill), my menstrual cramps became incredibly intense. When I was twenty-three, I was diagnosed with endometriosis. After nearly twelve years on and off the Pill, I stopped taking it and tried Lunaception. I've been amazed! For five months, I've ovulated within one or two days of the last day of sleeping with light, and I feel healthier than I have in years.

Ruth, thirty-one. I observe the Jewish laws of niddah, which means that my husband and I don't have sexual relations until seven days after my period ends—around Day 13. Once I started charting, I realized I was ovulating on Day 11. I wanted to conceive, and I wanted to continue following Jewish laws. I began taking vitamin supplements and doing yoga for about fifteen minutes three times a week, and almost immediately I started ovulating on Day 12. Then I tried Lunaception. We slept in darkness Days 1 through 12, then turned the light on Day 13 for three nights. I ovulated on Day 13—and conceived!

A truly good physician first finds out the cause of the illness,
and having found that, he first tries to cure it by food.
Only when food fails does he prescribe medication.

—SUN SSU-MO
(Tang dynasty physician, 590–692),
Precious Recipes

11. Food and Reproductive Health

So MUCH OF OUR WELLNESS, INCLUDING
our reproductive health, depends on how we feed ourselves. Food provides the
fuel our bodies use to move through the day; it also feeds the glands that secrete
the hormones necessary for reproductive health and fertility.

In the last one hundred years, as the world's population has exploded, most
Westerners have stopped growing their own food. We consume products that are
mass-produced with fertilizers and pesticides, nutritionally depleted, and genetically modified. I don't know of a large-scale solution to these problems. For each
of us, though, becoming educated about the situation is a first step.

If you're noticing menstrual problems and want to normalize your cycle, learning about the relationship between food and reproductive health can be a great place to start. Many of the women I see who have irregularities report that they eat a lot of white-flour products (cereal, bread, pasta, pastry, and cookies); soy products (including soy milk, soy burgers, protein bars, and tofu); potato and corn chips; and/or sugary snacks. Their diets often lack nutrient-dense foods and may be vegan or low fat.

While I have seen a lot of fertility charts show improved health after women decrease their consumption of fast foods and replace them with meals that are nutrient dense, expecting a quick fix isn't realistic. Shopping for and cooking with fresh food take money and time. Observing the effects of a new diet on your menstrual cycle takes patience. And no diet is right for everyone. While this chapter presents information about the nutrients that are essential to reproductive health, it does not offer menu plans or recipes.

Volumes of widely divergent ideas have been written about what constitutes healthy eating habits. I've chosen to focus on the research of Weston A. Price, a Canadian-born dentist who discovered dietary principles that conferred fertility and healthy babies, generation after generation. Dr. Price's research (conducted in the 1930s and '40s) presents what our ancestors knew about diet and sound health before vegetable oils, refined sugar, white flour, pesticides, processed foods, preservatives, and mass production of food became standardized.

Dr. Weston Price's Findings

In the early 1930s, dismayed by his patients' crowded, crooked teeth and frequent cavities, Weston Price left his dental practice in Cleveland, Ohio, to search for the keys to strong health. For ten years, he traveled to isolated communities where people ate food that was entirely indigenous—never imported—and studied their diets. On every continent, Dr. Price found dietary practices that created excellent health through old age. These diets all included substantial amounts of animal fat (butter, lard, tallow, fish oil, poultry fat) and/or cultured dairy products (such as yogurt and kefir made from unpasteurized whole milk). Price found that diets that avoided extremes of vegetarianism and carnivorism, and that were rich in vitamins A and D, resulted in excellent overall health, freedom from tooth decay, consistent fertility, and healthy offspring, generation after generation.

Dr. Price also found that if one or both parents raised on traditional diets ate processed foods before conceiving or during pregnancy, or if children ate poorly during their formative years (including food grown in depleted soil), then their children were typically born with health problems, including serious dental degeneration and pelvises too narrow for easy childbirth.

In *Nutrition and Physical Degeneration,* first published in 1939, Dr. Price wrote that in many of the groups he studied, "girls were not allowed to be married until after they had had a period of special feeding. In some tribes, a six-month period of special nutrition was required." This special nutrition was used to ensure the health of a couple's offspring with foods very high in vitamins A and D: liver, organ meats, butter from grass-fed cows, fish liver oils, shellfish, and fish eggs. The people Dr. Price studied told him they were conscious that "injuries (to children's health) would occur if the parents were not in excellent physical condition and nourishment."

None of the traditional peoples Price studied included processed or refined food or hydrogenated fats in their diets; and none of their food was grown with pesticides. (To clarify, canning or freezing green beans creates a processed food; milling wheat so that the outer hull and its nutrients are removed creates refined white flour.) In the United States, even by the 1930s, cake mixes made with refined flours and hydrogenated fats such as Crisco were common to the American diet; crops were frequently sprayed with the pesticide DDT.

Before packaged food and takeout became normal, elders taught adolescents how to grow food and prepare it for themselves and small children. Contemporary culture and processed foods have unfortunately discouraged us from transmitting this necessary information from one generation to the next. Still, like knowing how to chart and interpret your fertility signals, knowing what to eat and how to cook is a basic life skill.

Basic Nutrients for Reproductive Health

Information about the ingredients necessary for good health is often obscured by marketing of different food products. Based on Dr. Price's findings, foods that include the following nutrients are essential for fertility and reproductive health:

- Vitamin A
- Vitamin D

- Vitamin E
- Iodine
- Zinc

Vitamins and minerals work with other nutrients to direct chemical reactions in the body, including the production of hormones.[1] Because the body cannot manufacture most vitamins and minerals, they must be provided through food. Dr. Price found that fat-soluble vitamins (especially vitamins A and D) are catalysts on which all other biological processes depend.[2] "Fat-soluble" means that these vitamins can only be absorbed in fat.

Please note that the nutrients I describe are relevant to almost all bodily processes; my focus here is on their effects on reproductive health.

Vitamin A

Known commonly for its crucial role in eye development and health, vitamin A is also necessary for new cell growth and normal reproductive capabilities.[3] Without vitamin A, the body can't use protein.[4] According to Dr. Price, neither minerals nor water-soluble vitamins can be utilized by the body without vitamin A. "Water-soluble" means the vitamin's nutrients can be absorbed in water.

The first vitamin "discovered" was vitamin A—animals who lacked it were infertile. Vitamins A and D are necessary for the production of estrogen, progesterone, testosterone, and the adrenal hormones. Supplies of vitamin A are so vital to humans that we store large quantities of it in the liver. Stores of vitamin A can quickly be depleted by physical growth in infants and children as well as by pregnancy, lactation, and infection. All of these situations also require substantial quantities of vitamin A. An interval of three years between pregnancies allows mothers to rebuild vitamin A stores so that subsequent children will not suffer diminished vitality.[5]

Vitamin A is available only from animal sources. Provitamin A, also called carotene, is found in all yellow, red, orange, or dark green fruits and vegetables; and most adults can convert a small portion of these plant carotenes to vitamin A. However, many conditions interfere with this conversion: stress, cold weather, zinc or protein deficiency, low fat intake, diarrhea, being an infant or a child, diabetes, anorexia, poor thyroid function, and poor liver function.[6, 7, 8]

Vitamin A, iodine, and zinc are all necessary for thyroid health.[9] Vitamin A deficiency is associated with heavy menstruation,[10] PMS,[11] fibroids, and endometriosis. In *Fertility, Cycles and Nutrition,* nutritionist Marilyn Shannon explains that irregular patterns of cervical fluid can result from vitamin A deficiency.[12] While the recommended daily allowance (RDA) for vitamin A is 4,000 to 5,000 IU, in her classic *Nutrition Almanac,* Lavonne Dunne recommends that the vitamin A dose for preconception, pregnancy, and breast-feeding should be at least 20,000 IU per day from cod liver oil and other natural sources.

It's important to distinguish between vitamin A found naturally in foods and synthetic vitamin A, which is used in supplements and added to processed foods. The latter can be toxic and should be avoided—including when it's part of a multivitamin. Likewise, carotene supplements can have adverse effects and should be avoided.

Sally Fallon, founder of the Weston A. Price Foundation and author of *Nourishing Traditions,* explains: "While doctors may warn you that vitamin A is toxic, this

APPROXIMATE LEVELS OF VITAMIN A IN COMMON FOODS

Per 100 grams (100 grams equals about 3.5 ounces; 1 tablespoon equals about 15 grams)

High-vitamin cod liver oil: 230,000 IU
Regular cod liver oil: 100,000 IU
Beef liver: 35,000 IU
Chicken liver: 21,000 IU
Ghee (clarified butter): 3,800 IU
Butter: 3,100 IU
Egg yolk: 1,900 IU
Whipping cream: 1,500 IU

Depending on the season and the quality of the animals' feed, these amounts can vary. Research from the 1940s indicates that vitamin A is more easily absorbed from butter than from other foods—because vitamin A is fat soluble and butter is a fat. The U.S. Recommended Daily Allowance of vitamin A is currently only 5,000 IU. People from cultures Weston Price studied consumed at least 50,000 IU of vitamin A per day.[13] Accordingly, optimal reproductive health may require consuming levels of vitamin A well above the Recommended Daily Allowance.

is only true if the vitamin A is synthetic or taken in amounts exceeding 100,000 daily IU for months at a time. The foods that traditional societies gave to women and men preparing for childbearing and to pregnant women were packed with vitamin A: organ meats such as liver, cod liver oil, shellfish, egg yolks, and butterfat from grass-fed animals. These foods are absolutely essential for healthy reproduction and healthy offspring. In fact, Dr. Price discovered that the diets of healthy isolated peoples contained at least four times the minerals and at least *ten* times more vitamin A from animal sources than found in the American diet of his day."

Leah Morton, MD in family practice. If a woman comes to my office with a strong problem, I first ask about what she eats. If she's got a low-fat diet with lots of white-flour products and sugar, I'll suggest that she introduce fats from organically fed, free-range animals; make her own salad dressing with cold-pressed olive oil; and eliminate the sugar and white flour. People are often terrified that this will give them bad cholesterol. But our bodies need cholesterol to make hormones, and animal fats will provide it. Sugar and white flour will derange the cholesterol unfavorably. In fact, I've seen some people's unhealthy cholesterol levels improve dramatically when they apply Weston Price's discoveries to their diet.

Vitamin D

Recognized as essential for normal growth, including bone and tooth formation, vitamin D also supports the production of estrogen in men and women.[14] Another fat-soluble vitamin, it's necessary for the metabolism of minerals, and it's best utilized when combined with vitamin A.[15]

Butter, eggs, cod liver oil, liver, organ meats, marine oils, and seafood (especially shrimp and crab) are rich in vitamin D.

Vitamin D is also manufactured by your body with exposure to sunlight. However, to achieve optimal levels of vitamin D from sunlight, most of us aren't able to get enough exposure. To achieve optimal levels, 85 percent of your skin needs to be exposed to sunlight from 10 A.M. to 2 P.M. for 10 to 120 minutes. Lighter-skinned people require less exposure; darker-skinned people require longer exposure. Latitudes can also affect whether you can receive sufficient vitamin D from sunlight. For example, in parts of the United States that are between 30 and 45 degrees latitude, exposure to sunlight is insufficient to produce vitamin D for six months of the year.[16, 17, 18, 19, 20]

In *Fertility, Cycles and Nutrition,* Marilyn Shannon reports that menstrual cramps may result from vitamin D deficiency. PCOS (polycystic ovarian syndrome) has been corrected with vitamin D and calcium supplements.[21] Migraine headaches during menstruation have been linked with low levels of vitamin D and calcium.[22] PMS has been completely reversed by supplementing the diet with calcium, magnesium, and vitamin D.[23] And infertility is associated with low levels of vitamin D.[24] Vitamin D (and magnesium) are needed for calcium absorption; supplements (1,000 IU daily of vitamin D and 1 gram of magnesium) have relieved nervousness, irritability, insomnia, headaches, and depression in menopausal women who were calcium deficient.[25]

Excess levels of vitamin D (resulting from vitamin D therapy or lots of sunlight exposure) can be toxic. If you're concerned about this, nutritionist and vitamin D expert Krispin Sullivan advises requesting your physician to test your vitamin D levels.[26]

APPROXIMATE LEVELS OF VITAMIN D IN COMMON FOODS

Per 100 grams

Cod liver oil: 10,000 IU
Lard: 2,800 IU
Pickled Atlantic herring: 680 IU
Steamed eastern oysters: 642 IU
Water-packed sardines: 480 IU
One fresh egg yolk: 148 IU
Butter: 56 IU
Chicken livers: 12 IU

The Recommended Daily Allowance of vitamin D is 200 to 400 IU. Dr. Reinhold Vieth, a Canadian researcher, argues that the minimal daily requirement of vitamin D (from food sources and sunlight) should be 4,000 IU.[27] Dr. Vieth's findings match those of Weston Price.

Vitamin E

Vitamin E helps red blood cells carry oxygen to organs—including reproductive organs. When rats were given a diet lacking in vitamin E, the females miscarried their offspring, and the males eventually became sterile.[28] Conversely, in animal studies, vitamin E has had a dramatic effect on preventing miscarriages, increasing male and female fertility, and helping restore male potency.[29] In *Let's Have Healthy Children,* Adelle Davis explains that "vitamin E, essential to cell division . . . prevents the inactivation of vitamin A, which is necessary to maintain a healthy uterine lining to receive the newly fertilized egg." In other words, vitamin E works in concert with vitamin A to ensure reproduction.

Vitamin E is also fat soluble. It's found in butter, organ meats, unrefined vegetable oils, grains, nuts, seeds, legumes, and dark leafy vegetables. Consumption of commercial vegetable oils, which are invariably rancid, uses up vitamin E at a rapid rate, leading to depletion.

In human studies, vitamin E supplements significantly reduced breast tenderness and other PMS symptoms.[30] Vitamin E has been shown to regulate excessive

---

APPROXIMATE LEVELS OF VITAMIN E IN COMMON FOODS

1 tablespoon wheat germ oil: 34.6 IU

Almonds: 5 IU per ¼ cup

Hazlenuts: 7 IU per ¼ cup

Asparagus: 1.3 IU per ½ cup

Cucumber: 4.2 IU per ½ cup

Kale: 4 IU per ½ cup

Mangoes: 3 IU per mango

Liver: 1.6 IU per 4 oz.

Vitamin E can be toxic to people with high blood pressure and those with chronic rheumatic heart disease. Otherwise, it's considered nontoxic. If you decide to take supplements, begin with small doses and increase the amount gradually. Vitamin E supplements are frequently made from soy or wheat. If you prefer to avoid these products, look for labels that say "No soy; no wheat." For best absorption, most nutritionists recommend taking vitamin E along with fat (such as butter).

---

or scanty menstrual flows.[31] It can correct menstrual rhythm, ameliorate fibrocystic breasts,[32] help prevent miscarriage,[33] and diminish or remove hot flashes.[34] During pregnancy, vitamin E increases the elasticity and expandability of vaginal tissues; and it can help decrease sensitivity to pain during labor.[35] Vitamin E deficiencies have been linked to increased congenital heart defects.[36] During menopause, supplements of vitamin E (1,200 IU daily) have relieved nights sweats, hot flashes, backaches, fatigue, nervousness, insomnia, dizziness, shortness of breath, and heart palpitations.[37]

The RDA of vitamin E for adult women is 12 IU; for adult males, it's 15 IU. However, many nutritionists recommend considerably higher daily allowances for optimal health—from 400 to 800 IU daily. Realistically, such high amounts can only be consumed with supplements.

Iodine

Within the body, the actions of minerals are interrelated: no mineral can function without affecting others. Iodine plays an important role in regulating the body's production of energy and also promotes growth and development.

Along with vitamin A and zinc, iodine is critical to thyroid health; and thyroid health is critical to reproductive health. Excessive bleeding during menstruation may be caused by hypothyroidism due to iodine deficiency, as well as vitamin E and protein deficiency.[38] Lack of desire or strength for sex may result from a thyroid gland that's deficient in iodine, vitamin E, and B vitamins.[39] Iodine deficiency may result in cretinism, a form of retardation (including sexual retardation) in children whose mothers had limited iodine intake during adolescence and pregnancy. In animal studies, iodine and zinc have been linked to the prevention of miscarriage.[40]

Sources of iodine include most seafoods, unrefined sea salt, sea weed, pineapple, artichokes, asparagus, and dark green leafy vegetables. Surprisingly, butter is an excellent source of iodine. Some vegetables, such as cabbage and spinach, can prevent iodine absorption when they're eaten raw or unfermented.[41]

If your ancestors came from a coastal area, you may require more iodine than someone whose ancestors came from inland regions. To be utilized by the body, iodine requires vitamin A from animal fats. On the other hand, excesses of iodine can be toxic and can cause thyroid problems similar to iodine deficiency.[42] This can occur with overconsumption of seaweed or even iodized salt.

The Recommended Daily Allowance of iodine is 150 mcg.

Zinc

Zinc is required for normal growth, healing, production of estrogen and progesterone,[43] and sperm production.[44] Zinc increases the body's absorption of vitamin A.[45] The prostate gland includes high concentrations of zinc,[46] as does semen.[47] Vitamin A, vitamin E, and zinc may together relieve vaginal dryness.[48] Impotence (in men) and infertility or sterility (in men and women) can result from zinc deficiency.[49]

The best sources of zinc are oysters and red meat; it's also found in other fish, nuts, seeds, ginger, and colostrum, the first milk that a woman secretes after giving birth.

Oral contraceptives diminish zinc levels, and zinc deficiency during pregnancy can cause birth defects. It's therefore important for women to wait at least six months after discontinuing the Pill before trying to conceive—as pharmaceutical companies commonly advise. Phytic acid in grains and legumes can block absorption of zinc;[50, 51] proper soaking or fermenting of grains and legumes[52] can neutralize phytic acid. Physical and emotional stress as well as alcohol consumption can deplete zinc. Sugar depletes zinc levels, and zinc is necessary for metabolizing sugar.[53] White spots on the nails, small sex glands in boys, and loss of appetite and/or sensitivity to taste can all indicate zinc deficiency. Nutritionist Robert Crahyon, author of *Nutrition Made Simple*, reports that 90 percent of his clients do not have enough of this crucial mineral. Zinc supplements should be balanced with copper in a 15-to-1 ratio.

APPROXIMATE LEVELS OF ZINC IN COMMON FOODS

Oysters: 5.2 mg each

Clams: 3 mg per cup

Beef: 9.7 mg per 4 oz.

Chicken: 3.2 mg per 4 oz. dark meat

Cashews and sunflower seeds: 3 mg per ½ cup

Cooked lentils: 1.5 mg per cup

Sprouted mung beans: 1.89 mg per cup

Dairy products also include small amounts of zinc. The Recommended Daily Allowance of zinc is 12 mg per day for adult females, 15 mg per day for adult males, and 19 mg per day for nursing women.

Foods That Can Inhibit Reproductive Health

Commercial Oils

Around 1940, Weston Price and his colleagues predicted that as we increasingly substituted vegetable oils for animal fats, Westerners would develop more diseases, and reproduction would become increasingly difficult. Until after World War II, animal fats (such as butter, lard, and beef tallow) were commonly used for cooking; in many cultures, vegetable oils (such as olive, rapeseed, and sesame) were pressed in small batches as needed by street vendors with small stone presses. Frequent pressings ensured freshness.

Today's commercial vegetable oils (such as soy, canola, corn, safflower, and cottonseed) are processed by a combination of high-temperature mechanical pressing and solvent extraction, followed by refining, bleaching, and degumming. As the newly formed oil is exposed to light, heat, and oxygen, it turns rancid. Producers mask the "off" tastes and odors with a deodorizing process, but the oil is still rancid. When humans consume such vegetable oils, chain reactions are set off that destroy cells, damage DNA, promote disease, and accelerate aging.[54, 55, 56]

Canola oil has been shown to cause vitamin E deficiency in piglets.[57]

Trans-Fats

Trans-fats are found in hydrogenated vegetable oils such as margarine and vegetable shortening. Hydrogenation turns vegetable oils (normally liquid at room temperature) into solids by mixing them with small amounts of metal particles, then subjecting them to hydrogen in a high-pressure, high-temperature reactor. The oil's molecular structure is now rearranged. Emulsifiers, starches, and dyes give the final product (such as margarine) an attractive appearance.

Vegetable shortenings and margarines are commonly used in commercial baked goods, French fries, chips, cookies, crackers, commercial peanut butter, mayonnaise, and fast foods.

In *Know Your Fats,* nutritionist Mary G. Enig, PhD, explains that while trans-fats are good at keeping cookies from crumbling and peanut butter from separating, they can jeopardize human health. Nutritionist Kaayla T. Daniel, PhD, author of

The Whole Soy Story, explains that trans-fats "stiffen cell membranes, inhibit enzyme activity, block transport of nutrients and elimination of wastes. While they can fit into cell membranes, trans-fats operate like a key that slips into a lock but won't turn." Trans-fats have been linked to obesity, heart problems, cancer, infertility, lowered sperm counts, and low birth weight babies.[58, 59]

In a study of the effects of trans-fats in rats, ovulation became irregular, testosterone levels in males decreased, and abnormal sperm counts increased by 98 percent in the third generation.[60]

In 1994, the Danish Nutrition Council expressed concern that trans-fats could have a harmful effect on the growth of the fetus and that breast-fed babies are exposed to trans-fatty acids through breast milk when the mother consumes partially hydrogenated vegetable fats.[61] This exposure interferes with development of the nervous system and the growing infant's eyes.

Trans-fats lower the amount of fat in milk from lactating females in all species studied, including humans, thus lowering the overall quality of milk available to the infant.[62]

While the National Academy of Science's Institute of Medicine has declared that no level of trans-fat consumption is safe,[63] at this writing, the FDA unfortunately does not require producers to disclose trans-fat contents on food labels.

Sugar

Historically, people have considered sweets—such as a piece of fruit—an unusual treat. In 1821, Americans consumed, on average, ten pounds of sugar each year. Now, each person eats about 170 pounds per year—about half a pound of sugar every day.[64] Sugar is added to commercial breakfast cereals, coffee, bread, pastries, crackers, fruit-flavored yogurt, salad dressing, ketchup, canned vegetables, even "unsweetened" fruit juices.

Unfortunately, sugar not only lacks nutrients, it can also lead to blood sugar imbalances. Sugar consumption depletes your body of the vitamins, minerals, and enzymes you get from whole foods. While it might please your taste buds, sugar is a shock to the rest of your body, starting with your bloodstream. Nutritionist Krispin Sullivan likens the bloodstream to a flowing, twenty-four-hour smorgasbord. "Every cell and every organ in your body is fed by the nutrients available in your bloodstream," she says. "You want a diet that will provide nutrients throughout the day (and night) *steadily*, rather than in quick bursts." But sugar is absorbed suddenly by your bloodstream, causing a rise in blood sugar and a short-lived burst of energy. This rush is often followed by a period of letdown and exhaustion, which in turn may lead to craving for (and consumption of) more sugar, perpetuating an unhealthy cycle.

Eating a candy bar or muffin can raise levels of cortisol (the stress hormone) and deplete the adrenals—which in turn may affect other hormone levels.

Leah Morton, MD, explains one way that eating sugar can affect reproductive health: "If a woman eats excess sugar (and what constitutes excess sugar varies depending on the woman), she'll secrete excess insulin. Her ovaries will stop making estrogen and secrete testosterone instead. Ovulation and progesterone production will be greatly diminished or absent.[65] Repetition of this process can result in polycystic ovarian syndrome."

White Flour

In the modern process of milling and refining wheat, 50 percent or more of its crucial nutrients (B vitamins, vitamin E, calcium, zinc, copper, manganese, potassium) and fiber is lost. The lifeless white flour that remains will not go rancid; it therefore works well as a primary ingredient in products with extended shelf lives, such as pasta, bagels, and pretzels.

Nutritionist Lori Lipinski explains that "white flour breaks down in the body into glucose, which can lead to the very same problems caused by eating too much refined sugar."[66]

Soy

Soy products are now widely promoted from birth through old age as staples for a healthy diet. However, soy—including organic soy—has high levels of phytoestrogens. *Phytoestrogens* are estrogens found in plants (*phyto* means "plant-based"). Despite the current popularity of soy, numerous studies point to the harm of phytoestrogens in tofu, soy milk, soy margarine, edamame, soy-based protein powders, and soy-based protein bars. Soy products can disrupt endocrine functioning and digestion and have other harmful effects:

- Soy phytoestrogens are potent antithyroid agents, which can cause hypothyroidism.[67]
- Infants who are fed soy formula receive the equivalent of three to five birth control pills each day. A study of infants fed soy formula found that they had concentrations of estrogen compounds at levels 13,000 to 22,000 times higher than infants fed milk-based formula or breast milk.[68] Further, at this writing, every soy infant formula on the market is made from genetically modified soy.
- Large amounts of phytoestrogens in soy formula have been implicated in the current trend toward increasingly premature sexual development in girls (including breast development and pubic hair before the age of eight, sometimes before the age of three) and delayed or retarded sexual development in boys.[69] If you cannot breast-feed your baby, Sally Fallon's *Nourishing Traditions* offers recipes for homemade milk and meat-based formulas.
- In a recent study conducted at Johns Hopkins University, when female rats consumed low and high doses of genistein—the major type of phytoestrogen—during pregnancy, their male offspring were less likely to ejaculate after mounting female rats. Males exposed to the low dose were less likely to mount and begin intercourse than males whose mothers received the free- or high-genistein diets. While sperm counts were not affected by low or high doses, "the low dose led to alterations in male development of a greater degree than the high dose." Pregnant and nursing mothers are thereby advised to avoid all soy products.[70]

It's worth noting that the traditional Asian diet has primarily included soy as a condiment (no more than ¼ cup per day in Japan, much less in China), not as a replacement for animal protein.[71] If you do consume soy, miso and tempeh are safer choices because they're fermented. The fermentation process renders them more digestible, though it does not reduce their phytoestrogen levels.

More information and studies that show the adverse effects of soy can be found on www.westonaprice.org's Soy Alert, www.wholesoystory.com, and on www.soyonlineservice.co.nz.

Gretchen, twenty-two. I was raised on a vegetarian diet. Growing up, I ate tofu almost every day. I started menstruating at ten, and I usually had a period three or four times a year. About three years ago, I started eating meat once a week, and butter and eggs al-

most every day. But my menstrual cycles didn't become more normal in length until about six months after I stopped eating soy. Now I'm menstruating about every thirty-five to forty days; and I'm ovulating, too. I can't be sure, but I think that eating meat—and not eating soy—is making a difference for me.

Rhonda, thirty-four. *My temperatures are in the low 97s; at ovulation, they shift really slowly, in stairstep fashion; and I've never seen egg white. I've also got cold hands and feet. Given these symptoms, my doctor gave me a blood test that actually showed I lean toward* hyperthyroidism.

When I told her I'd been putting soy milk on my cereal every morning for about a year, she suggested I eliminate it. In the first cycle after I stopped the soy, my temperatures went up an average of about two-tenths of a degree. At ovulation, I had a crisp spike. And I reached 98.0 once in my luteal phase, which I've never done before. I didn't feel any differently, and I still didn't observe any egg white.

We've been trying to get pregnant for a year. Not conceiving has been really frustrating. But now I'm actually having fun experimenting with my diet and seeing what I can do to strengthen my cycles.

Too Much Protein

Traditionally, diets comprised about 15 percent protein, with the remainder coming from fats and carbohydrates. Energy bars, protein powders, milk powders added to low-fat milk, and lean meats can offset the balance of protein to fat and deplete the body of vitamin A.[72]

Organic cheese, cured sausage, and nuts that have been soaked and toasted make healthier snacks than energy bars.

Caffeine

While studies indicate that coffee drinking can inhibit reproductive health, other products that contain caffeine (dark chocolate, instant coffee, pain relievers such as Anacin and Excedrin, and tea and cola) are also not recommended.

Drinking just one cup of coffee daily can decrease your chance of conceiving by half.[73] Because caffeine delays conception, women who drink caffeinated beverages are three times as likely to have difficulty conceiving within one year as those who don't drink them.[74, 75] According to 1993 studies from McGill University, a woman who drinks two to three cups of coffee per day before conception can double the risk of miscarrying.

Problems with sperm count, sperm motility, and other sperm abnormalities also seem to increase by coffee drinking. The more a man drinks, the more his sperm health may be affected.[76]

What to drink? Clean water can't be overestimated. If you must have something flavorful, try squeezing a wedge of lemon or lime into your water.

And if you do decide to cut back on or eliminate caffeine, do so gradually so that your side effects will be minimized.

Foods Grown with Pesticides

Good food also requires sound soil. Plants grown on soil that lacks minerals (because of pesticides, synthetic fertilizers, and/or industrial farming practices) in turn offer minerally depleted vegetables. Most of the vegetables, fruits, and livestock raised today are done so with pesticides. Livestock grown in feedlots with grains (such as corn and soy) that have been sprayed with pesticides simply will not result in the nutrient-dense meat of livestock raised on organic pastures. Animals store fat-soluble chemicals in their fat. When you eat hamburger, chicken, or pork chops (as well as butter, cheese, ice cream, and eggs), you consume the same pesticides that the animal did. In fact, animal products can contain up to fourteen times more pesticides than plants.[77] Pesticides are also sprayed on seed oil plants that end up in vegetable oils.

Exposure to pesticides can be hazardous to hormonal, nervous, and respiratory systems; increase risk of cancer; and more.

Food labeled "organic" means that it came from seeds that were not genetically engineered and that it was farmed with natural pesticides (such as insects or crop rotation). An organic food label cannot be used on food treated with synthetic herbicides or fertilizers or sewage sludge fertilizer; it can't have been irradiated. Meat labeled "organic" means that the livestock were raised with organic feed and that the animals were not treated with antibiotics or hormones.

Some foods retain pesticides more than others. According to FDA and EPA data, the twelve vegetables and fruits most contaminated by pesticides (listed here in the order of the most contaminated) are: strawberries, bell peppers, spinach, cherries, peaches, cantaloupe, celery, apples, apricots, green beans, grapes, and cucumbers. According to the Environmental Working Group, baby foods, milk, and grains not marked "organic" are likely to contain high levels of pesticides.[78]

Fish

Cod liver oil and fish can provide essential nutrients for reproductive health, including vitamins A and D. But as demand for seafood has increased, so, too, have problems for human health and the environment. Unfortunately, the sparkling displays of fish in the marketplace can create a false impression. For example, mercury levels in tuna and mahi mahi have caused the FDA to advise pregnant women and children not to eat more than one small portion of these fish once a month.

Then, according to Mercedes Lee of the Blue Ocean Institute and editor of the National Audubon Society's *Seafood Lover's Almanac*, "Overfishing of Atlantic cod, Chilean seabass, snapper, sharks (and so many more) threatens world food security and ocean ecosystems." And while most types of shrimp are abundant, the way they're caught (some by nets that drag along the ocean's floor and catch large amounts of other marine life—most of which is then discarded and die) threatens habitat, sea turtles, and other creatures.

Fish farms also pose a threat: many fish farms are constructed at the shore, destroying wetlands, releasing waste, and spreading disease. When farm-raised salmon escape their nets (not infrequently), they can breed with wild salmon, which subsequently weakens the entire fish chain. This is a serious environmental hazard.

Additionally, farm-raised salmon are poor sources of vitamins A and D and omega-e fatty acids, since farming prevents the fish from feeding on algae—and algae allows them to store vitamin D in their fat.

At this writing, wild-caught salmon, sardines, striped bass, Alaskan halibut, and stone crab are choices recommended by the Blue Ocean Institute—though Mercedes Lee cautions that these choices would be for personal health, not ecosystem health.

Tom Cowan, MD, in family practice. I've seen countless people improve their health by applying the dietary principles Weston Price outlined. The diet is a whole program, a package deal. It means cutting out sugar, chips, and white-flour products. It means eating whole foods—including organic meat and animal fats, free-range eggs, fresh vegetables, and soaked grains; and supplementing with cod liver oil. In terms of reproductive health, I've seen women on the diet improve or reverse everything from PMS to anovulation, PCOS, hypothy-roidism, endometriosis, menopause problems, and inability to conceive or carry a pregnancy to term. Some people see results in a month; for others it can take a year. While not everyone's situation reverses, almost everyone who sticks to the diet shows improvement.

__Melanie, twenty-three.__ The first two cycles I charted, I didn't ovulate. I felt so frus-trated and hopeless. I'd learned the basics of how my body works only to find out that my body wasn't working well enough for me to use my charts confidently for birth control. As an experiment, I decided to cut white flour out of my diet. Within a couple of weeks, I could actually feel a buzz if I ate a piece of bread, so I kept with my experiment.

That first cycle I went without white flour, I ovulated! The next cycle, I didn't. But I'm still interested in this experiment. I love that it's totally free. I'm actually thinking of going completely without white flour or sugar for two or three months, then introducing them one at a time to see how my cycles are affected.

__Elena, twenty-three.__ I'm in school full time. I eat most of my meals in the school cafe-teria, and I drink coffee to keep myself going. I haven't had a period in six months. Since I learned Fertility Awareness and started facing the fact that I'm not ovulating, I've gotten concerned. I understand that my diet could have something to do with my not ovulat-ing. But it's just not realistic for me to start buying and cooking my own food. Until I finish school, I'll be eating in the cafeteria.

I've decided to cut back on sugar, tofu, and coffee, and to drink more water. I'll give this experiment two months. If I still don't ovulate, then I'll make time to see a doctor.

I'm also going to look into what happened to a committee we had last year that tried to get organically grown fruit available in the cafeteria.

Postscript: Within a month of changing her diet as she outlined above, Elena started ovulating. After eight months, she'd had six ovulatory cycles.

A Word About Veganism

While I have known women with vegan diets to have healthy charts, they more typ-ically indicate anovulation and thyroid problems. Key nutrients such as vitamins A and D are not available in a vegan diet. Sally Fallon explains that people can be healthy with lacto-ovo vegetarianism (which includes milk, milk products, and eggs) if the milk and eggs come from pasture-fed animals, if the milk and milk products are unpasteurized, and if grains and legumes are properly soaked and/or fermented. She also urges that vegetarians planning to have children add cod liver oil to their diets.

According to Krispin Sullivan, Certified Nutritionist, clinical researcher, and author of *Naked at Noon: Understanding Sunlight and Vitamin D,* "No matter what you eat, food is about communion: sharing nourishment with friends. The miracle of transmuting one form of life into another. When you're eating, don't watch the news, discuss grades or politics, or talk on the phone. If you're in fight or flight— if you're stressed out—digestive juices aren't activated. Just be with your meal. Gratitude improves digestion."

First Steps

There are enormous problems with the way our society grows and consumes food. Fortunately, even a little bit of change can make a difference. No diet is right for everyone. To create the meals that will give you increased health, familiarize your-self with this chapter's information, read more as you deem fit, and start cooking!

Meat, dairy products, poultry, fruits, and vegetables are available organically, and you can petition your grocers to sell local, organic products. Shop at your farmer's market, and encourage growers to farm organically. Consider joining a CSA (Community Supported Agriculture), a partnership between a farm and local consumers. Supporters generally cover part of a farm's yearly operating budget by purchasing a share of the season's harvest. In return, CSA members receive fresh produce throughout the growing season. An excellent search engine for locating sustainably grown organic food in your area is www.localharvest.org. Or, E-mail info@csacenter.org.

Lists of farmers who ship their produce are available on www.eatwild.org and through local chapters of the Weston Price Foundation (www. westonaprice.org). If they are not available in your area, organic vegetables, grains, and legumes can be purchased through www.diamondorganics.com (800-674-2642) and www.goldmine. com (800-475-3663).

Prominent "natural foods" stores may advertise a commitment to organic produce, while in fact they sell primarily commercially grown fruits, vegetables, and meat. Labels need to be read closely. Farmers who sell at local markets may also spray their produce with pesticides.

While eating organic food is more expensive, in the long run, it gives optimal health. Preparing your own food, rather than purchasing ready-made meals, is also more economical. Butchers and farmers often sell chicken backs and lamb bones (for example) quite cheaply; and these can be used to make healthful broths and stews.

To experiment with your diet and observe how your cycles are affected, you might eliminate something (like chips, caffeine, products with sugar or white flour), while adding butter, eggs, and organic greens. In your chart's miscellaneous section, you can check the days you eat sugar, and observe whether your mood, energy level, or the health of your cycle is affected.

I'll also put in a plug for the "80-20 Rule": 80 percent of the time, you eat well; 20 percent of the time, you do your best with what's available. Find out if any of the restaurants in your neighborhood have a commitment to organic or local food. And tell the owners of your favorite places that you'd love to see at least some choices on the menu available organically.

Let me say again that the information in this chapter is not meant to be comprehensive. It does not include information about many crucial aspects of modern food production, including:

- A hormone commonly given to cows to increase milk production, rBGH, which is then consumed by people who drink the cows' milk.
- The effects of pasteurization and homogenization on milk and milk products.
- Antibiotics that are commonly given to livestock. When these animals are consumed by people, the chance that human infectious diseases will develop resistance to available antibiotics increases.
- About 70 percent of our food supply is now genetically engineered (GE). GE foods are grown by injecting the gene of another plant or species to strengthen the first plant's ability to sustain frost or herbicides. For example, tomatoes might be injected with a frog gene to prevent them from withering at an early frost. The U.S. government does not require companies to label their food genetically modified; and proper studies about the effects of genetically modified organisms (GMOs) on people and the environment have not been conducted.

As the world's population has increased, we've become increasingly dependent on mass-produced food, which is denatured and grown with harmful pesticides and other chemicals. Farming practices that mass-produce livestock for consumption can be inhumane, unhealthy, and depleting of our planet's limited resources. The nutrient-dense foods necessary for reproductive health are increasingly at risk of extinction. While some individuals and families may be able to locate and afford organic food grown on small farms, the food available and affordable for most people is not conducive to reproductive health. What's our hope? We can continue to educate ourselves, make sustainable choices, take time to discover the diet that's right for us, and see whether our health—and that of the earth—is affected.

The first instinct should be to (see) if an operation can
be avoided, not to seek reasons for performing it.

—BRITISH MEDICAL JOURNAL, 1895

12. Natural Remedies for Reproductive Health Problems

ONCE WOMEN START OBSERVING PROB-
lems in their charts, they want to know their options; and many want to address
their concerns without pharmaceutical drugs. This chapter summarizes my findings about common gynecological problems over seven years of teaching Fertility
Awareness. You can find more thorough descriptions in chapters 8 through 11.

My aim is to present remedies that you can experiment with on your own, without harm. Educate yourself as well as you can before trying any of them. While
double-blind studies have not been conducted on many of these aids, clinical experience has found them to be helpful. To choose which of these options are

worth trying, refer to the resources listed throughout this book, search the Internet, talk with friends and health-care providers. Do what you're drawn to, what feels right for you.

Each of the following remedies can be tried at home to help strengthen reproductive health and address the specific health problems presented in this chapter:

- Lunaception, or sleeping in total darkness throughout your cycle (see chapter 10).
- Cut back on products containing commercial oils, trans-fats (commonly used in chips, cookies, crackers, commercial peanut butter, mayonnaise, and other fast foods), sugar, white flour, caffeine, pesticides, and unfermented soy (see chapter 11).
- Increase healthy fats and healthy cholesterol (the mother of lipid-based hormones, including nearly all the sex hormones) by eating organic butter, eggs from free-range chickens, organic lard, broth made from organic lamb, beef, chicken, or fish. If your budget requires that you choose between organic meat and dairy products and organic produce, go for organic meat and dairy (see chapter 11).
- Supplement your diet with cod liver oil, which has high levels of vitamins A and D (see chapter 11). High-quality cod liver oil is available from Radiant Life, 888-593-8333; Web site: www.RadiantLifeCatalog.com.
- Exercise encourages circulation of blood to the reproductive organs. Walk around your block or do fifteen minutes of yoga before you go to work. Bike to work. Take a dance class—belly dancing, known for being about fertility, encourages movement in the uterus.
- To address your *thinking* about your problem with your menstrual cycle, I highly recommend The Work of Byron Katie, described on page 154.

Different Kinds of Medicine

Like Fertility Awareness, I consider health care an educational process, an ongoing conversation with myself and others. Because every person is different, I'm suspicious of blanket remedies for specific problems. Each woman has a unique body that needs a unique diet and remedies.

In any case, your health care begins with your concerns and questions. The more you're involved in deciding how to address your concerns about your health, the more likely you'll be to get the care that feels right for you. If your charts indicate a situation that you'd like addressed by a health-care provider, consider what you might do with a diagnosis and the kind of treatment options you prefer. Bring your questions and your charts to your practitioner's office. Then take notes! When you seek health care, it's your responsibility to educate yourself so that you can make informed decisions.

Different kinds of medicine offer different ways of diagnosing and treating a problem. A medical doctor and an herbalist typically operate in very different paradigms. It's for you to choose which you prefer. And your rapport with the practitioner matters. I like feeling heard and kindly treated, and that there's enough time to consider my situation in all its complexity. I'm drawn to practitioners who love their work, whose relationship to the medicine they teach is passionate and personal, and whose care for themselves inspires me.

MEDICINAL SYSTEMS

The following list of health-care systems (presented in alphabetical order) is not meant to be comprehensive—it's an introduction. Just by bringing your charts to a practitioner's office, you're inviting integrative medicine that involves you.

Acupuncture
Also called doctors of Oriental medicine (DOMs), acupuncturists discern patterns in your health by an intake of your history and symptoms and by examining your pulse and tongue for the strengths and weaknesses in your *qi* (life force). DOMs look for the strength of a particular organ (i.e., the spleen) in relation to your overall system.

Doctors of Oriental medicine offer acupuncture, herbs, and/or nutritional counseling to address: PMS; anovulation; thyroid imbalances; progesterone deficiency; infertility; fibrocystic breasts; menopause problems (including low libido, night sweats, and hot flashes); restoring balance to a woman coming off hormonal drugs; increasing cervical fluid; strengthening overall health to prepare for and help sustain pregnancy;

continued

restoring balance after miscarriage, abortion, or childbirth; impotence and premature ejaculation; improving sperm count and motility.

Most states currently license or register acupuncturists. To find one, look in your Yellow Pages; or go to www.nccaom.org (National Certification Commission for Acupuncture and Oriental Medicine).

Herbalism

Herbalists can help the whole family for general and reproductive health issues. Herbalists who know plants well; who grow, harvest, and prepare their own remedies; who can provide alternatives to endangered herbs; and who live near you are often a good choice. Most herbalists learn from mentors and the plants themselves; except in the case of Oriental herbology, there is little formal training. Graduation from an herbal school is less important than clinical experience and personal reputation.

Herbalists are likely to collect information about your situation by asking about your history and symptoms, rather than by conducting tests. They can address menstrual cramps, anovulation, low progesterone levels, repeated miscarriage, vaginal and urinary tract infections, insomnia, menopause problems, and more; they can help you nourish yourself after coming off hormonal medication.

For some herbalists, their practice is a science, their work based not only on love for the plants but on appreciation for research, diagnostics, theories, and exact formulas. Others have a more spiritual approach.

Local herb shops often offer classes, herb walks, books, dried herbs, tinctures, and capsules, and referrals to herbalists in your area. You can also check your farmer's market and Yellow Pages, or phone the American Herbalists Guild at 770-751-6021.

Homeopathy

In one of his fifth-century writings, Hippocrates observed that medicinal systems can operate by "contraries" and by "similars." Homeopathy, founded by Samuel Hahnemann (1755–1843), is based on the law of similars—that like cures like. If a substance can *cause* symptoms in a healthy person, then the same substance can *treat* the symptoms in a sick person. For example, when cutting an onion, you might get watery eyes and a runny nose; when an onion is made into a homeopathic remedy, *Allium cepa*, and given to a person with a cold or hay fever, symptoms can be relieved. Homeopathic

continued

remedies are extremely dilute, safe, and inexpensive; and they're able to stimulate your vital force toward health.

Homeopathy is a complete medicinal system that can address all ailments and diseases. It considers the whole person, which means that in choosing a client's remedy, practitioners consider mental, emotional, and physical symptoms as well as individual habits and preferences. A long (one- to two-hour) initial interview is necessary to find a person's correct constitutional remedy. Because individuals are treated, rather than a "disease," two anovulatory women would probably be given different remedies.

Homeopathy can address a wide variety of situations, including PMS, irregular cycles, blocked fallopian tubes, repeated miscarriage, menopause complaints, and other problems. Most health-food stores carry remedies for acute situations. With a homeopathic reference book, which most stores keep on hand, you may be able to find a remedy that fits your acute ailment. For chronic conditions, it's best to consult a professional homeopath.

Classical homeopaths use one remedy at a time; others may use combinations of remedies in one treatment. Many MDs, naturopaths, and NPs use homeopathy as their primary medicinal system. While some practitioners are self-taught, formal training programs typically last four or five years.

To find a homeopath, consult the National Center for Homeopathy's Practitioner Directory, www.homeopathic.org. Their number in Alexandria, VA, is 703-548-7790 or 877-624-0613.

Naturopathy

Naturopathic physicians practice whole family medicine as primary care doctors. Naturopaths (NDs) often begin with gentle, slow-moving suggestions that encourage the body's overall health—such as changes in diet and exercise, herbal preparations, homeopathic remedies, and nutritional supplements. Some naturopaths are also practicing midwives; they may have additional certification in homeopathy, acupuncture, or Ayurvedic medicine. Some naturopathic schools include Fertility Awareness in their curriculum.

Naturopaths diagnose your situation primarily through an extensive interview of your history and symptoms, though they also routinely conduct blood tests and other diagnostics. They can conduct nearly all of the tests that MDs, NPs, and PAs can (including for cervical cancer, blocked fallopian tubes, endometriosis, fibroid tumors, ovarian

continued

cysts, sexually transmitted infections, etc.). For gynecological disorders such as an abnormal Pap smear, they can suggest nonpharmaceutical and nonsurgical treatments that you might opt for before trying more invasive procedures. They can fit you for a diaphragm or cervical cap.

Licensing of NDs differs from state to state. In licensed states, they can prescribe antibiotics, drugs for sexually transmitted infections, and hormones for contraception and menopause. NDs tend to work with compounding pharmacists for less synthesized hormones and to customize hormonal prescriptions. If necessary, they may refer you to an MD for a pharmaceutical prescription or surgery.

Lists of practicing naturopaths can be found at www.naturopathic.org. To find an ND in the Yellow Pages, look under Holistic Medicine, Homeopathy, or under Physicians and then Alternative Care, Complementary Medicine, or Naturopathy.

Deborah Keller, ND, and licensed midwife. I often find that clinical signs such as mucus and temperature are more important than lab tests, because the charts can show a trend toward a problem (such as polycystic ovarian syndrome, or hypothyroidism) before blood levels reach "abnormal" ranges. And it's much easier to address a problem before it falls outside the normal range.

Western Medicine

Medical doctors (MDs), nurse-practitioners (NPs), and physician assistants (PAs) can prescribe pharmaceutical drugs, which may be geared toward quick relief of symptoms and/or long-term resolution of a problem. They can conduct or prescribe tests (for cervical cancer, blocked fallopian tubes, endometriosis, fibroid tumors, ovarian cysts, thyroid problems and progesterone levels, sexually transmitted infections, etc.). These providers can also fit you for a diaphragm or cervical cap and provide intrauterine insemination. Some may offer menstrual extraction, an abortive procedure for very early pregnancies. When necessary, an MD can admit you to a hospital and perform surgery.

In the case of sexually transmitted infections, prescription drugs can cure gonorrhea, chlamydia, and syphilis. Drugs are also available to ease the symptoms of herpes, herpes simplex, warts, and infections associated with HIV; but these viruses have no known cures.

Reproductive endocrinologists (REs) offer in vitro fertilization and other high-tech reproductive procedures.

continued

MDs, NPs, and PAs can help in acute and chronic situations and when natural remedies fail. Their work is typically covered by insurance. Tax-exempt clinics that staff MDs,
NPs, and PAs offer care on a sliding scale. Increasingly, these conventionally trained
providers are offering a variety of holistic services.

Fertility Charts in the Doctor's Office

Whenever I walk into a health-care provider's office, take out my charts and my list of
questions, and hear, "This is very helpful," I start to feel better. I can't deny that. I also
think it's unrealistic to expect practitioners to read fertility charts. Most medical education—including alternative medical education—does not yet include Fertility Awareness.
Most health-care providers know little if anything about cervical fluid or how to read the
waking temperature to confirm ovulation; they are unaware of studies that show that FA
is virtually as effective as the Pill in preventing pregnancy when its rules are followed.

As a result, I've heard countless stories of women being told, "I don't look at charts,"
or, "You don't really believe this stuff, do you?" Until Fertility Awareness is routinely included in medical education, women who want their charts considered as data about their
health will have to scout around for providers who will at least value their observations, and
perhaps be open to learning FA. (If your practitioner wants to see studies that demonstrate
the effectiveness of Fertility Awareness, refer to page 236 in the appendix.)

I cannot emphasize enough that there's no such thing as a diet or remedy or health-
care system that works for everyone. Each person is unique and changing and requires
health care that addresses her uniqueness. The information offered here is by no means
exhaustive. May it inspire you to discover your own ways of strengthening your health.

Anovulation

The suggestions on page 186, along with homeopathy, herbs, or acupuncture can
be especially helpful in encouraging ovulatory cycles.

Eliminate unfermented soy, white flour, and sugar from your diet; eat foods
rich in vitamins A and D. Consider adding eggs and butter to your diet and supplementing with cod liver oil.

If you're anovulatory for six months or more, you might consider getting an
exam to rule out polycystic ovarian syndrome, diabetes, high prolactin levels (not
caused by breast-feeding), or other health problems.

Note that ibuprofen, a common ingredient in over-the-counter relief medicine, can prevent ovulation if a woman takes several pills daily. Ibuprofen prevents inflammation of irritated tissue; with repeated use, it can also prevent ovulation, which is actually inflammation of a follicle.

Low Progesterone Levels

Low progesterone can manifest in painful periods, miscarriage, and/or increased menopause problems. To strengthen progesterone levels:

• Decrease or eliminate your consumption of sugar and white flour. Sugar and white flour can cause blood glucose levels to increase, which in turn forces your pancreas to increase insulin production. Your adrenal glands then create more cortisols or stress hormones. Frequent production of cortisols can, in the long run, exhaust and deplete your adrenals. In turn, this can suppress progesterone levels.

• Decrease or eliminate your consumption of soy products. Soy's high levels of phytoestrogen can in turn diminish the benefits of the progesterone you do have.

• Nutritionist Krispin Sullivan says that women who repeatedly miscarry can normalize their progesterone levels by eating liver twice a week or by taking one teaspoon to one tablespoon of cod liver oil daily. (The amount depends on the quality of the brand and your own constitution and weight. Consult with a nutritionist.)

• Numerous progesterone creams and suppositories are now available over-the-counter and by prescription. Leah Shinbach, PA, likes to see "a definitive up and down" of progesterone levels (determined by saliva tests) when she prescribes natural progesterone for cycling women. Shinbach says, "It's difficult for over-the-counter progesterone creams and gels to provide this, so I prescribe 'human bio-identical progesterone,' which is prepared by compounding pharmacies and safer than synthesized progesterone." Human bio-identical progesterone (plant-sourced and molecularly identical to human progesterone) is prepared with a prescription by independent compounding pharmacists. It's available in a variety of forms: capsules, creams, lozenges, vaginal suppositories, and sublingual drops. Shinbach finds that the lozenges, or "troches," are the most effective form of all. Please note that naturally compounded progesterone needs to be prescribed by an MD, a nurse practitioner, a physician assistant, or a naturopath, and ordered from a compounding pharmacy.

Low Temperatures

Three or more temperatures in one cycle that are lower than 97.5 may indicate hypothyroidism (a sluggish thyroid).

- Naturopath Deborah Keller says that "stressed-out adrenals are often at the root of a thyroid disorder and unless the adrenals are addressed, remedies for the thyroid may not be helpful." To nurture your adrenals, stimulants such as coffee, tea, chocolate, sugar, and recreational drugs need to be eliminated; whole foods, a slower pace, and restful activities are helpful. Dr. Keller also suggests that at the end of a hot shower, rinse with cold water, including your whole head. This stimulates circulation, increases white blood cells, relaxes muscles, and moves *qi* (energy or vital force). All of this benefits the thyroid (and can also slow baldness).
- Some herbalists, notably Dr. Ryan Drum, treat hypothyroidism primarily with bladderwrack (also called *Fucus vesiculosis*), a kind of seaweed that contains Diiodotyrosine (Dit). The thyroid gland produces thyroxine from two Dits. Once consumed, Dit functions as a weakly active thyroid hormone and may be used as a supplement for T_3 and T_4 (thyroid hormones) when their production is inadequate. (Dit from seaweed can't provide enough thyroid hormone for those whose gland has been removed.) Drum suggests that people add small pieces of raw bladderwrack to their food or take it powdered in capsules. Ryan Drum also says that indulgent rest is imperative for people with a weak thyroid. You can order seaweed from: Ryan Drum, General Delivery, Waldron Island, WA 98297.
- Yoga postures, including shoulder stands, can be helpful. Note that many teachers advise not to do inversions (upside-down postures) while menstruating.
- Long periods of sadness can inhibit thyroid function. Because the thyroid is located in the throat, our avenue for expression, some people strengthen their thyroid by responding to emotional trauma with creative expression. I know a

woman who healed the grief she felt from a relative's molesting her by writing a play about it.

- Naturopaths and chiropractors can offer homeopathic thyroid remedies and thyroid glandulars (made primarily from ground-up pig and bovine thyroid). These remedies can encourage the thyroid to do its own work.
- Pharmaceuticals such as synthroid are available from MDs for severe cases unrelieved by natural options.

To read more about the thyroid, consider *Living Well with Hypothyroidism* by Mary Shomon. Shomon is a thyroid patient and a Fertility Awareness advocate. She explains what hypothyroidism is and why getting diagnosed is often a challenge. Shoman also addresses hyperthyroidism—wherein you're producing *too much* of the thyroid hormones and your temperatures may be above 98.0 throughout your follicular phase. In her book, she describes her personal experience with pharmaceutical and alternative therapies, the effects of hypothyroidism on infertility and pregnancy, and how to recognize a thyroid disorder in infants and children.

Coming Off the Pill

You might not notice anything unusual coming off the Pill; you might immediately resume a healthy, ovulatory cycle with a luteal phase of at least twelve days. About a third of my clients return quickly to healthy cycles. They may have "a weird one" (i.e., a very long cycle, or one with a very short luteal phase or an anovulatory bleed) about three or four months after coming off the Pill—and then resume normal cycles.

You might feel like lots of emotional and physical "stuff" suddenly surface when you come off the Pill. You may feel increasingly sensitive to certain foods, to bodily sensation and moods, to your partner's desires. Typically, the cycles of women coming off the Pill may take a while to show a discernible cervical fluid pattern, ovulation, and a healthy luteal phase. CF can be creamy and unchanging for months and months; you may not have any "dry" days, and you may not observe "tacky" cervical fluid or egg white. Unchanging mucus can be very frustrating if you want to prevent pregnancy—or to conceive. Also, you may have a very short luteal phase once you do begin ovulating.

According to Stephen Langer, MD, in *Solved: The Riddle of Illness,* the Pill can inhibit thyroid hormones (which in turn may create acne, hair loss, cold hands and feet, and/or fatigue); it can deplete B vitamins.

- Speak to a naturopath or herbalist about testing and strengthening your thyroid. Herbs can gently guide your body toward health.
- Eating unprocessed foods can help restore vitamins and minerals (including B vitamins and zinc) that the Pill depletes (see chapter 11).
- Acupuncture or homeopathy can help normalize your cycles.

Last, when you come off the Pill, your sexuality may seem especially unsettled. See Ondrea's story on page 58.

Follicular Phases Longer Than Twenty-one Days

Long follicular phases and frequent false peaks of cervical fluid can indicate a propensity for ovarian cysts. It is not unusual for a woman to have one "false peak" of cervical fluid once a year. If you observe this more frequently, you may be at risk for ovarian cysts or polycystic ovarian syndrome (PCOS). For some women, having long follicular phases does not pose a health problem. Consult with a knowledgeable practitioner.

- Eliminate sugar and white flour from your diet; increase whole, unprocessed foods and healthy fats such as organic butter; supplement with cod liver oil. Consult with a local chapter of the Weston A. Price Foundation (listed on www.westonaprice.org) about the steps you'll need to take to design menus that will work for you, and read *Nourishing Traditions* by Sally Fallon.
- Vitamin D and calcium supplements have been known to correct PCOS.

Lack of Cervical Fluid

First, do you have a vaginal infection? Are you coming off the Pill? Have your crypts been damaged from being on the Pill, an infection, or coning of your cervix? Also, women whose mothers took diethylstilbestrol (DES) during pregnancy to prevent miscarriage may lack cervical fluid. If you have one of these conditions, an acupuncturist, herbalist, or homeopath may be able to help you address it. Some infections only respond to allopathic (pharmaceutical) medications.

Some women's temperatures show a clear shift—indicating ovulation, but they don't have cervical fluid at their vulva. If this is true for you, try taking your CF sample from your cervix. According to nutritionist Marilyn Shannon, scant cervical fluid can also be related to vitamin A deficiency. (Heavy or prolonged menstrual periods can indicate this as well.) See page 168 for information about common foods that provide vitamin A.

Vaginal Dryness

Vaginal dryness, experienced by women of all ages, can make sexual intercourse very painful.

- Slow foreplay can encourage arousal fluid (produced like a sweat by your vaginal walls) to lubricate the vagina so that intercourse is not painful.
- Check with your local herbalist for lubricating creams. Note that such creams are likely oil-based and therefore can cause condoms to break and diaphragms or cervical caps to be ineffective. Over-the-counter, water-based lubricants are usually available at the drugstore; research their ingredients before you use them. Be wary of applying petroleum-based products to your mucous membranes.
- As we age, our muscles atrophy—if we don't use them. The good news is that the muscles of the pelvic floor respond quickly to exercise. Kegel exercises can strengthen your ability to produce lubricative fluid. *Very slow* Kegels (practiced for just a few minutes each day, while working at a computer, driving, or as meditation) can increase your vaginal walls' ability to become lubricated. Kegels can also help men to heal erectile dysfunction and to strengthen their prostate. (See page 22 for more information about Kegel exercises.)

Low Sperm Count

In *Our Stolen Future,* Theo Colburn reports that because of chemical toxins (such as pesticides, herbicides, and pollution) since the 1940s, men's sperm counts have been decreasing at the alarming rate of 2 percent each year. If your partner has a low sperm count, ask him to avoid marijuana, hot tubs, tight shorts, and cologne; to consider the dietary suggestions described in chapter 11 and at the start of this chapter; and to sleep in the absence of light (see chapter 10). Sperm counts can also be strengthened through acupuncture or Chinese or Western herbs.

Encouraging Awareness in Children

Children can be introduced to principles of Fertility Awareness before they become teenagers. Start simply by noticing the seasonal changes around your home. Plant vegetable and flower gardens. *A Kid's Herb Book* by Lesley Tierra includes how to identify plants you might find on a hike, how to dry the herbs, and how to make a tea from them. Visit farms so your children can see how food is grown. Notice how frost and hail affect the fruit trees in your area. Observing nature's cycles is part of observing fertility's cycles!

Research is the highest form of adoration.

—TEILHARD DE CHARDIN
Jesuit priest and scholar

13. Women Conducting Research

S**AY A WOMAN KNOWS HOW HER REPRODUC-**
tive system works and charts her fertility signals. She uses her charts to determine
whether she's ovulating, when she is fertile, if she may have a thyroid problem, and
more. She gets curious about how medications affect her menstrual cycles, how what
she eats affects her, curious to see if there's a pattern to her moods or her interest in
chocolate or sex. Every day, she collects data and observes her emerging patterns.
Dr. Justina Trott, President of the American College of Women's Health Physicians,
says, "Women who chart their fertility signals are doing clinical research."

This chapter presents charts from women in a variety of typical situations. It's an introduction to the kind of research women who practice Fertility Awareness can provide. It is not meant to show what charts *should* look like in these situations. My hope is that these fascinating charts will encourage more women to research their own gynecological health. My hope is that they will encourage further studies by other women, including students, biologists, medical researchers, health-care providers, and you!

Coming Off the Pill

Cathy, thirty-five, used the Pill for nine months. Here are her first four cycles off the Pill (figures 13.1 through 13.4). In her first cycle (see figure 13.1), Cathy didn't ovulate: she doesn't have a sustained rise in temperature.

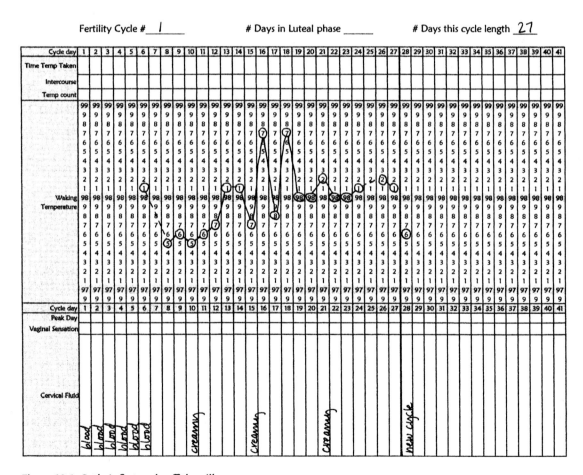

Figure 13.1. Cathy's first cycle off the pill.

Fertility Cycle # __2__   # Days in Luteal phase _____   # Days this cycle length __28__

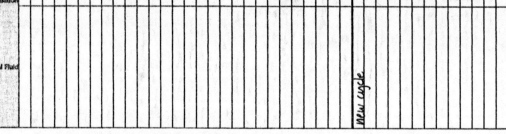

Figure 13.2. Cathy's second cycle off the Pill.
This cycle was twenty-eight days long. Again, she did not ovulate.

Because the Pill can encourage the cervical crypts to produce primarily thick fluid (impenetrable to sperm), it can take a while for a healthy mucus pattern to return after a woman comes off the drug. Typically, my clients who are coming off the Pill fail to discern any changes in their CF for at least several cycles. The mucus will simply read "creamy," and the lack of change often discourages women from charting it.

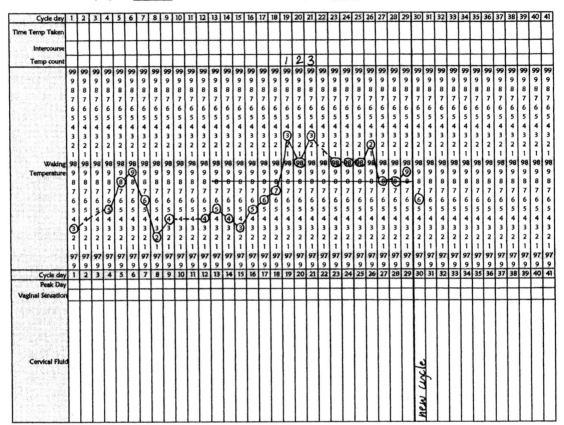

Fertility Cycle # _3_ # Days in Luteal phase _11_ # Days this cycle length _29_

Figure 13.3. Cathy's third cycle off the Pill.

She probably ovulated between Days 18 and 19. However, her luteal phase was short (only eleven days), and two of her temperatures fell on the coverline, indicating low progesterone levels for this cycle, and that she might have had difficulty sustaining a pregnancy at this point.

Fertility Cycle # __4__ # Days in Luteal phase __13__ # Days this cycle length __30__

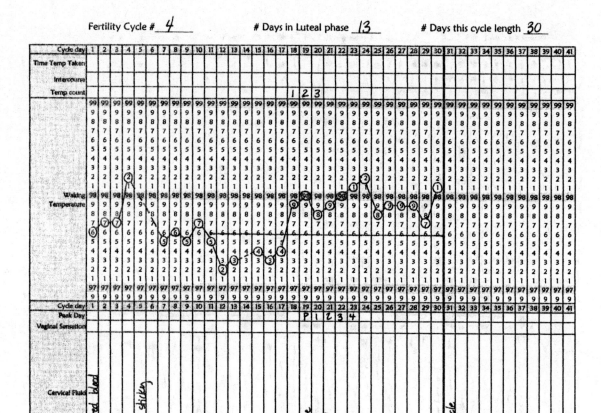

Figure 13.4. Cathy's fourth cycle off the Pill.

Her temperatures confirmed ovulation by the evening of Day 20; her CF did so by the evening of Day 23. By her temperature, she had a healthy, thirteen-day luteal phase. Her five temperatures below 97.5 suggest possible hypothyroidism. Her cervical fluid still didn't read crisply as her temperatures, but it looks like it's on the way.

I have seen several clients ovulate in their first cycle off the Pill, though typically it takes several months or longer.

I think it would be fascinating to compare women's fertility charts before and after being on the Pill. I'd also welcome seeing charts of women while they're *on* different kinds of oral contraceptives (the mini Pill, progestin-only Pill, etc.), and as they come off them. I don't know what version of the Pill Cathy took.

Hypothyroidism and Different Diets

Stephanie, thirty, was on the Pill for a year and a half when she was eighteen. A year before she began charting, she tested negative (through a blood test) for thyroid problems; but her low energy, sleep disorders, and increased weight indicated to her that she does have a thyroid problem. Her mother has been on thyroid medication since Stephanie was born. Once she began charting, Stephanie's low temperatures confirmed that despite the negative blood test, she needs to continue investigating what she suspects is hypothyroidism. (See figures 13.5 and 13.6.)

I suspect that improvements in fertility signals as a result of dietary and lifestyle changes may happen more slowly than the quick downturn Stephanie experienced in just one month of junk food. Again, these would make fascinating studies.

With an IUD

After her third child's birth, Connie opted for a progestin-emitting IUD. She attended my class after the IUD had been in place five and a half years. She wanted it removed because it gave her uncomfortable cramps. To gain confidence in her use of Fertility Awareness, she decided to chart for a cycle or two before she had the IUD removed. She turned thirty-two the month she began charting.

Connie reports, "Before my doctor put the IUD in, I asked him if I could conceive with it. He said he didn't believe so.

"But with my first fertility chart, I could see that whether or not other women ovulate with an IUD in place, I did. (See figure 13.7.) It was a major step for me to get this information, and to make decisions based on what I knew. I didn't think it could be healthy for my body to go through that every month. Also, while I'm pro-choice, I don't want to conceive with an IUD in place. For me, an IUD is simply not an option."

In her next cycle, Connie ovulated again, and she had the IUD removed. Her next three cycles, about thirty-six days each, were all anovulatory. Connie sensed that her body was adjusting to not having the IUD.

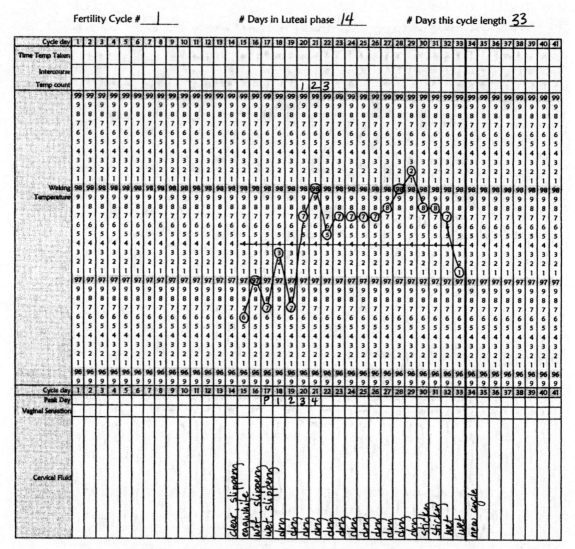

Figure 13.5. Stephanie's first chart (indicating possible hyperthyroidism).

Stephanie began charting while she was on a low-carbohydrate, low-sugar, high-protein diet. This was her first charted cycle. Her ovulation was crisp; her luteal phase was a healthy fourteen days; her cervical fluid and temperature nearly matched up exactly. Except for the lowness of her temperatures, she had a healthy-looking chart.

Fertility Cycle # __2__   # Days in Luteal phase __8__   # Days this cycle length __29__

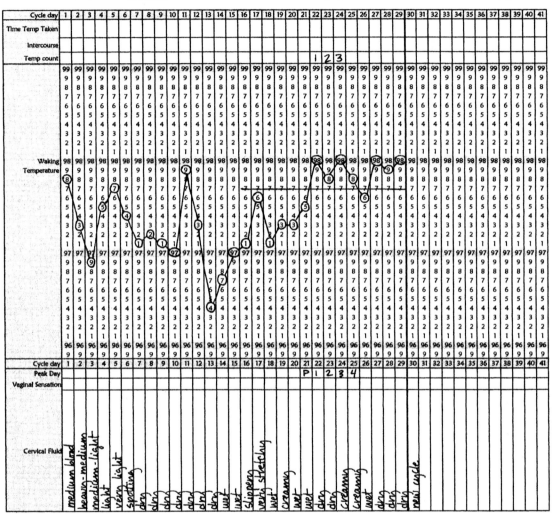

Figure 13.6. Stephanie's second chart.

This cycle showed progesterone deficiency because her luteal phase was only eight days long, and she dipped (Day 26) below her coverline. Stephanie "ate junk" this cycle. After comparing this chart to her previous one (when she was on the high-protein, low-carboyhdrate diet), she decided to go back on the diet.

Fertility Cycle # __1__   # Days in Luteal phase __9__   # Days this cycle length __36__

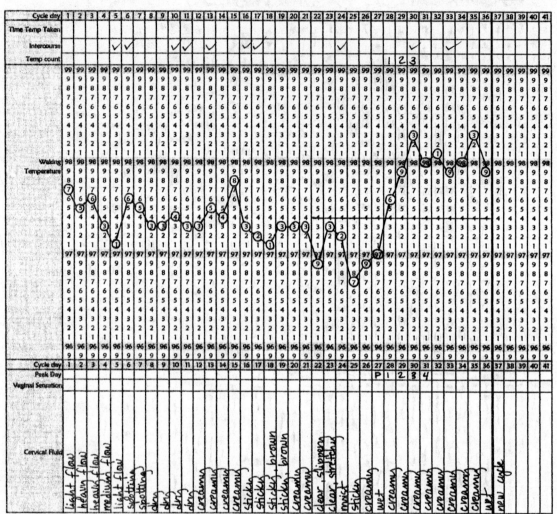

Figure 13.7. Charting fertility cycles with an IUD inserted.

During her first charted cycle, while an IUD was in place, Connie probably ovulated between Days 27 and 28. Her luteal phase was only nine days long—not enough to sustain a pregnancy.

After an Abortion

Eleanor took the Pill when she was twenty to twenty-five. When she came off it, her cycles varied from six weeks to three months long. She became a vegetarian and lost a lot of weight. At twenty-nine, she started eating chicken and fish; at thirty, she began using progesterone cream when her physician identified that she had a progesterone deficiency. She began charting just after her second abortion, when she was thirty-five. (She was thirty-two when she had her first abortion.)

Fifteen months after her second abortion, Eleanor, then thirty-six, contracted chlamydia from the same partner. She wasn't using anything to prevent pregnancy or sexually transmitted infections (and still did not know that her charts could tell her when she was fertile and infertile). Typically, women who contract chlamydia do not experience any symptoms. Eleanor's abdominal pain was unusual—and fortunate, in that it helped her to test for and treat the infection quickly.

"Clearly," Eleanor told me several years later, "I wasn't taking care of myself. I took the abortions and the chlamydia as opportunities to get honest with myself, and to take better care. The simple ritual of charting my fertility signals was my first step to connecting with my body in a positive way. I began asking why I behave so self-destructively."

Eleanor also began following a diet based on principles discovered by Weston A. Price (see chapter 11). She stopped eating soy products and hydrogenated fats, reduced her sugar intake, and focused on eating organic fruits and vegetables, meat, chicken, and dairy. She is now committed to using condoms and Fertility Awareness to prevent sexually transmitted infections and unintended pregnancy.

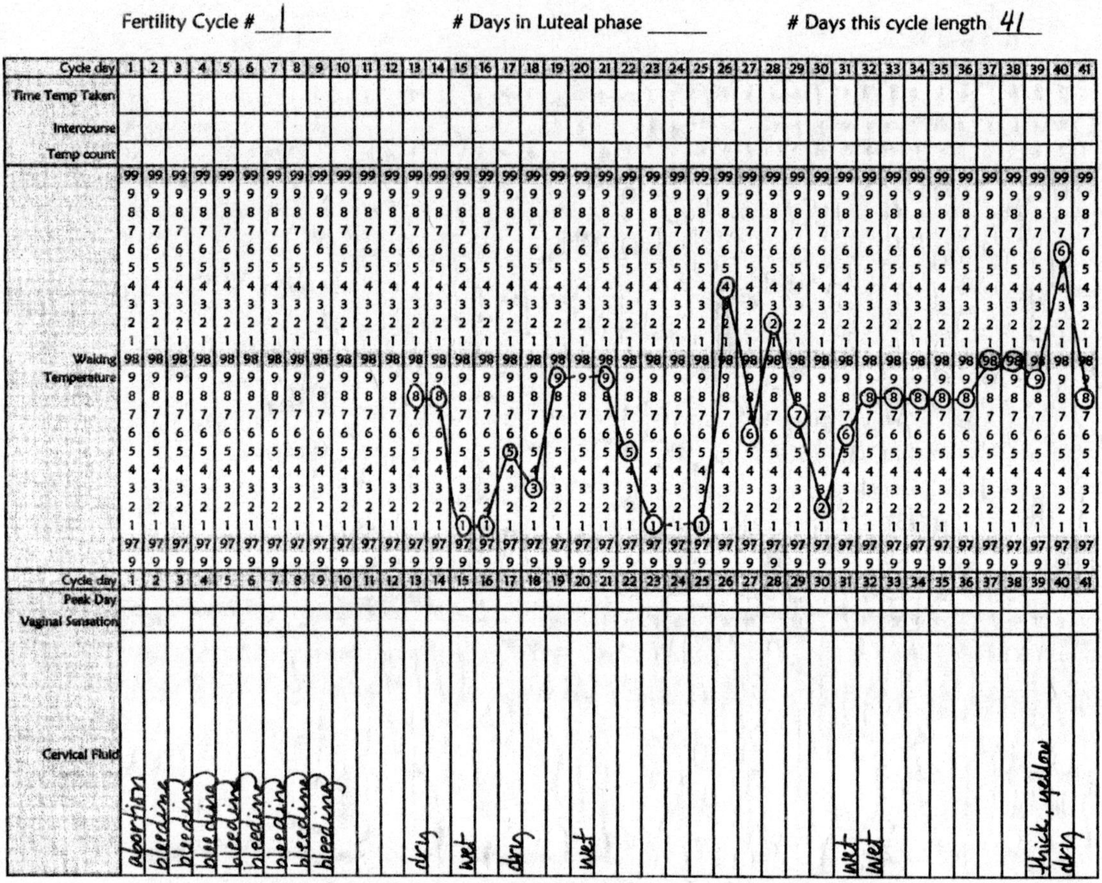

Fertility Cycle # __1__   # Days in Luteal phase _____   # Days this cycle length __41__

Cycle day	1	2	3	4	5	6	7	8	9	10	11	12	13	14	15	16	17	18	19	20	21	22	23	24	25	26	27	28	29	30	31	32	33	34	35	36	37	38	39	40	41
Time Temp Taken																																									
Intercourse																																									
Temp count																																									
Waking Temperature																																									
Cycle day	1	2	3	4	5	6	7	8	9	10	11	12	13	14	15	16	17	18	19	20	21	22	23	24	25	26	27	28	29	30	31	32	33	34	35	36	37	38	39	40	41
Peak Day																																									
Vaginal Sensation																																									
Cervical Fluid	abortion	bleeding	bleeding	bleeding	bleeding	bleeding	bleeding						dry		wet		dry			wet								wet	wet									thick, yellow	dry		

Figure 13.8. Eleanor's first charted cycle, following her second abortion.
The cycle was anovulatory.

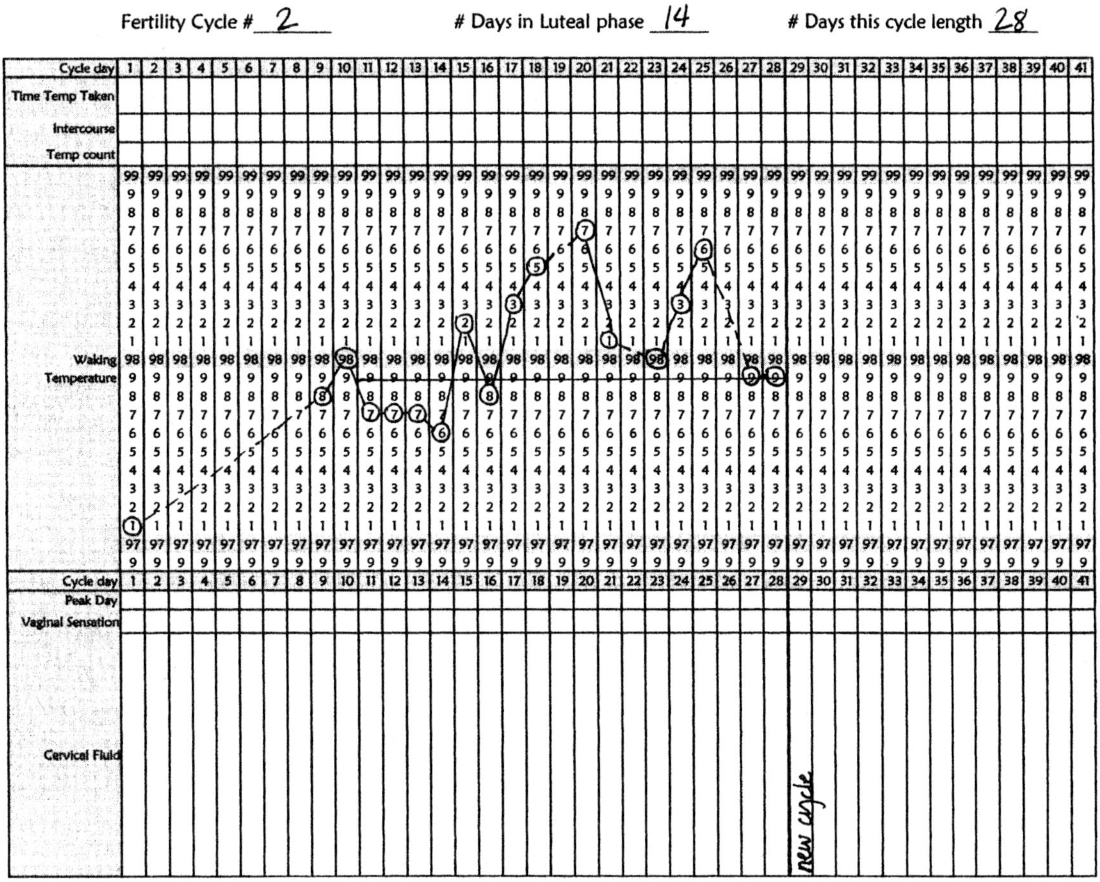

Fertility Cycle # __2__   # Days in Luteal phase __14__   # Days this cycle length __28__

Cycle day	1	2	3	4	5	6	7	8	9	10	11	12	13	14	15	16	17	18	19	20	21	22	23	24	25	26	27	28	29	30	31	32	33	34	35	36	37	38	39	40	41
Time Temp Taken																																									
Intercourse																																									
Temp count																																									
Waking Temperature																																									
Cycle day	1	2	3	4	5	6	7	8	9	10	11	12	13	14	15	16	17	18	19	20	21	22	23	24	25	26	27	28	29	30	31	32	33	34	35	36	37	38	39	40	41
Peak Day																																									
Vaginal Sensation																																									
Cervical Fluid																													new cycle												

Figure 13.9. Eleanor's second cycle after an abortion.

She probably ovulated sometime between Days 14 and 17. She indicated progesterone deficiency with the zigzag of temperatures on Days 15 and 16, around the time she ovulated; and also with the temperature dips to her coverline on Days 27 and 28. Eleanor continued with similar charts showing ovulation and progesterone deficiency.

Fertility Cycle # __3__   # Days in Luteal phase __16__   # Days this cycle length __33__

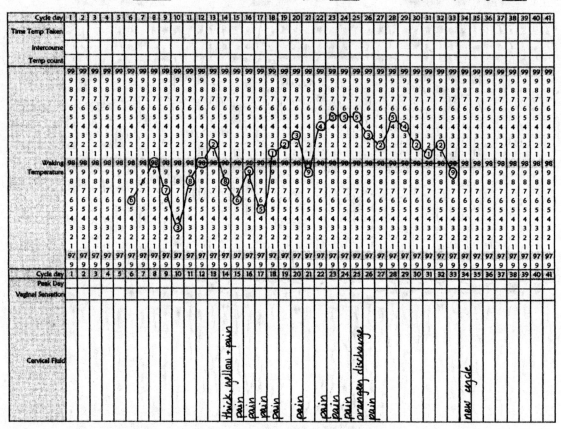

Figure 13.10. Eleanor's chart when she contracted chlamydia.

She probably ovulated between Days 17 and 18, although her high temperatures on Days 12 and 13 (high from the chlamydia infection?) fell on and above her coverline (at 98.0). Her luteal phase lasted an unusually long sixteen days, while the dip on Day 21 indicated slight progesterone deficiency. It is also possible that Eleanor didn't ovulate until Day 21, with an eleven-day luteal phase.

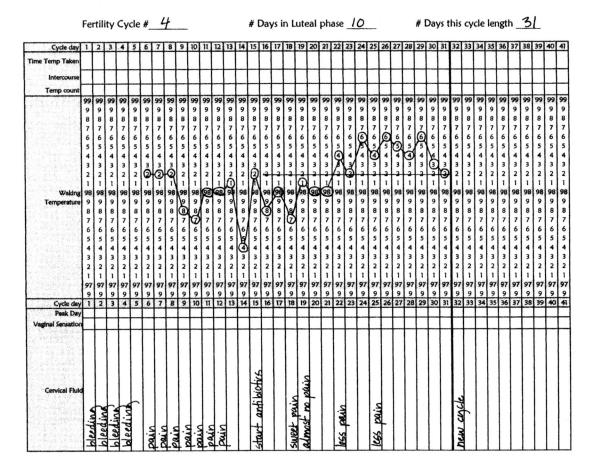

Fertility Cycle # __4__   # Days in Luteal phase __10__   # Days this cycle length __31__

Figure 13.11. Eleanor's chart when she began treatment for chlamydia.

Eleanor began antibiotic treatment for chlamydia about a month after she began feeling abdominal pain. She probably ovulated between Days 21 and 22, although Day 23's temperature fell on her coverline— and she therefore couldn't confirm ovulation until after 6 P.M. of Day 26, when she had three temps consecutively above her coverline. This cycle's short, ten-day luteal phase indicated progesterone deficiency.

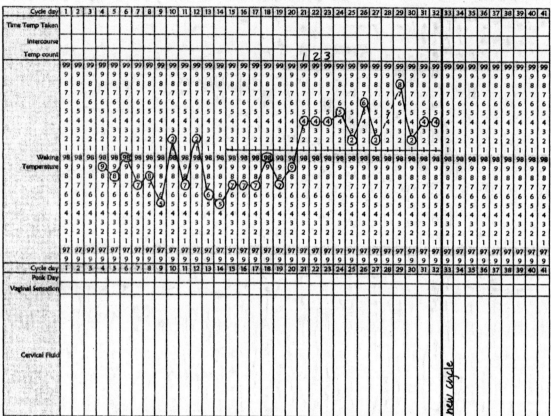

Fertility Cycle # _5_   **# Days in Luteal phase** _12_   **# Days this cycle length** _32_

Figure 13.12. Eleanor with a healthy chart.

This cycle, charted when she was thirty-eight, shows a crisp ovulation between Days 20 and 21, and a healthy twelve-day luteal phase.

After Depo-Provera

Diane started taking the Pill when she was sixteen, and stayed on it for four years. At twenty, she began taking Depo-Provera shots. For the seven years she continued with Depo (taking four shots each year), she never bled. Her doctor assured her that this was okay, though she sometimes felt nervous about it. Other than not bleeding, she didn't notice any unusual symptoms from the shots—until the last year or so, when her hair fell out in strange clumps, and she also had leg cramps. "I can't know for sure," Diane says, "but I felt these were both related to the Depo, partly because the symptoms went away once I stopped taking the shots."

She stopped taking Depo partly because of her symptoms and partly because she wanted to know if she could get pregnant. Six months after her last shot, she still hadn't menstruated. Her doctor honestly said she didn't know what to do. When Diane wondered if the Pill would "give her a period," the doctor gave her a prescription. "It seemed arbitrary to me," Diane explained later, "but nobody I knew had another option. I took the Pill for three months, and sure enough, I bled for a few days each month. I still didn't know that bleeding on the Pill isn't an actual period."

Diane took a Fertility Awareness class while she was still on the Pill, got off it, and started charting.

In eight months, Diane charted numerous "breakthrough bleeds": she spotted or bled, but never ovulated. At first, these breakthrough bleeds occurred every seven to seventeen days; and her mucus was usually dry, sticky, or creamy. After three months, her breakthrough bleeds began to space apart every twenty-five to thirty-six days. After seven months, her sense of smell—which she hadn't experienced for years—returned. She noticed an occasional day of "elasticy" mucus.

"We waited and waited and waited for my charts to look predictable," Diane said. "But the reality was that we couldn't make sense of them. We used condoms; we got creative. And I just had to get patient with my body to give me normal-looking charts."

I recently saw the first few charts of another woman coming off Depo-Provera (after one year of shots); and she, too, bled every week or two for a couple of months shortly after she stopped taking the Depo.

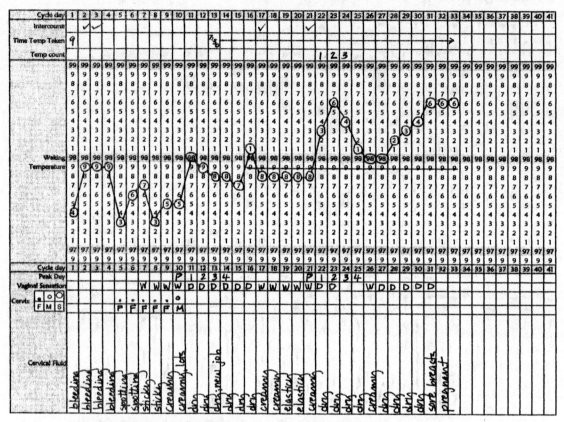

Fertility Cycle # __10__   # Days in Luteal phase _____   # Days this cycle length _____

Figure 13.13. Diane's first ovulatory cycle after Depo-Provera.

In her tenth cycle off Depo-Provera, she had an unusual split peak—unusual because her mucus dried up so definitively before it began building up again. Diane assumed that she was infertile, even though she could not confirm ovulation by her temperature. She also started a new job (and waking at a different time) on Day 13. She probably ovulated for the first time since she took Depo-Provera shots on Day 21. She confirmed pregnancy by a urine test on Day 32. At this writing, she's seven months pregnant.

When you're coming off hormonal medication (whether you want to avoid pregnancy *or* to conceive a healthy child), you need to use a combination of condoms and creativity and health-strengthening steps until you see regular, ovulatory cycles.

On Clomid

Charlene, thirty-seven, took the Pill for six months in her early twenties. She started charting when she married and began trying to conceive.

After four cycles of trying (unsuccessfully) to conceive, Charlene took Clomid (50 mg) for two cycles. She'd read that women over thirty-five who don't conceive after six months of trying should begin infertility treatment.

The next cycle, Charlene tried a stronger dose of Clomid.

After her fifth cycle with Clomid (now 150 mg), Charlene decided to take a break, because the drug "was doing such a number on my emotions." She had experienced flares of temper, intense crying, and strong feelings of inadequacy and hopelessness. "Because I hadn't conceived, I probably would've felt all of these things," she said. "But with the drug, they seemed exacerbated." In her third post-Clomid cycle, she conceived—and miscarried about a week after she confirmed that she was pregnant. Over the next half-dozen cycles, she tried progesterone suppositories, acupuncture, intra-uterine insemination, and two more doses of Clomid (one of which resulted in an anovulatory cycle).

Since beginning the Clomid treatments, Charlene, 5′3″, had gained fifty pounds. A new doctor explained that as she gained weight, doses of Clomid that worked before might not suffice, and the weight gain could indicate that she's hyperinsulinemic or even diabetic.

My heart broke for Charlene. She felt that all she had then was to trust that she's given what she needs and to turn her focus to her own health.

Fertility Cycle # _1_   # Days in Luteal phase _11_   # Days this cycle length _26_

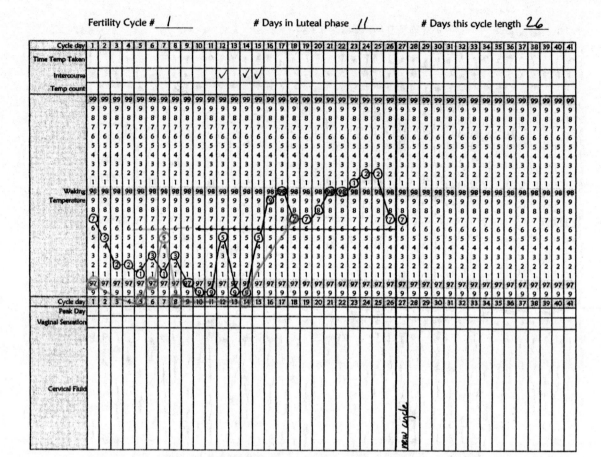

Figure 13.14. One of Charlene's first charted cycles, in which she tried to conceive.

Her cycle was ovulatory. It also indicated possible hypothyroidism (because of her eleven temperatures below 97.5) and progesterone deficiency (because her luteal phase was only eleven days long).

Fertility Cycle # __2__   # Days in Luteal phase __13__   # Days this cycle length __30__

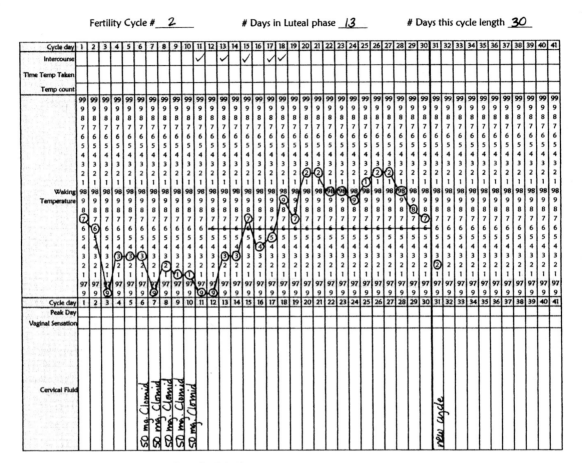

Figure 13.15. Charlene's first cycle with Clomid treatment.

It's difficult to tell when she ovulated in this cycle—some time between Days 14 and 20. The long "stairstepping" between her follicular and luteal phases (Days 12 to 20) suggested progesterone deficiency. She also still had low temperatures, indicating possible hypothyroidism.

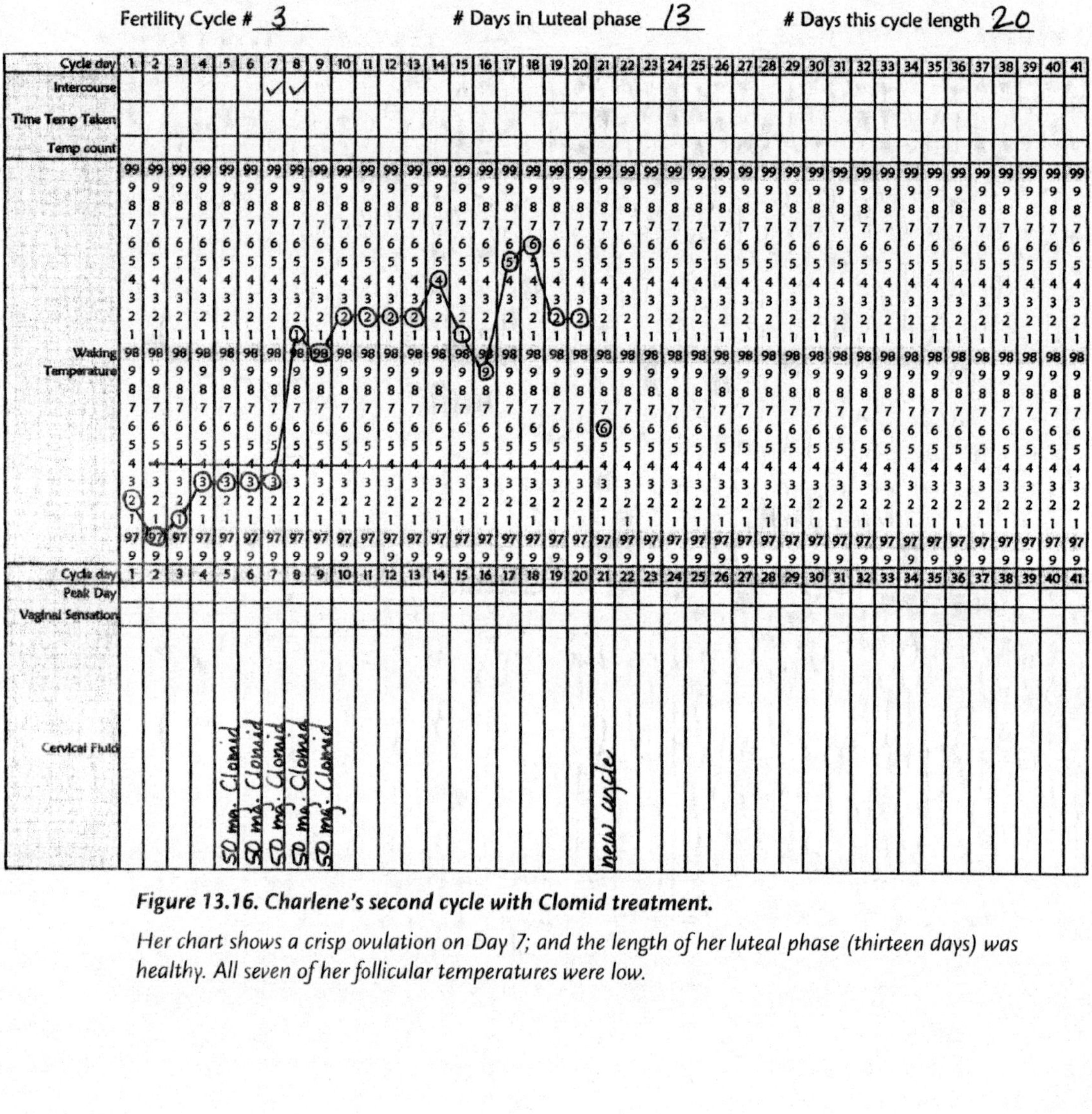

Fertility Cycle # __3__   # Days in Luteal phase __13__   # Days this cycle length __20__

Cycle day	1	2	3	4	5	6	7	8	9	10	11	12	13	14	15	16	17	18	19	20	21	22	23	24	25	26	27	28	29	30	31	32	33	34	35	36	37	38	39	40	41
Intercourse							✓	✓																																	
Time Temp Taken																																									
Temp count																																									

Waking Temperature chart (°F, 99 down to 97)

Cycle day	1	2	3	4	5	6	7	8	9	10	11	12	13	14	15	16	17	18	19	20	21	22	23	24	25	26	27	28	29	30	31	32	33	34	35	36	37	38	39	40	41
Peak Day																																									
Vaginal Sensation																																									
Cervical Fluid		50 mg. Clomid	50 mg. Clomid	50 mg. Clomid	50 mg. Clomid	50 mg. Clomid														new cycle																					

Figure 13.16. Charlene's second cycle with Clomid treatment.

Her chart shows a crisp ovulation on Day 7; and the length of her luteal phase (thirteen days) was healthy. All seven of her follicular temperatures were low.

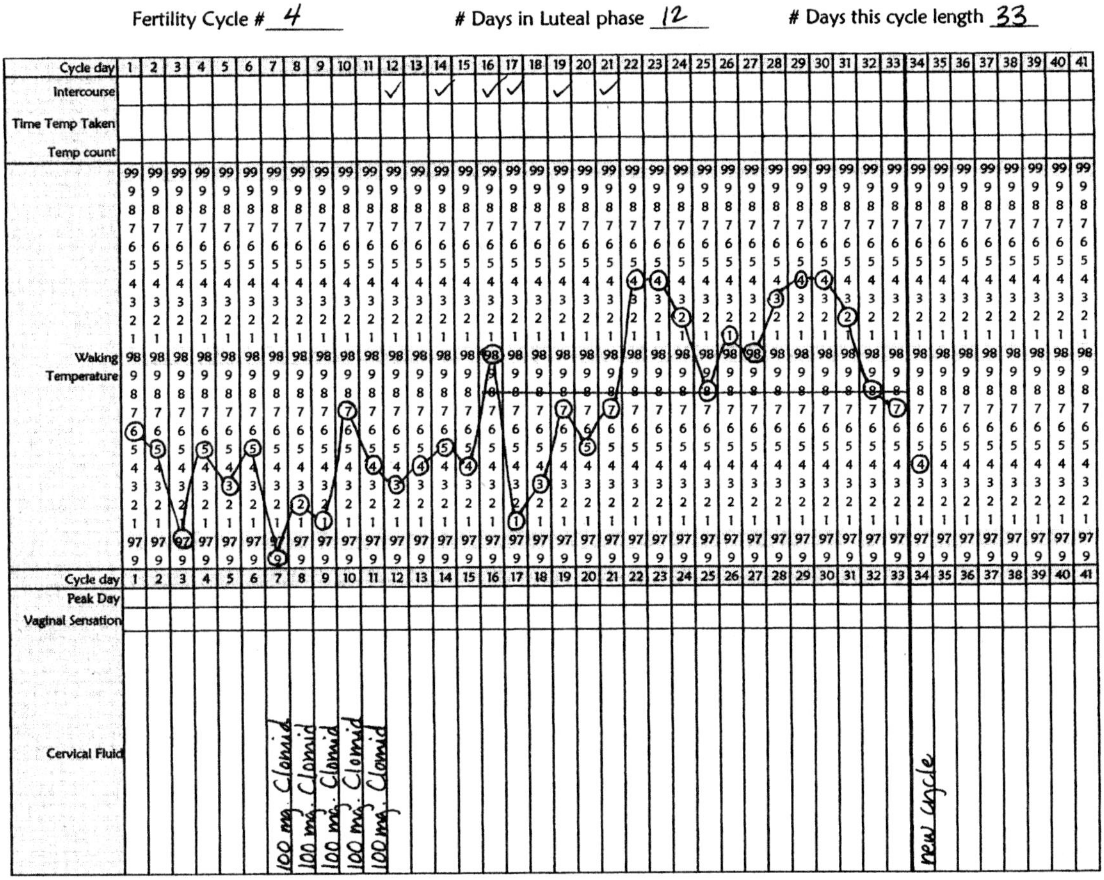

Fertility Cycle # __4__   # Days in Luteal phase __12__   # Days this cycle length __33__

Cycle day	1	2	3	4	5	6	7	8	9	10	11	12	13	14	15	16	17	18	19	20	21	22	23	24	25	26	27	28	29	30	31	32	33	34	35	36	37	38	39	40	41
Intercourse												✓		✓		✓	✓		✓		✓																				
Time Temp Taken																																									
Temp count																																									

Waking Temperature (chart grid, 97.9–99.9)

Cycle day	1	2	3	4	5	6	7	8	9	10	11	12	13	14	15	16	17	18	19	20	21	22	23	24	25	26	27	28	29	30	31	32	33	34	35	36	37	38	39	40	41
Peak Day																																									
Vaginal Sensation																																									
Cervical Fluid				100 mg. Clomid	100 mg. Clomid	100 mg. Clomid	100 mg. Clomid	100 mg. Clomid																										new cycle							

Figure 13.17. Charlene's third cycle with Clomid treatment.

I would guess that she ovulated on Day 21. Her luteal phase was twelve days long; the dips on Days 25, 32, and 33 suggested progesterone deficiency. Eleven temperatures were below 97.5 in her follicular phase.

Approaching Menopause

Ruby, forty-nine, wanted to use Fertility Awareness to prevent pregnancy because she didn't want to take hormonal drugs and her partner was allergic to latex (which a diaphragm is made of) and didn't like lambskin or polyurethane condoms, either. Ruby took the Pill for three years in her twenties. She has never been pregnant. When she began charting, she'd had very occasional premenopausal hot flashes. She didn't have enough cervical fluid to read it and felt the temperature gave her enough information to learn about her cycle and to know when she was not fertile.

Two charts later, Ruby didn't ovulate until around Day 28. Her luteal phase was only nine days long—not long enough to sustain a pregnancy.

Typically, premenopausal women can expect mucus to be less abundant and for the mucus they do have to be less stretchy and lubricative. The time between bleeds can become longer, with double or triple mucus peaks; and women are often anovulatory. Hypothyroidism is more common at this age, so temperatures are typically lower. Cervix changes can be especially helpful while approaching menopause. While a woman may bleed more heavily, she may also bleed for fewer days.

Deby Wood, goat farmer. I've kept goats for eight years. Our family drinks their milk; and I make soap with it, too.

Last July, Stella was freshening (giving birth) while we had a barn raising. All the women and girls gathered 'round. She actually gave birth in my lap. I'm forty-eight; I hadn't had a period in nine months, but I did two weeks after Stella's labor. That was my last period. It's been a year, and I haven't menstruated again, though I've been to other freshenings. The thing is, I bottle-fed that goat. We're bonded. When we evacuated during the Los Alamos fire, she rode with me in the front seat. When she gave birth, I figure Stella released some hormones, and I picked up on them. It showed me how we are all part of nature, and nature is part of us.

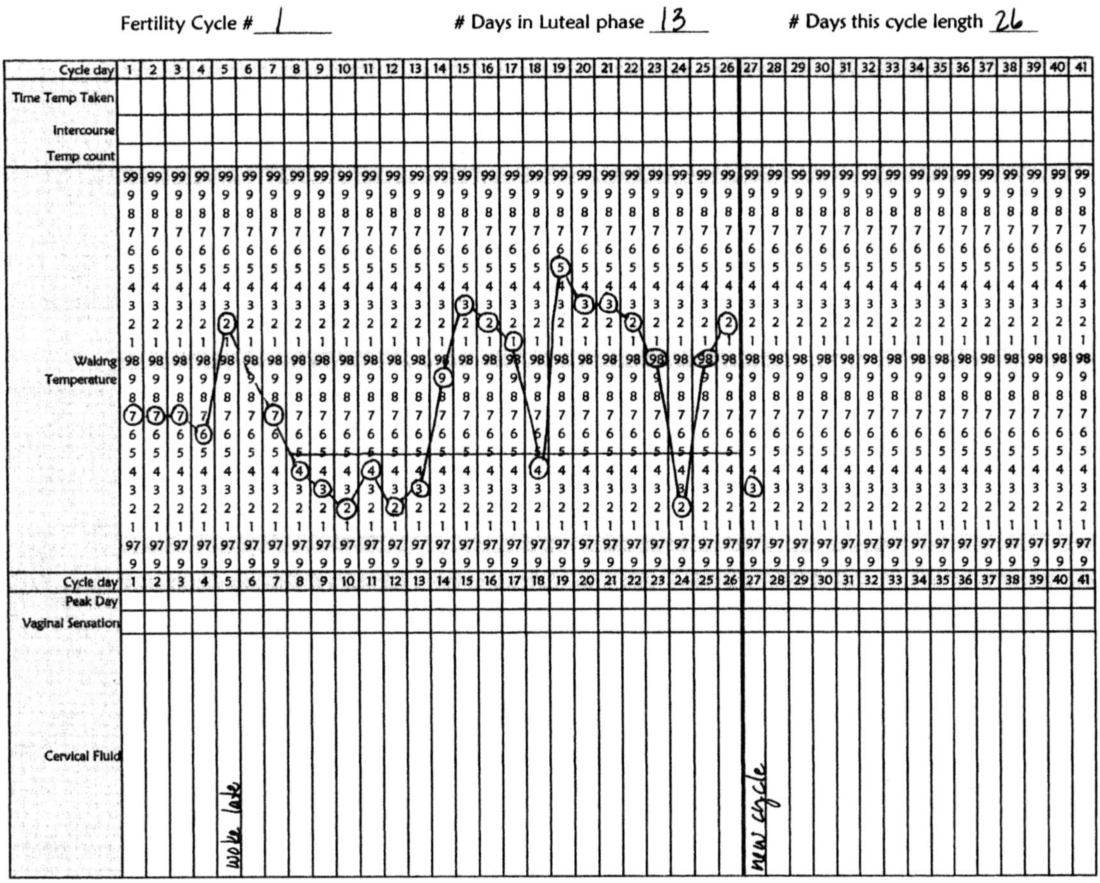

Fertility Cycle # _1_   # Days in Luteal phase _13_   # Days this cycle length _26_

Figure 13.18. Ruby's chart while she approaches menopause.

She probably ovulated on Day 13. Her eight temperatures below 97.5 suggest possible hypothyroidism; and the dips on Days 18 and 24 suggest progesterone deficiency. Still, Ruby could use her chart to prevent pregnancy. She entered her postovulatory infertile phase on Day 16 at 6 P.M.

More Women Conducting Research

I dream of a world where all women know that they can observe and chart their fertility signals. I dream of double-blind studies about the long-term effects of diet, of sleeping in the absence of light, and of fertility drugs on women's health and the health of their offspring and their children's offspring.

One of my students has begun observing if her occasional anxiety about sex connects to her hormonal cycle. Several women are observing improvements in their progesterone levels from taking herbal infusions. Some men notice that their interest in sex increases when their partner is fertile. One woman marks "UEEs" on her charts—unexplained explosions of emotion—and notices that they seem to occur just before she ovulates and gets her period. A woman who had a partial hysterectomy (she still has ovaries) wants to chart her BBT to see if she's still ovulating. A thirty-four-year-old woman with multiple sclerosis notices that she tends to lose her balance more often during her postovulatory phase, and even more so just before her period begins. An observant Jewish woman would like to know how fasting at different times of the cycle affects fertility—several Jewish holidays require fasting. An artist finds that learning about fertility cycles helps her to be gentler with herself when she's in an unproductive creative phase.

The observations and questions are endless. May medical researchers make use of the amazing data available from fertility charts. May high school and college students explore and write about topics related to Fertility Awareness in their classes. May research continue!

Appendixes

Since people began forming communities, guidelines have been created to encourage spiritual, emotional, and physical wellness—including sexual and reproductive wellness. While the aim of these guidelines has been for the health and sustenance of individuals and the community, the means to health are often very different from one culture to another. Laws related to menstruation, lovemaking, and reproduction can vary tremendously.

Why is this relevant to Fertility Awareness? I've heard many people say that once they learn reproductive anatomy and become intimate with their fertility signals, they become more appreciative of their desires. Sexuality and fertility become more integrated. This may be one of the juiciest aspects of charting. While FA is essentially a life skill, it also raises questions about core beliefs: Is sex for bonding or for reproduction or both? Is there a time when sex isn't appropriate? What would make me want to marry? What if I had an unintended pregnancy? If I gave birth, what factors would determine how long I would breast-feed? These questions are part of the beauty of charting: they give us the opportunity to know our thinking and our partner's thinking.

If you're heterosexual and you want to prevent pregnancy *and* make love during your fertile phase, what do you do? Do you abstain from sex altogether? Do you postpone intercourse and enjoy sexual massage and/or oral sex? Do you have intercourse and use a barrier method (such as a condom or diaphragm)?

Organizations that teach Fertility Awareness tend to advocate that each individual answer these questions for herself or himself. Organizations that teach Natural Family Planning tend to offer specific answers to these questions in a Catholic framework.

More than one woman has stormed out of my class after learning that she can't have unprotected intercourse every day if she practices FA and wants to postpone or avoid pregnancy. Often, these women say they have a lot of sexual energy, and they *need* intercourse every day.

I've come to think that having strong sexual desires is a gift, like having more money than you need. And I've come to see practicing Fertility Awareness as an opportunity to discover your own rhythm, and that of your partner, without the influence of artificial birth control.

Almost everyone I know who practices Fertility Awareness or Natural Family Planning feels that charting enhances their appreciation of the sacredness of sex and fertility. People can have very different definitions, however, about what constitutes sacred, blasphemous, and even necessary sex.

To encourage discussion about all these issues, this section clarifies some of the terms and organizations involved:

Names for Different Methods

The *Calendar* or *Rhythm Method* is based on the discovery made simultaneously in the 1920s by surgeons from Austria and Japan (Hermann Knaus and Kyusaku Ogino)—that women typically ovulate about fourteen days before the onset of their next period. John Smulders, a Dutch, Roman Catholic physician, applied the results of this discovery and published them with the Dutch Roman Catholic medical association in 1930. Smulders wrote that his motivation to encourage natural family planning came from wanting a method that "first did no harm" and that recognized periodic fertility "as a gift from the Creator."

When rules of the Rhythm Method are followed, the probability of pregnancy during the first year of perfect use is about 13 percent.[1]

Here's how the Rhythm Method works: to determine the first day of your fertile phase, observe the number of days in your previous twelve cycles, and subtract eighteen from the length of your shortest cycle. To determine the last day of your fertile phase, subtract eleven from the length of your longest cycle. For example, if your shortest cycle was twenty-six days long, and your longest was thirty-four days long, your first fertile day would be Day 8, and your last fertile day would be Day 23.

Essentially, this method makes predictions about future cycles based on past cycles. It doesn't require knowledge about the reproductive system or the self-observations that charting requires. For women with regular cycles, it can be somewhat reliable. For women with irregular cycles, it's unreliable.

The *Ovulation Method* uses observations of cervical fluid and vaginal sensation to determine when a woman is fertile or infertile. It does not include observations of the basal body temperature (BBT). It may include observations of cervix changes. The first-year probability of pregnancy for couples using the Ovulation Method is about 3 percent among perfect users and 20 percent among typical users who abstain during the fertile phase.[2]

The *Standard Days Method (SDM)* was developed in 1999 at the Institute for Reproductive Health at Georgetown University to increase choice and address the large unmet need for family planning. SDM is inspired by surveys that show that well over 60 million women worldwide use periodic abstinence to avoid pregnancy—though they don't know when they are fertile. By using CycleBeads, a color-coded string of beads, women whose cycles are usually twenty-six to thirty-two days long are able to identify the days when they can conceive and the days when conception would be very unlikely. SDM takes about twenty minutes to learn and is more than 95 percent effective when used correctly. It's currently offered by state health departments, Planned Parenthood clinics, church-based groups, and private providers in the United States and internationally. For more information, contact the Institute for Reproductive Health of Georgetown University, 4301 Connecticut Ave. NW, #310, Washington, DC 20008; 202-687-1392; www.irh.org; www.cyclebeads.com.

The *Sympto-Thermal Method* integrates observations of cervical fluid and cervix changes (sympto) and the waking temperature (thermal) to determine when a woman is fertile or infertile. Charting cervix changes is considered optional.

Discovery of a slight but distinct rise in the body's waking temperature after ovulation is credited to J. Ferin, a Belgian physician, and Wilhelm Hillebrand, a German Catholic priest, around 1935. John and Evelyn Billings, Australian MDs, have brought attention to the mucus changes during a woman's cycle since the sixties. J. Roetzer, a physician from Austria, advocated for the Sympto-Thermal Method from the sixties.[3] The first-year probability of pregnancy among couples who use the Sympto-Thermal Method is about 2 to 3 percent among perfect users, and as high as 13 to 20 percent among typical users.[4]

Cultural Terms

Fertility Awareness (FA) practitioners use the Ovulation Method or the Sympto-Thermal Method. FA teachers may discourage couples from using barrier methods during the woman's fertile phase, because the risk of unintended pregnancies increases slightly. However, they will inform clients how to use such methods effectively in conjunction with charting. Fertility Awareness teachers tend to support individual choice around sexual and reproductive matters. Many FA teachers are also counselors, doulas, herbalists, or lactation consultants; and they integrate this work with their teaching. Training is usually conducted in a mentoring fashion, one on one. For more information, see headings under the Fertility Awareness Institute, the Fertility Awareness Network, and Justisse.

Natural Family Planning (NFP) practitioners use the Ovulation Method or the Sympto-Thermal Method to determine when a woman is fertile or infertile. They tend to be practicing Catholics and to perceive NFP as part of their religious practice. NFP organizations typically advocate for abstinence during the fertile phase if a couple wants to avoid or postpone pregnancy, openness to the child (throughout a marriage), and breast-feeding. Their guidelines may state that their teachers cannot recommend contraception, abortion, masturbation, oral sex, premarital sex, homosexual behavior, or sterilization. NFP organizations have conducted the most comprehensive medical research in the field. For more information, see headings under the Billings Method, the Couple to Couple League, Families of the Americas Foundation, and Serena Canada.

Organizations

The *Billings Ovulation Method Association* offers classes, conferences, teacher training, and research in the Ovulation Method. Drs. Evelyn and John Billings, Australian MDs, began developing it in 1953; research has continued since then, and currently the Billings Method is practiced and taught in 120 countries. While the Billingses' orientation is Catholic, their classes and annual conferences are open to people of all faiths. Their international website (www.woomb.org) provides current research about the Ovulation Method. Dr. Evelyn Billings's book, *The Billings Method,* Penguin Books/Australia, can be ordered in the United States from the St. Paul office, BOMA-USA, PO Box 16206, St. Paul, MN 16206; 651-699-8139; Web site: www.boma-usa.org.

The *Couple to Couple League* teaches the Sympto-Thermal Method of Natural Family Planning. Founded in 1971 by John and Sheila Kippley, the CCL is staffed primarily by volunteers who are practicing Catholics. Over 700 CCL teaching couples offer NFP throughout the world. The CCL's publications include *The Art of Natural Family Planning: Breast-feeding and Natural Child Spacing*; *Fertility, Cycles and Nutrition*; and a bi-monthly journal. The CCL offers teacher training; information on charting for teenagers; and conferences for families, doctors, and clergy. Many of their materials are available in Spanish. The mission of the Couple to Couple League is to promote marital chastity through the teaching of NFP in a Christian context. PO Box 111184, Cincinnati, OH 45211; 513-471-2000; Web site: www.ccli.org.

Family of the Americas Foundation, founded by Mercedes Arzu Wilson in 1977, teaches the Ovulation Method of Natural Family Planning. FAF has developed a charting system that is used worldwide and is easily understood even by those who don't read or write. Their educational materials are available in twenty-one languages, and they conduct teacher-training programs internationally. FAF recently completed comparative studies about how the practice of NFP affects the duration of marriages, communication between wives and husbands, church attendance, etc. PO Box 1170, Dunkirk, MD 20754; 800-443-3395, 301-627-3346; Web site: www. FamilyPlanning.net.

The *Fertility Awareness Institute*, founded by Katie Singer in 2002. For a listing of current offerings, please refer to FAI's Web site: www.gardenoffertility.com.

The *Fertility Awareness Network*, founded in 1990, provides a list of Fertility Awareness teachers in the United States and Canada (and occasionally other countries) and offers classes and consultations in New York City. PO Box 1190, New York, NY 10009; 800-597-6267, 212-475-4490; Web site: www.fertaware. com/fan_resources. html.

Justisse, founded by Geraldine Matus in 1986, provides classes, private sessions, and teacher training in the Ovulation and Sympto-Thermal Methods, with a focus on holistic, reproductive health care that respects individual choices. 8621 104th St., Edmonton, AB T6E 4G6 Canada; 780-420-0877; Web site: www.justisse.ca.; info@justisse.ca.

Serena Canada, founded by Gilles and Rita Breault in 1962, provides classes and teacher training in the Sympto-Thermal Method in English and French. It teaches NFP couple to couple and in groups. 151 Holland Ave., Ottowa, Ontario K1Y OY2 Canada; 613-728-6536, 888-373-7362; Web site: www.serena.ca; serena@on.aibn.com.

Every person I've met who practices and/or teaches Fertility Awareness or Natural Family Planning treasures the information these methods provide, wants as many people as possible to know it, and wants women and families around the world to be healthy. For the record, this book could not have been written without the contributions of people who align with each of the groups listed here.

To find a fertility awareness teacher, contact the Fertility Awareness Network or Justisse (see page 230). Your local women's clinic, Planned Parenthood clinic, or an herb shop may also be able to refer you to someone in your neighborhood. Many teachers provide consultations by phone—you can mail or fax them your charts.

To find a teacher in your area with a Catholic orientation, contact the Billings Ovulation Method Association, the Couple to Couple League, or Serena Canada (see pages 229–230); or ask your local diocese.

IF YOU FEEL MOVED TO TEACH THIS MATERIAL, start reading! Familiarize yourself with the resources described in this book.

To teach effectively, you'll need thorough knowledge of reproductive anatomy and the ability to describe it well—along with information about how to chart, how to interpret charts, and where to refer women with problematic cycles. You'll need clear handouts for your workshops and an experienced teacher to call on when your students ask questions you can't answer.

Most Fertility Awareness teachers have been trained one on one. Because of limited funding, nonsectarian programs have been available sporadically. Programs in Natural Family Planning often require students to agree to moral principles before beginning to train.

Geraldine Matus, Fertility Awareness teacher since 1978, founder of Justisse, midwife and psychologist. When I first started teaching FA, my students usually had charts that reflected healthy menstrual cycles—and the rules were easily learned. Twenty-five years later, I rarely see women with normal-looking charts. I think this reflects the use of hormonal birth control (by today's women and their mothers). The typical North American diet (which includes hormonally treated animal products, fast foods, and a deficit of whole, fresh, nonprocessed foods) also interferes with the normal functioning of male and female reproductive systems. Sexual abuse, sexually transmitted infections, the use of alcohol and recreational drugs, increased stress—all of these affect reproductive health and can make charts challenging to interpret.

A good Fertility Awareness teacher conveys information clearly. She can help a woman understand that her chart reflects not only her reproductive health but her overall health and life choices as well. She can interpret a problematic chart and knows where to refer a woman to help restore normal cycling.

By all means, more Fertility Awareness teachers are needed!

Principles of the Fertility Awareness Institute

1. Fertility Awareness means having a basic understanding of how female and male reproductive systems work, how to observe and chart a woman's fertility signals, how to determine whether a woman is fertile or infertile, and how to use charts to gauge gynecological health. This knowledge is a fundamental life skill.

2. For anyone who wants to learn it, this life skill should be widely available at an affordable cost.

3. Fertility Awareness is an excellent tool for encouraging a woman's friendly relationship with her body, regardless of her sexual preference or marital status.

4. The method is an excellent tool for encouraging understanding, communication, and appreciation about the differences between female and male fertility and sexuality.

5. Reproductive health is an environmental issue: human fertility is one part of nature's wide web. If the earth's fertility is compromised (through soil depletion, air or water pollution, etc.), human fertility will also be compromised. How we feed and medicate ourselves affects our reproductive health and that of our children; so does the air we breathe, the water we drink, and the soil in which we grow our food. Our attitudes about the menstrual cycle and how we prevent or achieve pregnancy may parallel our attitudes about the earth and her cycles. Fertility Awareness encourages awareness of our connectedness to other living systems along with appreciation of each person's uniqueness.

6. Fertility is a privilege, not a right.

7. Fertility and sexuality are deeply personal and sacred. Each person's choices deserve respect.

8. As women and men approach new stages of their fertile lives (adolesence, young adulthood, desire to parent or not to parent, pregnancy, menopause), education about their options, including nonpharmaceutical options, should be easily accessible.

9. A woman has the right to keep or terminate a pregnancy. For the optimum health of individual women, their families and communities, educational efforts need to be focused on *pre*-choice: on a woman knowing when she is fertile and not fertile and how to act on her desires so that she has the best chance of welcoming pregnancy when she finds herself pregnant.

10. Fertility Awareness is an exceptional tool for researchers who seek to test the effects of diet; light; herbal, pharmaceutical, and homeopathic remedies; exercise; and more on gynecological health.

CONTRACEPTIVE TECHNOLOGY REPORTS THAT given perfect use, the probability of becoming pregnant by the Sympto-Thermal Method in the first year of use is 2 percent. If women make love only during their postovulatory phase, only 1 percent will experience unintended pregnancy.

Studies about typical user effectiveness (wherein rules are *not* followed perfectly) with Fertility Awareness show failure rates of 10 to 25 percent. These studies are inconsistent because different systems (mucus-only, temperature-only, and the Sympto-Thermal Method) are used and because not all users adhere to the same guidelines. The method's effectiveness may also be affected by teaching quality.

Method failure with the diaphragm and the cervical cap (when spermicide is used) is about 9 percent; typical user failure with these methods is about 20 percent. With a male condom, method failure is about 3 percent; typical user failure is 14 percent. The Pill's method failure rate is about .5 percent; typical user failure is 5 percent.

To be effective, each of these methods for preventing pregnancy depends on the user. With Fertility Awareness, the key is to chart every day, to know the rules well, and to follow them.

Guida, M., "An Overview of the Effectiveness of Natural Family Planning," *Gynecological Endocrinology* (June 1997): 203–19.

Keefe, Edward F., MD, "Self-Obervation of the Cervix to Distinguish Days of Possible Fertillty," *Bulletin of the Sloane Hospital for Women,* 1962.

Lamprecht, V. and J. Trussel, "Natural Family Planning Effectiveness: Evaluating Published Reports," *Advances in Contraception* 13 (1997): 155–65.

Qian, Shao-Zhen, De-Wei Zhang, et al., "Evaluation of the Effectiveness of a Natural Fertility Regulation Programme in China," presented at the Centre for Study and Research in the Natural Regulation of Fertility, Università Cattolica del Sacro Cuore, Italy, September 2000. This study of 1,654 healthy women found the Billings Ovulation Method more effective (99.5%) than the IUD (98%).

Rice, Frank J., PhD, Claude A. Lanctot, MD, and Consuelo Farcia-DeVesa, PhD, "Effectiveness of the Sympto-Thermal Method of Natural Family Planning: An International Study," *International Journal of Fertility* 26 (1981): 222–30.

Trussell, James and Laurence Grummer-Strawn, "Contraceptive Failure of the Ovulation Method of Periodic Abstinence," *Family Planning Perspectives* 22 (March/April 1990): 65–70.

Wade, Maclyn E., MD, et al., "A Randomized Prospective Study of the Use-Effectiveness of Two Methods of Natural Family Planning," *American Journal of Obstetrics & Gynecology* 141 (October 1981): 368–76.

World Health Organization, Task Force, "A Prospective Multicentre Trial of the Ovulation Method of Natural Family Planning. II. The Effectiveness Phase," *Fertility and Sterility* 36 (November 1981): 591–98.

———, "A Prospective Multicentre Trial of the Ovulation Method of Natural Family Planning. III. Characteristics of the Menstrual Cycle and of the Fertile Phase," *Fertility and Sterility* 40 (December 1983): 773–78.

THIS TEST IS DESIGNED TO HELP YOU CLAR-ify what you need to know about the method in order to use it effectively and confidently. If you're partnered, you might each take the test, then go over your answers together. If you still have unanswered questions, call a Fertility Awareness teacher. (See "How to Find a Teacher" on p. 231.)

1. *Explain the difference between Fertility Awareness and the Rhythm Method.*

The Rhythm Method determines fertility by observations of *past* cycles. For most women, it is not effective for preventing pregnancy. In contrast, Fertility Awareness determines fertility by daily charting of a woman's current fertility signals. If its rules are followed, Fertility Awareness is virtually as effective as the Pill in preventing pregnancy.

2. *In the context of the menstrual cycle, define the word* period; *define the word* cycle.

The *period* refers to the days of menstrual bleeding at the beginning of the cycle. A *cycle* starts on the first day of menstrual bleeding and ends the day before you begin bleeding again.

3. *How do you determine the first day of your cycle?*

The day you begin bleeding bright red blood is the first day. Brownish spotting belongs to the cycle that's ending.

4. *Explain the differences between cervical fluid (CF) and arousal fluid.*

Cervical fluid is produced in the cervix's crypts. It can keep sperm alive for up to five days, filter out impaired sperm, alkalinize the vagina, and provide a conduit for sperm to swim from the cervix to the outer edge of the fallopian tube at ovulation. Arousal fluid can't perform these functions. It's produced like a sweat in the vaginal walls; it lubricates the woman so that intercourse isn't painful.

5. *What is the life span of a mature egg?*

Twelve to twenty-four hours.

6. *What behaviors could affect your waking temperature?*

The BBT can be affected if, before taking it, you make love, eat or drink, climb stairs, have a bowel movement, sleep on a heated waterbed or with an electric blanket, sleep embraced with a partner or child, drink alcohol the night before, if you're ill, or if you take it later or earlier than usual.

7. *If you don't check your morning temperature until later that evening, your thermometer will retain your temperature. True or False?*

True—assuming you've got a working thermometer!

8. *How and when do you check for cervical fluid and vaginal sensation?*

Three times a day, before urinating, wash your hands and take a mucous sample from just inside the vagina. Observe its consistency and color. For vaginal sensation—sense if it's wet or dry. (Wiping yourself after urinating, sometimes you may notice a dry sensation—though you've just urinated. Other times, you may notice a slippery sensation—though you're not aroused.)

9. *When recording your mucus and vaginal sensation at the end of the day, what do you write down?*

A description of the day's wettest sample.

10. *If, after your period, you have a moist sensation on your vaginal lips but no mucus, would you consider yourself fertile or infertile?*

Fertile.

11. *What is the Peak Day?*

The *last* day of observing wet vaginal sensation or wet mucus before your mucus begins to transition to a dryer quality (not the day of the most mucus). Typically, ovulation occurs on the Peak Day.

12. *Can you have more than one Peak Day in a cycle? Explain.*

Yes. It's possible for cervical fluid to build up to a wet consistency, then dry up without your ovulating. Mucus can build up to a peak several times before you confirm ovulation with four consecutive dry days after the peak and a sustained temperature rise. Of course, it's also possible to have false peaks followed by anovulatory bleeding.

13. *What is the follicular phase?*

The fertile preovulatory phase, while follicles (unripe eggs in sacs) are maturing.

14. *What hormone dominates the follicular phase?*

Estrogen. The ripening follicles emit estrogen.

15. *What is the luteal phase?*

The postovulatory phase.

16. *What hormone dominates the luteal phase?*

Progesterone. The corpus luteum (the sac formerly called the follicle that released a mature egg at ovulation) emits progesterone.

17. *Name four reasons to chart your BBT every day.*

a. It can confirm that ovulation has taken place.
b. If your temperatures are below 97.5, it can indicate that you may have a thyroid problem.
c. It can show that you may have low progesterone levels (if your luteal phase is eleven days or less, or if your luteal phase temperatures dip onto or below your coverline).
d. It can confirm pregnancy.

18. *A woman can ovulate more than once in a menstrual cycle. True or False?*

False. Even when two eggs are released (as with fraternal twins), it's still considered one ovulation for that cycle.

To Prevent Pregnancy

19. *How do you determine if you're fertile or infertile while menstruating?*

The period is potentially fertile because it's possible to have cervical mucus present while you're bleeding; and this mucus could keep sperm alive until you ovulate. While you're bleeding, you can't tell whether you have cervical fluid present. During the first twelve cycles that you chart, consider yourself fertile during menstruation. Once you've observed twelve cycles that are all twenty-six days or longer, you can consider yourself infertile during the first five days of your cycle. If one of your previous twelve cycles was shorter than twenty-six days, you can consider yourself infertile during your cycle's first three days.

20. *Before ovulation, the basal body temperature (BBT) can let you know what days you're fertile or infertile. True or False?*

False! Before ovulation, the waking temperature can*not* let you know whether you're fertile.

21. *After your period and before ovulation, how do you determine whether you're fertile?*

By observing your vaginal sensation and cervical fluid. If you've observed dryness all day, you are considered infertile after 6 P.M. The next day, you need to observe dryness all day again in order to consider yourself infertile that evening. Once you observe a moist sensation and/or cervical mucus, your fertile phase has begun.

Also, if you observe that your cervix is soft, higher in the vaginal canal, and/or your os is open, consider yourself fertile.

22. *Using the rules for cervical mucus, how do you determine the end of your fertile phase?*

a. Locate your Peak Day.
b. You need four consecutive days of mucus and vaginal sensation that are dryer than they were on the Peak Day.
c. After 6 P.M. on the fourth consecutive day of mucus that is dryer than the Peak Day's mucus, your fertile phase ends, and your postovulatory infertile phase begins.

23. *Using the BBT, how do you confirm that you've ovulated and you're infertile?*

a. When you see a rise in temperature, count back six temperatures, starting with the first low temperature before the rise.
b. Draw a coverline one-tenth of a degree above the highest of the six low temperatures.
c. You need three consecutive temperatures above the coverline. After 6 P.M. of the third consecutive evening above the line, you can confirm that your egg is dead and gone and that your infertile phase has begun.

24. *Why do you need to wait so many days until after your Peak Day to consider yourself infertile?*

It's possible that you don't ovulate until forty-eight hours after the Peak Day. Then it's possible to release two eggs. If each of these eggs lives the maximum of twenty-four hours, that adds up to four days after the Peak Day when an egg could be available for fertilization.

25. *Why do you need to wait so many days until after your BBT rises to consider yourself infertile?*

It's possible that you don't ovulate until twenty-four hours after your temperature rises. Then it's possible to release two eggs. If each of these eggs lives the maximum of twenty-four hours, that adds up to three days above the coverline when you could have an egg ready to be fertilized.

26. *If you use a diaphragm (or any other birth control that requires spermicide), how will your fertility signals be affected?*

Spermicide can obscure your reading of cervical fluid. You can only use the waking temperature to determine whether you've ovulated.

27. *Sticky or creamy mucus before ovulation signals that you're fertile; after ovulation, the same kind of mucus can signal that you're infertile. True or False? Then, why is this so?*

True. Once you've had four days of mucus that is dryer than your Peak Day mucus, you can consider yourself infertile after 6 P.M. of that fourth day. So if your Peak Day mucus was like egg white, creamy and sticky mucus (which are dryer than egg white) would therefore indicate (after four days) that you'd entered your postovulatory, infertile phase.

28. *Explain how it's possible to conceive without genital-genital contact or ejaculation.*

Say pre-ejaculate lands on the man's thigh, the woman wraps her legs around his thigh—and she has fertile CF. Mucus can provide a conduit for the pre-ejaculate's sperm to swim to the cervix and keep it alive there until she ovulates.

29. *Lambskin condoms prevent pregnancy and sexually transmitted infections. True or False?*

False. They can prevent pregnancy; they are not effective in preventing STIs. Latex or polyurethane condoms can prevent pregnancy *and* STIs.

30. *How can you use your chart to confirm that you're pregnant?*

When you've got eighteen temperatures above your coverline, you're probably pregnant. Eighteen high temps are needed because you might not have conceived until a second egg was released (two days after the rise in temperature); and the luteal phase is never longer than sixteen days—unless you're pregnant. In a very rare case, eighteen high temperatures (and no menstruation or pregnancy) might indicate a corpus luteum cyst.

To Conceive

31. *What are the best days to have intercourse if you want to conceive, and your partner has a normal sperm count?*

When the man's sperm count is normal, have intercourse each day once you observe wet mucus and wet vaginal sensation. The Peak Day (the day before your mucus begins drying up) signals that ovulation is imminent; it's the best day to try.

32. *What are the best days to have intercourse if you want to conceive, and your partner has a low sperm count?*

When the man's sperm count is low, have intercourse every other day once you observe wet mucus and wet vaginal sensation. The Peak Day (the day before your mucus begins drying up) signals that ovulation is imminent; it's the best day to try.

Using Charts to Gauge Gynecological Health

33. *What does an anovulatory chart look like?*

The mucus is continuously dry or sticky; it typically doesn't get slippery. Also, there's no sustained temperature shift. So—the temperature might rise, but it won't stay up.

34. *Healthy progesterone levels are needed for what? Name five things.*

a. To make the uterine lining spongy for implantation of a fertilized egg.
b. Easy menstruation (i.e., menstruation without intense cramps).
c. To sustain a pregnancy.
d. Easy menopause.
e. Breast cancer prevention.

35. *How can you determine if you may have progesterone deficiency? Describe four ways.*

a. If the luteal phase lasts eleven days or less.
b. If the transition between the follicular phase and the luteal phase takes more than three days.
c. If the transition between the luteal phase and the follicular phase takes more than three days.
d. If the luteal phase temperatures dip onto or below the coverline.

36. *How can you determine if you've miscarried?*

If you begin bleeding after you've confirmed pregnancy with eighteen temperatures above your coverline.

37. *How can charts help you determine if you may be at risk for ovarian cysts or polycystic ovarian syndrome?*

If, more than once a year, your cervical fluid indicates a "false" peak. This signals that your follicles are maturing—but not releasing an egg.

38. *What is hypothyroidism, and how can charts help you determine if you may be at risk for it?*

Hypothyroidism is a sluggish thyroid. Temperatures below 97.5 can indicate that you may have this condition. Other symptoms include cold hands and feet, mild depression, and unexplained weight gain.

Questions Only You and Your Partner Can Answer
39. *Most women are fertile for one third to one half of their cycle. If you want to make love while you're fertile and you don't want to conceive, what are your options?*

40. *If you follow the rules, Fertility Awareness is virtually as effective as the Pill in prevent-ing pregnancy. If you conceive unintentionally while using this method, what options would you consider?*

41. *If you have difficulty conceiving, what measures do you think are appropriate?*

42. *When do you think hormonal drugs for preventing or achieving pregnancy are appropriate?*

43. *Would you encourage children to learn Fertility Awareness? Starting when?*

For Each of the Following Charts:

Is the woman infertile before ovulation? If so, when?

When does her fertile phase begin?

Which is her Peak Day?

Where is her coverline?

When does her postovulatory infertile phase begin?

How many days long is her luteal phase?

How many days long is her cycle?

If she wants to conceive (and assuming her partner's sperm count is normal), when are the best days to try?

What do you observe about her gynecological health?

Several of these charts aren't exactly "textbook." Indeed, most women's charts aren't. To use Fertility Awareness effectively, you need to be able to apply the rules when idiosyncracies appear.

If you like, put a clean sheet of paper over each chart, and uncover each day one at a time to simulate how you would answer these questions as a cycle evolved.

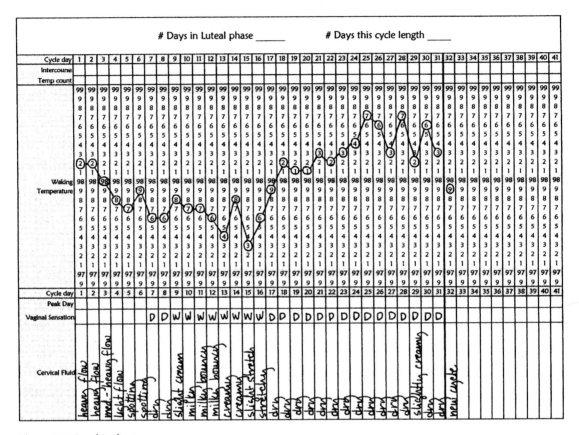

Figure A.1. Sarah's chart.

She's infertile after 6 P.M. on Days 7 and 8. Her fertile phase begins on Day 9. Her Peak Day is Day 16. Her coverline is at 98.0. Her postovulatory infertile phase begins at 6 P.M. on Day 20. (Her CF and temperature match up exactly.) Her luteal phase is fourteen days long. Her cycle is thirty-one days long.

If she wants to conceive, Sarah's best days to try in this cycle are Days 14, 15, and 16.

Gyn health-wise, the stair-stepping transition between her preovulatory and postovulatory phases may indicate a very slight progesterone deficiency.

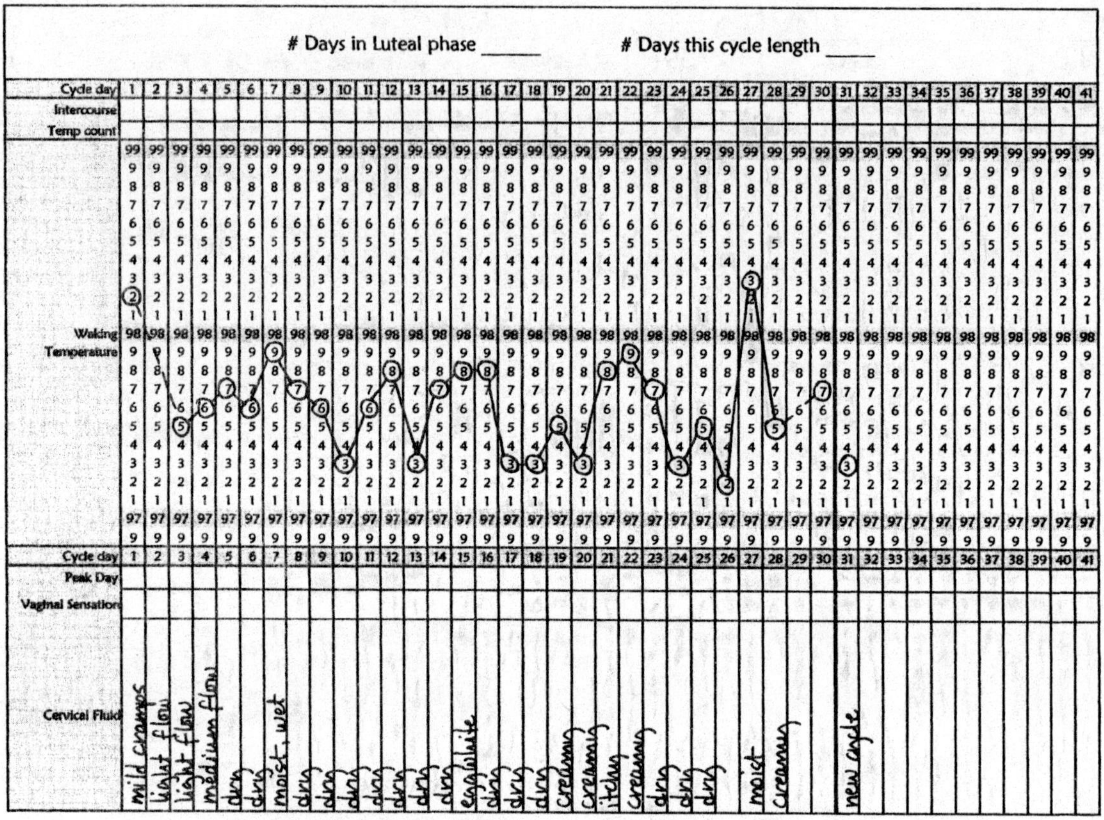

| # Days in Luteal phase _____ | | | | | | | | | | # Days this cycle length _____ | | | | | | | | | | | | | | | | | | | | | | | | | | | | | |

Cycle day	1	2	3	4	5	6	7	8	9	10	11	12	13	14	15	16	17	18	19	20	21	22	23	24	25	26	27	28	29	30	31	32	33	34	35	36	37	38	39	40	41
Intercourse																																									
Temp count																																									

Figure A.2. Gabrielle's chart.

Gabrielle is infertile after 6 P.M. on Days 5 and 6. Day 7 is a false Peak Day. Because of the four dry days that follow, she's infertile after 6 P.M. on Day 11. She can also consider herself infertile on Days 12 through 14 after 6 P.M.. Day 15 is another false Peak Day—although she didn't build up to it, and on Day 19 she starts developing wetter mucus again. She therefore can't consider herself infertile in the evening of Day 19. Day 22 is her third false Peak Day; because she didn't observe her mucus on Day 26, she can't consider that evening infertile, either.

There's no place for a coverline, because her temperature doesn't go up and stay up.

In this cycle, Gabrielle did not ovulate. Also, eight of her temperatures are below 97.5, indicating she may have hypothyroidism.

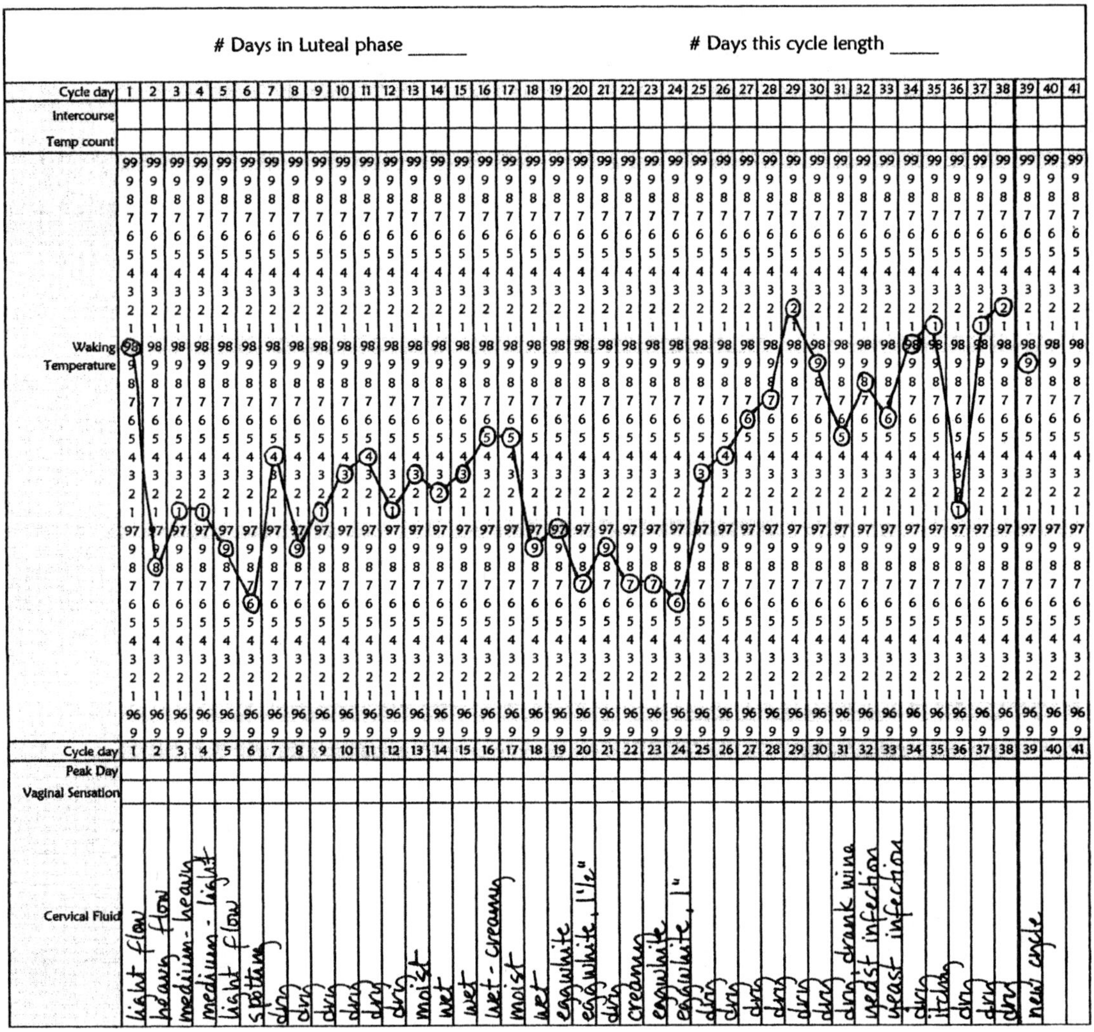

Figure A.3. Stephanie's chart.

She's infertile after 6 P.M. on Days 7 through 12. Her fertile phase begins on Day 13. She has a false peak Day on Day 20; her true Peak Day is Day 24. Her coverline is at 97.1. Her postovulatory infertile phase begins at 6 P.M. on Day 28 by her CF and Day 27 by her temperature. To be cautious, she should wait until the evening of Day 28 to consider herself infertile. Her luteal phase is fourteen days long; her cycle is thirty-eight days long.

To conceive, Stephanie's best days to try are Days 22, 23, and 24 in this cycle—although she might have thought Days 17 through 20 were best while her first (false) peak was building up.

Stephanie's very low temperatures indicate she may be hypothyroid. If she has more than one false peak each year, she might get tested for PCOS. Also, her temperature on Day 36 falls onto her coverline, indicating possible (slight) progesterone deficiency.

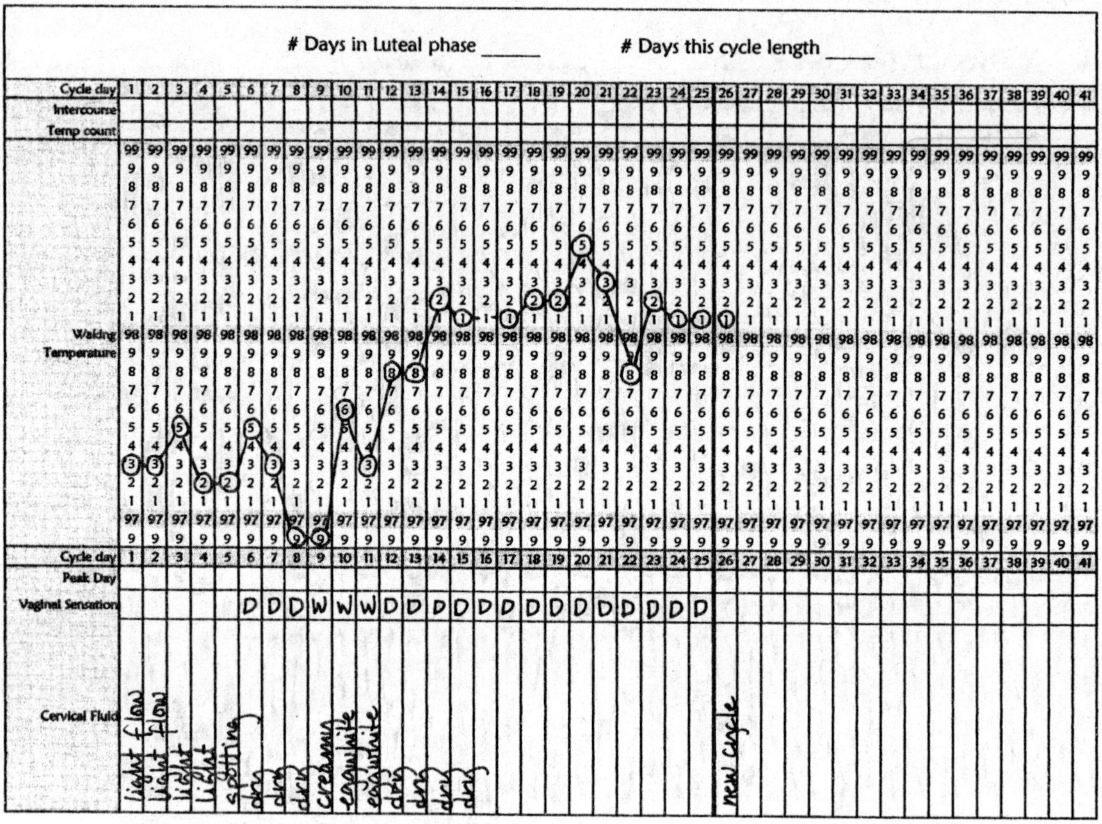

 # Days in Luteal phase _____   **# Days this cycle length** _____

Cycle day	1	2	3	4	5	6	7	8	9	10	11	12	13	14	15	16	17	18	19	20	21	22	23	24	25	26	27	28	29	30	31	32	33	34	35	36	37	38	39	40	41
Intercourse																																										
Temp count																																										

(Waking Temperature grid, Cycle day row, Peak Day row)

| Vaginal Sensation | | | | | | | D | D | D | W | W | W | D | D | D | D | D | D | D | D | D | D | D | D | D | | | | | | | | | | | | | | | | |

Cervical Fluid: light flow, light flow, light, light, spotting, dry, dry, dry, creamy, eggwhite, eggwhite, eggwhite, dry, dry, dry ... new cycle

Figure A.4. Elsa's chart.

She's infertile after 6 P.M. on Days 6, 7, and 8. Her fertile phase begins on Day 9. Her Peak Day is Day 11. Her coverline is at 97.7. By her mucus, her postovulatory infertile phase begins at 6 P.M. on Day 15. By her temperature, her postovulatory infertile phase begins at 6 P.M. on Day 14. To be conservative, she should wait to consider herself infertile until after 6 P.M. on Day 15. Because of the short length of her cycle (twenty-five days), she can consider only the first three days of her period safe for unprotected sex if she wants to prevent pregnancy. Elsa's luteal phase is fourteen days long; her cycle is twenty-five days long.

To conceive, her best days to try in this cycle are Days 9, 10, and 11.

She has eight temperatures below 97.5, indicating possible hypothyroidism.

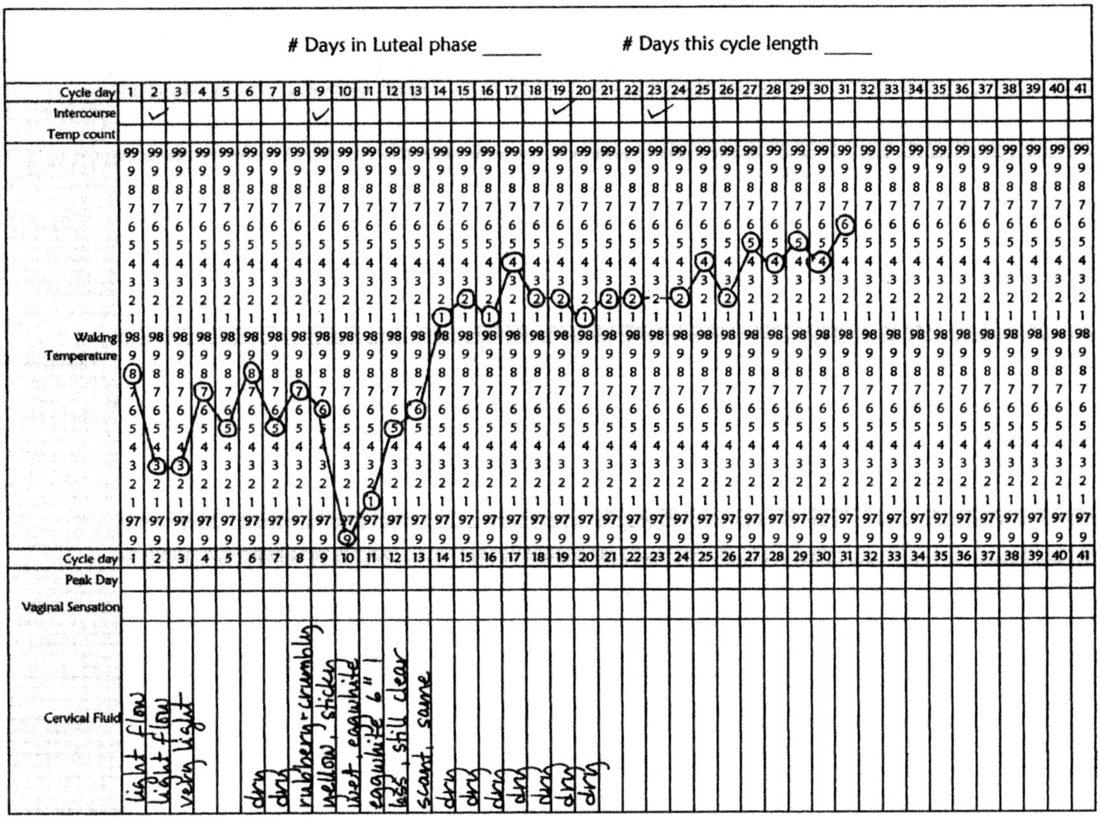

Days in Luteal phase _____   # Days this cycle length _____

Cycle day	1	2	3	4	5	6	7	8	9	10	11	12	13	14	15	16	17	18	19	20	21	22	23	24	25	26	27	28	29	30	31	32	33	34	35	36	37	38	39	40	41
Intercourse		✓							✓										✓				✓																		
Temp count																																									

Waking Temperature (chart grid, values 99 down to 97.9)

Cycle day	1	2	3	4	5	6	7	8	9	10	11	12	13	14	15	16	17	18	19	20	21	22	23	24	25	26	27	28	29	30	31	32	33	34	35	36	37	38	39	40	41

Peak Day

Vaginal Sensation

Cervical Fluid:
light flow, light flow, very light, dry, dry, rubbery-crumbly, yellow/sticky, wet eggwhite, eggwhite 6", less still clear, scant, same, dry, dry, dry, dry, dry, dry

Figure A.5. Linda's chart.

Because she didn't chart her CF on Days 4 and 5, she should consider herself potentially fertile until she observes four days of mucus that are dryer than her Peak Day. Her Peak Day is Day 13, the last (not the most) day of wet mucus. Her coverline is at 97.8. By her mucus, her postovulatory infertile phase begins at 6 P.M. on Day 17. By her temperature, her postovulatory infertile phase begins at 6 P.M. on Day 16. To be conservative, she should wait to consider herself infertile until after 6 P.M. on Day 17.

To conceive, her best days to try are Days 10, 11, 12, and 13.

Linda became pregnant this cycle because of intercourse she had on Day 9, the second day into her fertile phase, four days before she (probably) ovulated. She confirmed the pregnancy on Day 31, with eighteen temperatures above her coverline.

Resources

Fertility Awareness

Dr. Evelyn Billings and Ann Westmore, *The Billings Method: Using the Body's Natural Signal of Fertility to Achieve or Avoid Pregnancy,* Rev., Penguin Books/Australia, 2000. Since the early sixties, Drs. Evelyn and John Billings have dedicated their lives to research and international teaching of the Ovulation Method, which exclusively uses mucus and vulva sensation to determine when a woman is fertile. In the United States, their materials (including *The Billings Method*) can be ordered from the St. Paul office. BOMA-USA, PO Box 16206, St. Paul, MN 16206; 651-699-8139; Web sites: www.boma-usa.org and www.woomb.org.

Elizabeth Clubb, MD, and Jane Knight, *Fertility: Fertility Awareness and Natural Family Planning*, David & Charles, 1997. An excellent presentation of the Sympto-Thermal Method by a British physician and nurse; includes a wonderful chapter on FA during premenopause. Web site: www.fertilityUK.org.

Barbara Kass-Annese, RN, CNP, *Natural Birth Control*, Hunter House, 2003. Barbara has taught and written about Fertility Awareness for twenty-five years.

John and Sheila Kippley, *The Art of Natural Family Planning*, 4th ed., Couple to Couple League, 1996. The guide presents thorough information about how to observe fertility signals to avoid or achieve pregnancy. A Spanish edition is available. Please note that strong Catholic morals are woven throughout the text. Also, the CCL can refer you to a (CCL) teaching couple in your area. Order from the CCL, PO Box 111184, Cincinnati, OH 45211; 513-471-2000; Web site: www.ccli.org.

Toni Weschler, *Taking Charge of Your Fertility*, Rev., Quill, 2001. Where would we be without Toni's book? For anyone who charts, it's a necessary resource. Includes a thorough presentation of reproductive anatomy from the perspective of a Fertility Awareness teacher—and the rules for preventing or achieving pregnancy. Web site: www.TCOYF.com.

Pregnancy, Breast-feeding, and Parenting

The Compleat Mother: The Magazine of Pregnancy, Birth and Breast-feeding. Packed with heartfelt stories and excellent tips for pregnant and breast-feeding women. PO Box 209, Minot, ND 58702; Web site: www.CompleatMother.com. For a similar publication from Britain, check out www.themothermagazine.co.uk.

Thomas Hale, *Medications and Mothers Milk*, Pharmasoft Publishing, 2002. An annually published resource for health-care providers to determine if a medication is safe for nursing mothers; it also provides alternatives.

Kathleen Huggins, RN, MS, *The Nursing Mother's Companion*, 4th ed., Harvard Common Press, 1999. Packed with clearly written, practical suggestions for all sorts of breast-feeding situations and problems.

Sheila Matgen Kippley, *Breast-feeding and Natural Child Spacing*, 4th ed., Couple to Couple League, 1999. Sheila Kippley advocates for breast-feeding, the family bed, daily naps, and allowing the baby to direct weaning. Includes numerous practical tips on delaying or encouraging fertility and stories from nursing mothers.

Sheila Kitzinger, *Breast-feeding Your Baby*, Rev., Knopf, 1999. An excellent how-to, with clear, sympathetic advice and two hundred photographs by Nancy Durrell

McKenna. A comprehensive and wonderfully illustrated book by a widely admired and prolific social anthropologist. Web site: www.sheilakitzinger.com.

Nan Koehler, *Artemesia Speaks: VBAC Stories and Natural Childbirth Information,* Jerald Brown Inc., 1985. VBAC stands for vaginal birth after cesarean section. This book is packed with practical and heartfelt information for anyone preparing for childbirth. It also includes essays by numerous people in the childbearing community on circumcision, children and herbs, vaginitis and herpes, herbal abortion, and more.

Lact-Aid; 423-744-9090; www.lact-aid.com, for women to "nurse" while giving their baby a supplemental feeding. Ideal for women with adopted babies, or those without sufficient breast milk.

La Leche League, the international resource for breast-feeding mothers. Call 847-519-7730 to find a group in your area. Web site: www.lalecheleague.org.

Jean Liedloff, *The Continuum Concept,* Perseus Books, 1975. An anthropologist, Liedloff describes Venezuelan Indians' babies receiving constant physical contact with their mothers (or another familiar caregiver as needed) while the mother goes about her life until the baby is able to crawl, practicing the family bed, and caregivers immediately responding to squirming and crying without making the baby the constant center of attention. An exceptional and provocative book for anyone interested in parenting and human nature. Web site: www.continuum-concept.org.

Barbara Luke and Tamara Eberlein, *When You're Expecting Twins, Triplets or Quads: A Complete Resource,* Quill, 1999.

Mothering Magazine. A fabulous bi-monthly magazine with articles about breast-feeding, the family bed, cloth vs. plastic diapers, circumcision, the connection between autism and vaccines, encouraging children's creativity, and more. *Mothering* advocates fiercely for children's needs and rights while it recognizes parents as the experts, and encourages decision making that considers all members of the family. PO Box 1690, Santa Fe, NM 87504-1690; 800-984-8116; Web site: www.mothering.com.

Meredith F. Small, *Our Babies, Ourselves: How Biology and Culture Shape the Way We Parent,* Anchor Books, 1998. A mother and an anthropologist, Small explores how parenting is often based on cultural tradition, which may run counter to our babies' biological needs. In this context, she considers whether children should be encouraged to sleep alone from an early age, if breast-feeding really is better than bottle-feeding, how to respond to a crying baby, and more.

Sandra Steingraber, *Having Faith: An Ecologist's Journey to Motherhood,* Perseus, 2001. This beautiful book held me like a good novel. Steingraber, a poet and biologist, lovingly describes discovering her pregnancy, giving birth, and breastfeeding while she also attends to her career; these narratives are woven with biological descriptions of the developing baby, the transformation of the mother's body, and the alarming extent to which environmental hazards—from industrial poisons found in amniotic fluid to toxic contamination of breast milk—now threaten each crucial stage of infant development. Steingraber concludes with a call for "the world's feast [to] be made safe for women and children. May mother's milk run clean again. May denial give way to courageous action." Web site: www.steingraber.com.

Tine Thevinin, *The Family Bed: An Age Old Concept in Child Rearing,* Avery, 1987. Thevenin describes the benefits of the family bed, tactfully addresses some parents' hesitations, and also presents a fascinating history of childhood and family sleeping customs.

Kim Toevs and Stephanie Brill, *The Essential Guide to Lesbian Conception, Pregnancy and Birth,* Allyson, 2002.

General Health

Boston Women's Health Book Collective, *Our Bodies, Ourselves for the New Century,* Simon & Schuster, 1998. This book is a bible for women wanting clear information about reproductive anatomy, sexuality, birth control, pregnancy, childbearing losses, menopause, sexually transmitted infections, and more. A Spanish edition, *Nuestros Cuerpos, Nuestras Vidas,* was issued in 2000 by Seven Stories Press. Web site: www.ourbodiesourselves.org.

Bonnie Bainbridge Cohen, *Sensing, Feeling, and Action: The Experiential Anatomy of Body-Mind Centering,* Contact Editions, 1993. Body-Mind Centering (BMC) is an experiential study of the major body systems—skeletal, muscular, fluid, organ, neuroendocrine. A necessary book for anyone who wants to explore anatomy in depth. Web site: www.bodymindcentering.com.

D. Ehling and K. Singer, "Gauging a Woman's Health by Her Fertility Signals: An Introductory Synthesis of Western and Traditional Chinese Medical Principles," *Alternative Therapies* 5(6): 70–83. Also available on www.gardenoffertility.com and www.OrientalHealthSource.com.

Federation of Feminist Women's Health Centers, *A New View of a Woman's Body,* Feminist Health Press, 1995. An indispensable guide to female anatomy, illustrated by

Suzann Gage, L Ac, RNC, NP (whose drawings grace this book, too); it presents self-exam and self-help techniques. Order from Feminist Health Press, 8240 Santa Monica Blvd., Los Angeles, CA 90046; Web site: www.womenshealthspecialists.org.

Stephen Langer, M.D., and James Scheer, *Solved: The Riddle of Illness—Your Amazing Thyroid and How You Can Work with It*, Keats Publishing, 2000.

Lennart Nilsson, *A Child Is Born: New Photographs of Life Before Birth*, Dell, 1977. Nilsson was the first to photograph a live fetus in the womb.

Mary J. Shomon, *Living Well with Hypothyroidism*, Quill, 2000. Written by a hypothyroid patient, this excellent book is packed with info about the symptoms, diagnoses, and (conventional and alternative) treatments for thyroid imbalances.

Elizabeth Lee Vliet, MD, *Screaming to Be Heard: Hormonal Connections Women Suspect and Doctors Still Ignore*, Rev., Evans, 2000. Describes how estrogen, progesterone, and other hormones affect your heart, bladder, metabolism, sleep, pain regulation, and more.

Sexually Transmitted Infections

American Social Health Association (ASHA) operates hot lines and publishes numerous materials. Several of their publications, including *Questions and Answers About Chlamydia, PID, Herpes* (etc.) are available for free. Their National Herpes Hotline operates Monday through Friday, 9 A.M. to 7 P.M., EST, at no charge: 919-361-8488. PO Box 13827, Research Triangle Park, NC 27709; 919-361-8400; Web site: http://sunsite.unc.edu/ASHA.

Planned Parenthood: www.plannedparenthood.org. Your local office is listed in the White and Yellow Pages.

Project Inform is a nationwide referral organization for HIV/AIDS treatment. 1965 Market St., San Francisco, CA 94103; 415-558-8669; Treatment Hotline: 800-822-7422; Web site: www.projinfo.org.

The Safer Sex Page!: www.safersex.org.

STIs: www.igc.apc.org/ppfa/stis/sti_facts_main.html offers factual info on STIs.

Healing Childbearing Losses

Ellen Bass and Laura Davis, *The Courage to Heal: A Guide for Women Survivors of Child Sexual Abuse*, 3rd ed., HarperPerennial, 1994. A comprehensive guide offering hope and encouragement to every woman who was sexually abused as a child— and to those who care about her.

Compassionate Friends offers friendship and understanding for bereaved families who have lost a child of any age to any cause of death. PO Box 3696, Oak Brooke, IL 60522; 877-969-0010; Web site: www.compassionatefriends.org.

The Federation for Children with Special Needs, based in Boston, provides networking and training for families with children with special needs. 617-236-7210; Web site: www.fcsn.org.

Bert Hellinger, Gunthard Weber, and Hunter Beaumont, *Love's Hidden Symmetry: What Makes Love Work in Relationships,* Zeig, Tucker, 1998. In his books and videos (available through Zeig, Tucker), Hellinger addresses abortion, adoption, artificial insemination, incest, serious illness, and more. His provocative work aims to create a family dynamic that supports the flow of love. I've found Hellinger's work challenging, clarifying, and healing. Web site: www.Hellinger.com.

Byron Katie with Stephen Mitchell, *Loving What Is,* Harmony Books, 2002. Called inquiry, or The Work of Byron Katie, the tool offered here provides a way to become the teacher or healer you've been waiting for. The audio presentations are especially potent. Web site: www.TheWork.org.

Claudia Panuthos and Cathy Romeo, *Ended Beginnings: Healing Childbearing Losses,* Bergin & Garvey, 1984. This timeless book presents practical and loving suggestions and first-person narratives for healing from all kinds of childbearing losses, including miscarriage, abortion, release to adoption, stillbirth, and traumatic delivery.

Niravi Payne, *The Whole Person Fertility Program: A Revolutionary Mind-Body Process to Help You Conceive,* Three Rivers, 1998. Payne explains how generationally held family beliefs and behavior patterns can affect fertility and presents techniques for discovering and working through psychological barriers to conceiving and carrying a baby to term.

Nancy Verrier, *The Primal Wound: Legacy of the Adopted Child,* Gateway Press, 1991. Calling on her experiences as an adoptive mother and therapist, Verrier describes the unique challenges of children who lose their mothers at birth. Website: www.primalwound.com.

RESOLVE, 1310 Broadway, Somerville, MA 02144; 617-623-0744; Web site: www.resolve.org.

Herbs, Homeopathy, and Oriental Medicine

Harriet Beinfield and Efram Korngold, *Between Heaven and Earth: A Guide to Chinese Medicine*, Random House, 1992. Explains the philosophy behind Chinese medicine, how it works, and what it can do.

Miranda Castro, *Homeopathy for Pregnancy, Birth and Your Baby's First Year*, St. Martin's, 1993.

Rosemary Gladstar, *Herbal Healing for Women*, Fireside, 1993. A classic presentation of how to make herbal teas, salves, pills, and tinctures to address PMS, skin problems, endometriosis, vaginal infections, pregnancy, and menopause. Gladstar founded United Plant Savers, a nonprofit organization dedicated to the conservation and cultivation of at-risk medicinal plants. Web sites: www.plantsavers.org and www.traffic.org/news/medicinal_plants.html.

James Green, *The Male Herbal*, Crossing Press, 1991. Green's book includes a wealth of natural remedies for men, including specific herbs for addressing low sperm count and low sperm motility, impotence, and descriptions of how diabetes, hypothyroidism, and other conditions can affect male fertility. Green also lists other books that address male sexuality and fertility naturally.

Ted Kaptchuk, OMD, *The Web That Has No Weaver*, Contemporary Books, 2000. A comprehensive guide to the theory and practice of Chinese medicine.

Deborah Soule, *The Woman's Book of Herbs*, Citadel Press, 1998. Lovingly written. Includes attention to lesbian health. Order herbal remedies, books about herbs, and take classes at Soule's farm. Avena Botanicals, 20 Mill St., Rockland, ME 04841; Web site: www.avenaherbs.com.

Dana Ullman, *Homeopathy: Medicine for the Twenty-first Century*, North Atlantic Books, 1988. Strong overall book about homeopathy and how to use it for acute problems.

Susun Weed, *Wise Woman Herbal for the Childbearing Year*, Ash Tree Publishing, 1985. A classic. *New Menopausal Years the Wise Woman Way: Alternative Approaches for Women 30–90* was published in 2002. Along with the Six Steps of Healing, this book presents remedies for menstrual cramps, thyroid problems, vaginal dryness, fertility after forty, and much, much more. Website: www.susunweed.com.

Night-Lighting

Joy DeFelice, RN, BSN, PHN, *The Effects of Light on the Menstrual Cycle: Also Infertility*, 2000. Based on twenty-seven years of clinical research, DeFelice's booklet includes a bibliography of studies and books about the effects of darkness and artificial light on human health. Order from the Couple to Couple League, 513-471-2000.

Louise Lacey, *Lunaception: A Feminine Odyssey into Fertility and Contraception,* Coward, McCann & Geoghegan, 1975. This fascinating story is no longer in print, but a revised edition should be available in 2004. For details, write Louise Lacey, PO Box 489, Berkeley, CA 94701.

Gay Gaer Luce, *Biological Rhythms in Human and Animal Physiology,* Dover, 1971. Citing hundreds of scientific studies, Luce presents a survey of everything known about biological rhythms as of 1970, including chapters on food and stress (within the compass of a day), dreams, the rhythm of various illnesses, newborns and sleep, work-rest schedules, the impact of light, and much, much more. A necessary book for anyone who wants to know more about biological rhythms and light.

John Ott, *Health and Light: The Effects of Natural and Artificial Light on Man and Other Living Things,* Pocket Books, 1976. A banker who developed his hobby of time-lapse photography into a full-time career in photobiology, Ott explains that light is a nutrient. Like food, the wrong kind of light can make us ill, while the right kind can cure many ills. For example, sunglasses may provoke illness and eye disease; fluorescent lighting can create fatigue and hyperactivity; arthritis can respond to a treatment of full-spectrum light.

Jane Wegscheider Hyman, *The Light Book: How Natural and Artificial Light Affect Our Health, Mood, and Behavior,* Tarcher, 1990. This excellent book explains circadian rhythms and how sleep, fertility, eating disorders, alcoholism, and depression can all be linked to light.

Food and Reproductive Health

Kaayla T. Daniel, *The Whole Soy Story,* New Trends, 2004. A devastating description of why farmers have gone from producing virtually no soybeans in 1900 to hundreds of millions of tons annually; and a thorough report on the studies that indicate the dangers of soy products to basic and reproductive health. Website: www.thewholesoystory.com.

Sally Fallon, *Nourishing Traditions,* New Trends Publishing, 1999. Based on the research of Weston A. Price, this book explains why nutrient-dense foods are necessary for women before conception, during pregnancy, and while breast-feeding. Packed with great recipes, a chapter on feeding babies, and recipes for feeding those who don't nurse. Can be ordered from www.RadiantLifeCatalog.com; 888-

593-8333; or www.westonaprice.org; PMB 106-380, 4200 Wisconsin Ave., NW, Washington, DC 20016; 202-333-HEAL.

FAO. Web site: www.FAO.org. Presents UN–funded studies on food and agriculture.

www.farmedanddangerous.org. Explains the hazards of farmed salmon to personal health and wild ecosystems.

Susan Kano, *Making Peace with Food,* HarperCollins, 1989. Presents a method for overcoming compulsive eating, chronic dieting, yo-yoing weight, food and body anxieties; advice for loved ones who want to help, and workbook pages.

Mercedes Lee, ed., *Seafood Lover's Almanac,* Audubon's Living Ocean Programs, 2000. This exceptionally beautiful book is packed with info about the health benefits of seafood, how specific fish are caught or farmed, how (given the high level of pollution in our waterways) individual species are doing, and alternative choices to species in trouble. A must-read for seafood lovers. Website: www.blueoceaninstitute.org.

The Price-Pottenger Nutrition Foundation. Francis Pottenger, an MD, studied the effects of giving several generations of cats pasteurized and unpasteurized (raw) milk and cooked and uncooked meats. The cats that ate raw milk and meat thrived and had sweet dispositions; the cats that ate cooked (pasteurized) milk and meat were sickly and had aggressive dispositions. The Foundation provides educational materials about Pottenger's and Weston Price's work. PO Box 2614, La Mesa, CA 91943-2614; 619-462-7600; Web site: www.price-pottenger.org.

www.rawmilk.org; www.realmilk.com. These sites speak to the hazards of pasteurization and homogenization and the benefits of raw milk.

Marilyn Shannon, *Fertility, Cycles and Nutrition,* 3rd ed., Couple to Couple League, 2001. Shannon explains how anovulation, frequent miscarriage, hypothyroidism, vaginal infections, male infertility, and more can be remedied through improved nutrition and vitamin supplements.

Krispin Sullivan, *Naked at Noon: Understanding Sunlight and Vitamin D,* Basic Health Publishing, 2003. A nutritionist and researcher, Sullivan explains the necessity of vitamin D, how it affects overall and reproductive health, and how it's available only from sunlight and certain animal foods (such as cod liver oil, lard, herring, butter, and eggs). Sullivan's article in *Wise Traditions'* Fall 2000 issue, "The Miracle of Vitamin D," is an excellent introduction to this material. Website: www.krispin.com.

www.truefoodnow.com. Presented by Greenpeace, this website offers information about the hazards of genetically modified (GM) foods, a list of products that contain them, and suggestions for lobbying for better testing and labeling of GM foods.

Union of Concerned Scientists. The Union's Food and the Environment program addresses numerous issues including the overuse of antibiotics in agriculture. 2 Brattle Square, Cambridge, MA 02238; Web site: www.ucsusa.org.

Wise Traditions in Food, Farming, and the Healing Arts. This excellent quarterly includes accessible articles about treating various ailments with sound nutrition, ecological and nutritional farming practices, the benefits of raw milk, the hazards of soy, and more. Each issue (and the website) includes a list of chapters that can help you find locally and organically grown meat, dairy products, and produce, as well as farmers who ship. Weston A. Price Foundation, PMB 106-380, 4200 Wisconsin Ave., NW, Washington, DC 20016; 202-333-4325; Web site: www. WestonAPrice.org.

Reproductive Technology

Gay Becker, *The Elusive Embryo: How Women and Men Approach New Reproductive Technologies,* University of California Press, 2000. An exceptional (and readable) anthropological study based on hundreds of interviews about being named "infertile" and not feeling normal because of not conceiving quickly. The book presents women's and men's psychological and physical experiences when reproductive technologies do and don't work. I consider this book a must for anyone considering fertility treatment. Website: www.ucpress.edu/books/pages/9014.html.

Susan Martha Kahn, *Reproducing Jews: A Cultural Account of Assisted Conception in Israel,* Duke University Press, 2000. Israel has more fertility clinics per capita than any other country in the world and the highest per capita rate of in-vitro fertilization procedures. Fertility treatments are fully subsidized by national health insurance and available to all Israelis. Kahn's book is an amazing ethnographic study of the Israeli embrace of reproductive technologies.

Judith Turiel, *Beyond Second Opinions: Making Choices About Fertility Treatment,* University of California Press, 1998. Turiel, a consumer-health activist and a veteran herself of fertility treatments, exposes the risks, errors, and distortions surrounding fertility medicine. Her book provides hard data on diagnostic methods and treatments. If you are considering reproductive technology to help you conceive a child, please read this book first. Website: www.ucpress.edu/books/pages/6983.html.

Common Products That Can Be Hazardous to Reproductive Health

Lindsey Berkson, *Hormone Deception: How Everyday Foods and Products Can Disrupt Your Hormones—and How to Protect Yourself and Your Family,* Contemporary Books, 2000. Explains how common items like plastic, paint, soap, and pesticides can disrupt men's and women's hormones; and how to reduce your exposure to harmful chemicals. Berkson is a DES daughter, and her observations and resources about this (still used) drug are also part of her excellent book. Web site: www.HormoneDeception.com.

The Bioneers. This organization includes activists, scientists, entrepreneurs, farmers, and prophets with a vision of the future guided by the principles of nature, kinship, interdependence, cooperation, and community. The Bioneers host an awesome annual national conference, radio shows, and more. 901 W. San Mateo, Suite L, Santa Fe, NM 87505; 877-246-6337; Web site: www.bioneers.org.

Chemical Injury Information Network. Publishes *Our Toxic Times,* an excellent newsletter for people with chemically induced immune system disorders—and for those who aim to prevent the release of more toxic chemicals to our earth, air, and waterways. PO Box 301, White Sulphur Springs, MT 59645; Web site: www. ciin.org.

Theo Colborn, Dianne Dumanoski, and John Peterson Myers, *Our Stolen Future,* Plume, 1997. Picking up where Rachel Carson's 1962 *Silent Spring* left off, this groundbreaking and gripping book traces birth defects, sexual abnormalities, and reproductive failures in wildlife to their source: synthetic chemicals that mimic natural hormones. The book includes studies that show that sperm counts have decreased internationally as much as 50 percent in recent decades. Website: www.ourstolenfuture.com.

Debra Lynn Dadd, *Home Safe Home: Protecting Yourself and Your Family from Everyday Toxics and Harmful Household Products,* Tarcher, 1997. Filled with hundreds of tips for making or buying inexpensive, safe products to replace the harmful ones we may be exposed to—for everything from washing windows and clothes to toys, art supplies, and pet products. Dadd is also the author of *Nontoxic, Natural & Earthwise* and *The Nontoxic Home & Office.*

Environmental Causes of Infertility looks at studies concerning miscarriage and/or infertility due to environmental factors. Website: www.chem-tox.com/infertility/.

Kim Erickson, *Drop-Dead Gorgeous: Protecting Yourself from the Hidden Dangers of Cosmetics,* Contemporary Books, 2002. Reveals the dangers of common over-the-counter beauty products, shows how to read and interpret misleading product labels, and offers recipes for creating your own cosmetics at home.

Health Care Without Harm (HCWH). This international coalition focuses on reducing the environmental impact of the health-care industry. HCWH works to phase out PVC (polyvinyl chloride) plastic, which creates hormone-disrupting carcinogenic chemicals when it's made and burned and also leaches toxic phthalates during use. 1755 S St., NW, Suite 6B, Washington, DC 20009; 202-234-0091; www.noharm.org.

Barbara Seaman, *The Greatest Experiment Ever Performed on Women: Exploding the Estrogen Myth,* Hyperion, 2003. Since the 1950s, researchers have known about the harmful effects of hormone therapy, and yet estrogen continues to be prescribed. A cofounder of the National Women's Health Network, Seaman has shed light on the hazards of the Pill since the late sixties. Here she illuminates today's "menopause industry."

For Kids and Teenagers

Ruth Bell and members of the Teen Book Project, *Changing Bodies, Changing Lives,* 3rd ed., Times Books, 1998. Coauthored by members of the Boston Women's Health Book Collective, this outstanding book includes chapters called "Changing Bodies, Changing Relationships," "Changing Sexuality," "Emotional Health Care," "Eating Disorders," "Sexually Transmitted Diseases," "Safer Sex and Birth Control," and "So You Think You Might Be Pregnant."

Robie Harris and Michael Ember, *It's So Amazing: A Book About Eggs, Sperm, Birth, Babies and Families,* Candlewick Press, 2002. In a reassuring tone, this book provides clear, accurate answers to nearly every conceivable question and encourages children to have a healthy understanding of their bodies. Harris and Ember also wrote *It's Perfectly Normal: Changing Bodies, Growing Up, Sex and Sexual Health,* for ages ten and up.

Ellen Evert Hopman, *Walking the World in Wonder: A Children's Herbal,* Healing Arts Press, 2000. A lovely book that introduces the medicinal and magical aspects of sixty-seven common herbs, color photos for identification, simple recipes for treating minor ailments, and more. Ages five to ten.

Catherine Paladino, *One Good Apple: Growing Our Food for the Sake of the Earth,* Houghton Mifflin, 1999. A beautiful book that explains what happens to an apple grown with pesticides and waxed for market—and how farm workers, consumers, and the environment are affected. Organic farms are presented as habitats for wildlife. The book also includes an excellent list of ideas for helping grow good food, including apprenticing at an organic farm and making compost. Ages ten and up.

Eric Schlosser, *Fast Food Nation*, Perennial, 2001. Schlosser outlines the economic structure of the fast-food business, then describes what really goes into those famous cheeseburgers and tacos. I recently met a teenager who was reading this book for a course requirement, and he was *riveted*.

Lesley Tierra, *A Kid's Herb Book*, Robert Reed Publishers, 2000. Connecting with the earth through herbs is a great way for children of all ages to begin learning the principles of Fertility Awareness. This lovely book explains differences between herbs and weeds; gives recipes for making flower vinegar, compost, and simple medicinal teas; lists novels for kids who love herbs; and more. Tierra and her husband, Michael, are well-known herbalists who've written for adults as well. Website: www.planetherbs.com.

Glossary

Amenorrhea. Prolonged absence of menstruation (and ovulation). While this is normal and healthy among women who are pregnant, breast-feeding, or menopausal, amenorrhea can also be caused by a metabolic disorder (such as diabetes, malnutrition, or obesity); emotional disorders (such as anorexia); endocrine disorders (including problems of the pituitary, thyroid, and adrenal glands); and hormonal contraceptives..

Anovulation. Lack of ovulation.

Arousal fluid. Lubricates the woman so that intercourse is not painful; produced by a sweat of the vaginal walls. Though it may look and feel like cervical fluid, it can't nourish or provide a conduit for sperm.

Assisted reproductive technology (ART). Used to enhance a woman's chance of conceiving or carrying a pregnancy to term with drugs and/or surgeries—in vitro fertilization (IVF), for example.

Barrier method. A contraceptive device that prevents sperm from reaching a ripe egg by creating a physical barrier—e.g., a condom, diaphragm, or cervical cap.

Basal body temperature (BBT). The waking temperature, before activity begins.

Basic infertile pattern (BIP). A pattern of dry or sticky mucus that does not change. It typically indicates low estrogen levels and anovulation.

Breakthrough bleeding. Bleeding that occurs in the absence of ovulation, caused by insufficient estrogen or an unfavorably high ratio of progesterone to estrogen.

Cervical fluid (CF). Produced in the crypts of the cervix, it can nourish sperm for up to five days, filter out impaired sperm, and provide a conduit for sperm to swim to the ripe egg at ovulation.

Cervical mucus. Another name for cervical fluid.

Cervix. The base of the uterus that extends slightly into the vaginal canal. Its crypts produce cervical fluid. Through its os (opening), menstrual blood (and babies) pass through to the vaginal canal.

Chlamydia. A prevalent sexually transmitted infection that can scar the fallopian tubes and cause infertility.

Cilia. The hairlike lining of the fallopian tubes, which moves the fertilized egg toward the uterus.

Clitoris. Comparable to the glans of the penis, it's the organ of female orgasm, located inside the clitoral hood, where the lips of the vagina join.

Clomid. An ovulation-enhancing drug that binds to estrogen receptors in the brain, so that more estrogen is produced and more eggs are matured in a given menstrual cycle.

Conception. When egg and sperm unite, usually in the outer edge of a fallopian tube.

Conceptus. The fertilized egg, implanted in the uterine lining; not yet an embryo or a fetus.

Corpus luteum. The sac that, having released a ripe egg, remains in the ovary after ovulation and secretes progesterone for about twelve to sixteen days. With its demise, a new menstrual cycle begins. If pregnancy occurs, the corpus luteum will live for three months, at which time the placenta takes over production of progesterone.

Coverline. The line drawn to confirm ovulation and distinguish a cycle's pre-ovulatory and postovulatory phases, based on the BBT.

Cowper's glands. Located below the prostate, these two glands secrete lubricative, pre-ejaculatory fluid.

Crypts. The parts of the cervix that produce cervical fluid.

Cyst. An abnormal sac containing fluids or semisolids; it does not dissolve. While most cysts are benign and cause no discomfort, they can be cancerous.

Depo-Provera. An injectable hormonal contraceptive that lasts three months.

Donor insemination (also called *alternative* or *artificial insemination*). When donor's sperm is inserted into (or just outside) the cervix by a syringe.

Dry Day Rule. A rule for preventing pregnancy by charting observations of cervical fluid and vaginal sensation. It states that after the period, a woman who does not want to conceive is safe for unprotected intercourse after 6 P.M. if she has observed dry CF and dry vaginal sensation throughout the day.

Ejaculation. The penis' release of seminal fluid during orgasm.

Embryo. Developmental stage that begins shortly after fertilization until around week eight.

Endocrine system. The hormone-producing glandular system.

Endocrinologist. An MD who specializes in the glandular, hormonal system.

Endometriosis. Growth of tissue in areas other than the uterus, such as the fallopian tubes or ovaries. It may create pain during menstruation, pain during intercourse, or long periods.

Endometrium. The uterine lining, which is shed (if pregnancy does not occur) when the corpus luteum dies and menstruation begins, about two weeks after ovulation. Pregnancy occurs when the conceptus implants in the endometrium.

Epididymis. Attached to the testicles, the duct in the scrotum where sperm are matured and stored, and from which they are transported to the vas deferens.

Estrogen. Primarily produced in the ovaries, the hormone that dominates the pre-ovulatory phase of the menstrual cycle. Among other things, estrogen causes the crypts to produce cervical fluid; the body's waking temperature to cool; and the cervix to soften, open, and rise.

Fallopian tubes. A pair of tubes connected to either side of the uterus. A ripe egg is fertilized in a tube's outer third; the conceptus then travels down the tube toward the uterus for implantation (pregnancy).

Ferning. Fertile cervical mucus contains high levels of estrogen; when dried on a glass slide, it looks like the leaves of a fern plant.

Fertile phase. The days of the menstrual cycle during which cervical fluid is produced and capable of keeping sperm alive.

Fetus. Medical name for the developing human from three months after conception until birth.

Fimbria. The fingers of the fallopian tubes.

Follicle. A sac that surrounds an oocyte through to its development as an ovum.

Follicle-stimulating hormone (FSH). Secreted by the pituitary gland, FSH stimulates follicles (unripe eggs) to ripen in an ovary. In men, FSH regulates sperm formation in the testicles.

Follicular phase. The menstrual cycle's pre-ovulatory phase, when estrogen is dominant.

Hormone. A messenger secreted by one gland and received by another; it travels through the blood.

Human chorionic gonadotropin (HCG). The only hormone that healthy men and women don't have in common. Once a woman becomes pregnant (the conceptus implants in her uterine lining), HCG is activated and signals the corpus luteum to continue producing progesterone to sustain the pregnancy. Pregnancy tests test for the presence of HCG.

Hyperthyroidism. A condition where the thyroid is overactive, which typically manifests in high temperatures, difficulty conceiving, etc.

Hypothyroidism. A condition where the thyroid is underactive, or sluggish, which typically manifests in low temperatures, mild depression, unexplained weight gain, low energy, difficulty conceiving, etc.

In vitro fertilization (IVF). A medical procedure in which a woman is given a fertility drug to increase her production of mature eggs, these eggs are "harvested" through surgery, then mixed with her partner's (or a donor's) sperm in a petri dish. Two days later, fertilized eggs are surgically implanted in her uterus.

Kegel exercises. Involve contracting and relaxing of the vaginal muscles. Kegels can strengthen the pelvic floor in preparation for childbirth; they can also push semen out of the vagina after intercourse.

Labia. The lips to the vagina.

Lactational amenorrhea. Lack of ovulation and menstruation due to breast-feeding.

Libido. Sex drive.

Lunaception. Based on experiments conducted by John Rock, MD, and developed by Louise Lacey, a method of encouraging regular, ovulatory cycles wherein a woman sleeps in the absence of light on all but three nights each cycle.

Luteal phase. The postovulatory phase of a menstrual cycle, dominated by progesterone, and normally lasting twelve to sixteen days. It begins on the first day of
the thermal shift; it ends on the day before menstruation begins.

Luteal phase deficiency (LPD). When, in a given cycle, a woman's luteal (postovulatory) phase is eleven days long or less. This signals that she may have difficulty
becoming pregnant or sustaining a pregnancy because of low progesterone
levels.

Luteinizing hormone (LH). Released by the pituitary gland, it causes ovulation and
transformation of the follicle into a corpus luteum.

Menopause. When a woman has not menstruated or ovulated for a year or longer;
usually begins around age fifty.

Menstruation. Cyclic shedding of the endometrium, about two weeks after ovulation.

Mittelschmerz. Pain in the lower abdomen felt by some women around the time of
ovulation.

Mucus. Another name for cervical fluid.

Night-lighting. The absence or presence of any light while sleeping, which can affect the menstrual cycle, emotional wellness, and other aspects of health.

Norplant. A contraceptive in which six matchstick-size hormone-releasing capsules
are inserted under the skin of a woman's upper arm to prevent pregnancy for
five years.

Oocyte. An unripe egg.

Oral contraceptive (OC). The Pill.

Os. An opening, as the cervical os is the opening to the uterus.

Ovarian cyst. A follicle that began maturing but did not disintegrate or release a
ripe egg, and then forms a fluid-filled cyst on the ovarian wall.

Ovulation. The release of a ripe ovum (egg) by an ovarian follicle; the egg is typically taken by the fimbria into the outer edge of the fallopian tube. Ten percent
of the time, women release two eggs at ovulation. This is still considered one
ovulation: a woman ovulates only once each cycle.

Ovum. A mature, ripe egg. Ova is the plural form of ovum.

Oxytocin. The hormone released to letdown breastmilk and to activate an orgasm.

Peak Day. The *last* day of slippery mucus or wet vaginal sensation in a given cycle.

Peak Day Rule. A woman can confirm ovulation and consider herself infertile after
6 P.M. of the fourth day of mucus that is dryer than her Peak Day mucus.

Period. Cyclic bleeding that results from shedding the uterine lining after ovulation.

Phytoestrogen. A plant-based estrogen (*phyto* means plant).

Pituitary gland. The master gland, located in the brain, which produces many hormones, including FSH and LH.

Placenta. The sac that nourishes the growing baby in the womb.

Polycystic ovarian syndrome (PCOS). A common disorder whereby developing follicles remain trapped in the ovary and later become cysts. Thought to be related to insulin-resistance.

Pre-ejaculate. A small amount of fluid that the penis releases when aroused, before ejaculation, to provide lubrication for lovemaking. It can contain enough sperm to cause a pregnancy or an STI.

Pregnancy. When a fertilized egg implants in the uterine lining, about five to seven days after conception.

Progesterone. This hormone dries up cervical fluid, raises a woman's temperature, firms and lowers the cervix in the vaginal canal, closes the os, and prepares the uterine lining (the endometrium) for possible pregnancy. Progesterone is secreted by the corpus luteum; around the third month of pregnancy, it's secreted by the placenta.

Progesterone deficiency. Low progesterone levels. This can lead to menstrual cramps, miscarriage, and menopause problems. Progesterone also contributes to bone building, a balanced libido, efficient fat burning, and more.

Prolactin. The hormone that stimulates production of breastmilk and inhibits estrogen production.

Prolactinemia. In a non-nursing woman, elevated levels of prolactin, the hormone that causes production of breastmilk and can inhibit ovulation

Prostate gland. Located at the base of the male bladder, its secretions form a significant portion of seminal fluid.

Qi. Chinese term for the body's life force or essence.

Reproductive endocrinologist (RE). An MD who specializes in reproductive hormones.

Rhythm Method. Also called the Calendar Method, an unreliable method of natural family planning determined by the lengths of previous cycles.

Scrotum. The pouch that carries the testicles.

Semen. The fluid ejaculated from the penis during orgasm, comprised of sperm and secretions from the seminal vesicles and the prostate gland.

Seminal fluid. The fluid ejaculated from the penis during orgasm, without sperm (as when a man has a vasectonomy).

Sexually transmitted infection (STI). An infection that is transmitted through sexual contact, such as HIV, chlamydia, gonorrhea, or herpes.

Split peak. Occurs when the body prepares to ovulate (demonstrated by a buildup of mucus, a Peak Day, and drying up of mucus), but ovulation can't be confirmed by a temperature shift. Mucus then builds up again, with or without ovulation. Split peaks are normal and healthy while breast-feeding and/or shortly after weaning. Among non-nursing women, frequent split peaks can indicate a propensity for polycystic ovarian syndrome (PCOS).

Temperature Shift Rule. When a woman has three consecutive temperatures above her coverline, she can confirm ovulation.

Ultrasound. A diagnostic technique that uses sound waves (not X-rays), to see inside the body.

Unambiguous infertility. Infertility achieved after childbirth as a result of frequent nursing, characterized by dry cervical fluid and dry vaginal sensation.

Uterine lining. See *endometrium.*

Uterus. A sterile muscle, shaped like an upside-down pear. A fertilized egg implants in its lining for pregnancy. The uterus's muscular contractions push the baby out through the birth canal during labor.

Vagina. The muscular canal that extends from the cervix to the vulva.

Vaginal sensation. Sometimes described as *vulva sensation,* it's charted as being wet or dry to help determine when a woman is in a fertile or infertile phase.

Vas deferens. A pair of tubes that carry sperm from the testicles to the urethra. They're snipped for a vasectomy.

Vulva. The external female genitalia, including the labia (lips), the clitoris, and the vagina's opening.

Withdrawal bleeding. Bleeding that occurs in the absence of ovulation.

Blank Charts

The following charts can be enlarged and photocopied. They can also be down-loaded from www.gardenoffertility.com.

Fertility Cycle #_____

Start Date _____   # Days in Luteal phase _____   # Days this cycle length _____

Cycle day	1	2	3	4	5	6	7	8	9	10	11	12	13	14	15	16	17	18	19	20	21	22	23	24	25	26	27	28	29	30	31	32	33	34	35	36	37	38	39	40	41
Date																																									
Intercourse																																									
Time Temp Taken																																									
Temp count																																									

(Waking Temperature grid: rows from 99 down to 97, repeated across cycle days 1–41)

Cycle day	1	2	3	4	5	6	7	8	9	10	11	12	13	14	15	16	17	18	19	20	21	22	23	24	25	26	27	28	29	30	31	32	33	34	35	36	37	38	39	40	41
Peak Day																																									
Vaginal Sensation																																									
Cervix																																									
Cervical Fluid																																									

Cervix legend: F M S

Cycle day	1	2	3	4	5	6	7	8	9	10	11	12	13	14	15	16	17	18	19	20	21	22	23	24	25	26	27	28	29	30	31	32	33	34	35	36	37	38	39	40	41
Miscellaneous:																																									

Low-Temperature Chart

Fertility Cycle #_____

Start Date _____   # Days in Luteal phase _____   # Days this cycle length _____

Cycle day	1	2	3	4	5	6	7	8	9	10	11	12	13	14	15	16	17	18	19	20	21	22	23	24	25	26	27	28	29	30	31	32	33	34	35	36	37	38	39	40	41
Date																																									
Intercourse																																									
Time Temp Taken																																									
Temp count																																									

Waking Temperature

(temperature grid chart)

Cycle day	1	2	3	4	5	6	7	8	9	10	11	12	13	14	15	16	17	18	19	20	21	22	23	24	25	26	27	28	29	30	31	32	33	34	35	36	37	38	39	40	41

Peak Day

Vaginal Sensation

Cervix ● o O   F M S

Cervical Fluid

EGG BROWN

BSE

Cycle day	1	2	3	4	5	6	7	8	9	10	11	12	13	14	15	16	17	18	19	20	21	22	23	24	25	26	27	28	29	30	31	32	33	34	35	36	37	38	39	40	41

Miscellaneous:

Celsius Chart

Fertility Cycle #_____

Start Date _____   # Days in Luteal phase _____   # Days this cycle length _____

Cycle day	1	2	3	4	5	6	7	8	9	10	11	12	13	14	15	16	17	18	19	20	21	22	23	24	25	26	27	28	29	30	31	32	33	34	35	36	37	38	39	40	41
Date																																									
Intercourse																																									
Time Temp Taken																																									
Temp count																																									

Waking Temperature (scale repeated across all days): 10, 5, 37, 95, 90, 85, 80, 75, 70, 65, 60, 55, 50, 45, 40, 35, 30, 25, 20, 15, 10, 5, 36, 95, 90

Cycle day	1	2	3	4	5	6	7	8	9	10	11	12	13	14	15	16	17	18	19	20	21	22	23	24	25	26	27	28	29	30	31	32	33	34	35	36	37	38	39	40	41
Peak Day																																									
Vaginal Sensation																																									
Cervix ● ○ ◯ / F M S																																									
Cervical Fluid																																									

(BSE noted at cycle day 7)

Cycle day	1	2	3	4	5	6	7	8	9	10	11	12	13	14	15	16	17	18	19	20	21	22	23	24	25	26	27	28	29	30	31	32	33	34	35	36	37	38	39	40	41
Miscellaneous:																																									

Endnotes

Introduction

1. Marshack, Alexander, *The Roots of Civilization: The Cognitive Beginnings of Man's First Art, Symbol, and Notation,* McGraw-Hill, 1972.

2. *The Lunar Calendar,* Luna Press, PO Box 15511, Kenmore Station, Boston, MA 02215-0009; www.thelunapress.com.

3. Mucharski, Jan, *History of the Biologic Control of Human Fertility,* Married Life Information, 1982.

4. "Doctors Prescribe New Methods to Eliminate Women's Periods," by Tara Parker-Pope, *The Wall Street Journal,* June 25, 2002.

Chapter 1. A Woman Is Like the Earth: Reproductive Anatomy and Physiology

1. Reid, Daniel P., *The Tao of Health, Sex & Longevity: A Modern Practical Guide to the Ancient Way,* Fireside, 1989.
2. Green, James, *The Male Herbal,* The Crossing Press, 1991.
3. Winkler, Gershon, *Sacred Secrets: The Sanctity of Sex in Jewish Law and Lore,* Jason Aronson, 1998.
4. Engel, Cindy, *Wild Health,* Houghton Mifflin, 2002.
5. Steingraber, Sandra, *Having Faith,* Perseus, 2001.
6. "Older bull elephants control young males: orphaned male adolescents go on killing sprees if mature males aren't around," *Nature,* November 23, 2000.
7. Line, Les, "onepicture," *Audubon,* May–June 2001.
8. Engel, *Wild Health,* Houghton Mifflin, 2002.
9. Steingraber, *Having Faith,* Perseus, 2001.
10. Masson, Jeffrey Moussaieff, *The Emperor's Embrace: Reflections on Animal Families and Fatherhood,* Pocket Books, 1999.
11. Buford, Bill, "Rats," *The New Yorker,* October 13, 1997.
12. Steingraber, *Having Faith,* Perseus, 2001.

Chapter 4. Fertility Awareness While Breast-feeding

1. Price, Weston A., *Nutrition & Degeneration,* Price-Pottenger Foundation, 1939.
2. Hrdy, Sarah Blaffer, *Mother Nature: A History of Mothers, Infants, and Natural Selection,* Pantheon, 1999.
3. Taylor, H. William, M. Vazquez-Geffroy, S. Samuels, and D. M. Taylor, "Continuously Recorded Suckling Behaviour and Its Effect on Lactational Amenorrhoea," *Journal of Biosocial Science* 31(1999): 289–310.
4. Brazelton, T. B., MD, John S. Robey, MD, et al., "Infant Development in the Zinacanteco Indians of Southern Mexico," *Pediatrics* 44(1969): 274–90.
5. Konner, M., and C. Worthman, "Nursing frequency, gonadal function, and birth spacing among ¡Kung hunter-gatherers," *Science* 207(1980): 788–91.
6. Small, Meredith F., *Our Babies, Ourselves: How Biology and Culture Shape the Way We Parent,* Anchor, 1988.

Chapter 5. Enhancing Your Chances of Conceiving

1. Stanford, Joseph B., MD, MSPH, George White, Jr., PhD, MSPH, et al., "Timing Intercourse to Achieve Pregnancy," *Obstetrics and Gynecology* 100(2002): 1333–41.

Chapter 7. Common Products That Can Be Hazardous to Reproductive Health

1. Montague, Peter, "The Precautionary Principle," *Rachel's Environment and Health Weekly* 586 (Feb. 19, 1998). A description of a new principle for preventing harm to the environment and human health, defined at Wingspread in Wisconsin in January 1998. Web site: www.biotech-info.net/rachels_586.html.

2. Whittemore, A., et al., "Characteristics relating to ovarian cancer risk; collaborative analysis of twelve U.S. case-controlled studies, collaborative ovarian cancer group," *American Journal of Epidemiology* 136(10): 1175–220.

3. Rossing, Daling, and Weiss Rossing, "Ovarian tumors in a cohort of infertile women," *New England Journal of Medicine* 331(1994): 12, 771–76.

4. Anteby, I., E. Cohen, E. Anteby, and D. BenEzra, "Ocular manifestations in children born after in vitro fertilization," *Archchives of Opthalmolmology* 119(10)(2001): 1525–29. Ocular anomalies (eye problems) were frequently observed in this cohort of offspring born after in vitro fertilization.

5. Hansen, M., J. J. Kurinczuk, C. Bower, and S. Webb, "The risk of major birth defects after intracytoplasmic sperm injection and in vitro fertilization," *New England Journal of Medicine* 347(18)(Oct. 31, 2002): 1449–51. Infants conceived with use of intracytoplasmic sperm injection or in vitro fertilization have twice as high a risk of a major birth defect as naturally conceived infants.

6. Koivurova, S., A. L. Hartikainen, M. Gissler, et al., "Neonatal outcome and congenital malformations in children born after in vitro fertilization," *Human Reproduction* 17(5)(2002): 1391–98. Neonatal outcome after IVF is worse than in the general population with similar maternal age, parity, and social standing, mainly due to the large proportion of multiple births after IVF. The higher prevalence of heart malformations does not solely arise from multiplicity but from other causes.

7. Weschler, Toni, *Taking Charge of Your Fertility*, Rev., Quill, 2001.

8. Scholes, D., A. Z. LaCroix, et al., "Bone mineral density in women using depot medroxyprogesterone acetate for contraception," *Obstetrics and Gynecology* 93(2)(1999): 233–38.

9. Cromer, B. A., J. M. Blair, et al., "A prospective comparison of bone density in adolescent girls receiving depot medroxyprogesterone acetate (Depo-Provera), levonorgestrel (Norplant), or oral contraceptives," *Journal of Pediatrics* 129(5)(1996): 671–76.

10. Skegg, D. C. G., E. A. Noonan, et al., "Depot medroxprogesterone acetate and

breast cancer: A pooled analysis of the World Health Organization and New Zealand studies," *Journal of the American Medical Association,* (1995): 799–804.

11. Partsch, C.-J., M. Audkamp, and W. G. Sippell, "Scrotal Temperature Is Increased in Disposable Plastic-Lined Nappies," *Archives of Disease in Childhood* 83(2000): 364–68. Male infertility and testicular cancer, which are increasing, may be related to baby boys wearing disposable plastic diapers in their first six months of life. The plastic diapers raise the temperature of baby boys' scrotums, thereby affecting their development at a crucial time. With cloth diapers, temperatures are not raised. www.archdischild.com.

12. Reingold, A. L., "Toxic shock syndrome: An update," *American Journal of Obstetrics and Gynecology* 165 (4)(1991): 1236–39.

13. Philipp, R. A. Hughes, et al., "Getting to the bottom of nappy rash," *British Journal of General Practice* 47(1997): 493–97.

14. Heal, Carrie, "The Many Evils of Disposables," *Archives of Disease in Childhood* 85: 268d.

15. Chang, L. W., and P. R. Wade, "Prenatal and neonatal toxicology and pathology of heavy metals," *Advances in Pharmacology and Chemotherapy,* vol. 17, Academic Press, 1980.

16. Cordier, S., et al., "Paternal exposure to mercury and spontaneous abortions," *British Journal of Industrial Medicine* 48(1991): 375–81.

17. Houlihan, Jane, Charlotte Brody, et al., "Not Too Pretty: Phthalates, Beauty Products & the FDA," July 2002, a report by the Environmental Working Group and HCWH; www.NotTooPretty.org.

18. Duty, Susan M., Narendra P. Singh, et al., "The relationship between environmental exposures to phthalates and DNA damage in human sperm using the neutral comet assay," *Environmental Health,* December 6, 2002.

19. DiGangi, Joseph, PhD, Ted Schettler MD, MPH, et al., "Aggregate Exposure to Phthalates in Humans" published in 2002 by Health Care Without Harm, 1755 S St., NW, Suite 6B, Washington, DC 20009; www.noharm.org.

20. Billings, Evelyn, MD, *The Billings Method,* Penguin Books Australia, 2000, pp. 164–65.

21. Hatcher, R. A., F. Guest, et al., "Hormonal Overview," *Contraceptive Technology,* 14th ed., Irvington, 191–92.

22. Larimore, Walter, MD, and Joseph Stanford, MD, MSPH, "Postfertilization Effects of Oral Contraceptives and Their Relationship to Informed Consent," *Arch Fam Med* 9(23)(Feb. 2000).

23. Moreno, Victor, and F. Xavier Bosch, et al., "Effect of Oral Contraceptives on Risk of Cervical Cancer in Women with Human Papilloma Virus Infection: The IARC Multicentric Case-Control Study," *Lancet* 359(2002): 1085–92.

24. Lidegaard, O., "Oral contraceptives, pregnancy, and the risk of cerebral thromboembolism: The influence of diabetes, hypertension, migraine and previous thrombotic disease," *British Journal of Obstetrics and Gynaecology* 102(2)(1995): 153–59.

25. Thorogood, M., J. Mann, et al., "Is oral contraceptive use still associated with an increased risk of fatal myocardial infarction? Report of a case-control study," *British Journal of Obstetrics and Gynaecology,* 98(1991): 1245–53.

26. Thorogood, M., and M. Vessey, "An epidemiologic survey of cardiovascular disease in women taking oral contraceptives," *American Journal of Obstetrics and Gynecology* 163(1)(1990): 274–81.

27. Researchers, including Dr. Merethe Kumle of Community Medicine in Tromso, Norway, followed 103,027 women between the ages of thirty and forty-nine from 1991 to 1999 and reported their findings at the Third European Breast Cancer Conference, 2002.

28. Caruso, S., and C. Grillo, et al., "A Prospective Study Evidencing Rhinomanumetric and Olfactometric Outcomes in Women Taking Oral Contraceptives," *Human Reproduction* 16(11)(Oct. 2001): 2288–94.

29. Ilyia, Elias F., PhD, Deborah McLure, BS, and Michel Y. Farhat, PhD, "Long-Term Effects of Topical Progesterone Cream Application: A Case Study," *International Journal of Pharmaceutical Compounding,* June 1998.

Chapter 9. Healing Childbearing Losses

1. Walker, Barbara, *The Women's Encyclopedia of Myths and Secrets,* Harper & Row, 1983, p. 220.

Chapter 10. Fertility, Light, and Darkness

1. Marieb, Elaine N., *Human Anatomy and Physiology,* 4th ed., Addison Wesley Longman, 1998.

2. Ayre, E. A., and S. F. Pang, "Iodomelatonin binding sites in the testis and ovary: Putative melatonin receptors in the gonads," *Biological Signals* 3(1994): 71–84. Abstract: Through the synthesis and secretion of the hormone melatonin, the pineal has been assigned the role of synchronizing a reproductive response to appropriate environmental conditions. Theoretical melatonin target sites may

occur at several levels of the hypothalamic-pituitary-gonadal hierarchy, including a direct action on the gonads.

3. Dewan, E. M., PhD, Miriam Menkin, MA, and John Rock, MD, "On the Possibility of a Perfect Rhythm of Birth Control by Periodic Light Stimulation," *American Journal of Obstetrics and Gynecology* 99(1967): 1016–19.

4. Lacey, Louise, *Lunaception: A Feminine Odyssey into Fertility and Contraception,* Coward, McCann & Geoghegan, 1975.

5. Kippley, John F., "By the Light of the Silvery Moon: Report #R2," Couple to Couple League, 1976.

6. DeFelice, Joy, RN, BSN, PHN, *The Effects of Light on the Menstrual Cycle: Also Infertility,* 2000.

Chapter 11. Food and Reproductive Health

1. Dunne, Lavonne, *Nutrition Almanac,* 3rd ed., McGraw-Hill, 1990, p. 11.

2. Price, Weston A., *Nutrition and Physical Degeneration,* Price-Pottenger, 1939.

3. Marieb, Elaine, RN, PhD, *Human Anatomy and Physiology,* 4th ed., Benjamin Cummings Science Publishings, 1998.

4. Balch, Phyllis, CNC, *Prescription for Nutritional Healing,* 3rd ed., Avery, 2000, p. 15.

5. Fallon, Sally, and Mary G. Enig, PhD, "Vitamin A Saga," *Wise Traditions* (Winter 2001): 24–34.

6. Dunne, Lavonne.

7. Jennings, I. W., *Vitamins in Endocrine Metabolism,* Heineman, 1970.

8. Rao, C., and B. Rao, "Absorption of dietary carotenes in human subjects," *Am J. Clin. Nutr* 23(1970): 105–109.

9. Berger, S., MD, *What Your Doctor Didn't Learn in Medical School,* Avon Books, 1988: 103–104.

10. Lithgow, D., and W. Politzer, "Vitamin A in the treatment of menorrhagia," *South African Medical Journal,* 51(1977): 191ff.

11. Balch, p. 589.

12. Shannon, Marilyn, *Fertility, Cycles and Nutrition,* 3rd ed., Couple to Couple League, 2001, p. 128.

13. Fallon, Sally, and Mary G. Enig, PhD, "Vitamin A Saga," *Wise Traditions,* Winter 2001.

14. Kinuta, K, H. Tanaka, et al., "Vitamin D is an important factor in estrogen

biosynthesis of both female and male gonads," *Endocrinology* 141(2000): 1317–24.

15. Dunne, p. 80.

16. Glerup, H., K. Mikkelsen, et al., "Commonly recommended daily intake of vitamin D is not sufficient if sunlight exposure is limited," *Journal of Internal Medicine* 247(2000): 260–68.

17. Glerup, H., and E. F Eriksen, "Vitamin D deficiency: Easy to diagnose, often overlooked," *Ugeskrift for Laeger* 161(1999): 2515–21.

18. Pettifor, J. M., G. P. Moodley, et al., "The effect of season and latitude on in vitro vitamin D formation by sunlight in South Africa," *South African Medical Journal.* 86(1996): 1270–72.

19. Webb, A. R., L. Kline, et al., "Influence of season and latitude on the cutaneous synthesis of vitamin D3: Exposure to winter sunlight in Boston and Edmonton will not promote vitamin D3 synthesis in human skin," *Journal of Clinical Endocrinology and Metabolism.* 67(1988): 373–78.

20. Sullivan, Krispin, CN, "The Miracle of Vitamin D," *Wise Traditions,* Fall 2000.

21. Thys-Jacobs, S., D. Donovan, et al., "Vitamin D and calcium dysregulation in the polycystic ovarian syndrome," *Steroids* 64(1999): 430–35.

22. Thys-Jacobs, S., "Vitamin D and calcium in menstrual migraine," *Headache* 34(1994): 544–46.

23. Thys-Jacobs, S., "Micronutrients and the premenstrual syndrome: The case for calcium," *Journal of American College of Nutrition* 19(2000): 220–27.

24. Uhland, A. M., G. G. Kwiecinski, et al., "Normalization of serum calcium restores fertility in vitamin D–deficient male rats," *Journal of Nutrition.* 122(1992): 1338–44.

25. Dunne, p. 226.

26. Sullivan, Krispin, CN, "Vitamin D Update—A Warning," *Wise Traditions,* Fall 2002.

27. Vieth, R., "Vitamin D supplementation, 25-hydroxyvitamin D concentrations, and safety," *American Journal of Clinical Nutrition* 69(1999): 842–56.

28. Ballentine, Richard, MD, *Diet and Nutrition,* Himalayan International Institute, 1982, p. 210.

29. Dunne, p. 53.

30. London, R., MD, G. Sundaram, et al., "Evaluation and treatment of breast symptoms in patients with the premenstrual syndrome," *Journal of Reproductive Medicine* 28(1983): 503ff.

31. Ebon, Martin, *The Truth of Vitamin E,* Bantam, 1972, p. 80.

32. Dunne, p. 55.

33. Davis, Adelle, and Marshall Mandell, MD, *Let's Have Healthy Children*, Signet, p. 43.

34. *Journal of the American Medical Association*, vol. 167, p. 1806, 1958, as reported in Rodale, *The Encylopedia for Healthful Living*, 1970, p. 980.

35. Dunne, p. 223.

36. Davis, Adelle, revised by M. Mandell, MD, *Let's Have Healthy Children*, Signet, p. 25.

37. Dunne, p. 226.

38. Dunne, p. 225.

39. Dunne, p. 226.

40. Davis and Mandell, pp. 22–23.

41. Fallon, Sally, *Nourishing Traditions*, New Trends, 1998, p. 44.

42. Ensminger, A. H., et al., *The Concise Encylopedia of Foods & Nutrition*, CRC Press, 1995, p. 586.

43. Dunne, p. 226.

44. Marieb, p. 922.

45. Balch, p. 33.

46. Berger, S., MD, *What Your Doctor Didn't Learn in Medical School*, Avon, 1988, p. 143.

47. Balch, p. 463.

48. Shannon, p. 109.

49. Dunne, p. 227.

50. Reinhold, John G., *Ecology of Food and Nutrition*, Vol. 1, 1972, pp. 187–92.

51. Reddy, N. R., et al., *Phytates in Cereals and Legumes*, CRC Press, 1989.

52. Fallon, Sally, *Nourishing Traditions*, New Trends Publishing, 1999.

53. Goei, G., MD, and J. Ralston, et al., "Dietary patterns of patients with premenstrual tension," *Journal of Applied Nutrition* 34(1982): 9.

54. Pinckney, Edward R., MD, and Cathey Pinckney, *The Cholesterol Controversy*, Sherbourne Press, 1973.

55. Enig, Mary G., PhD, et al., *Federation Proceedings* 37(9)(1998): 2215–20.

56. Machlin, I. J., and A. Bendich, *FASEB Journal* 1(1987): 441–45.

57. Enig, Mary G., PhD., and Sally Fallon, "The Great Con-ola," *Wise Traditions*, Summer 2002.

58. Enig, Mary G., PhD, *Trans Fatty Acids in the Food Supply: A Comprehensive Report Covering 60 Years of Research*, 2nd ed., Enig Associates Inc., 1995.

59. Koletzko, B., and J. Muller, "*Cis-* and *Trans-*Isomeric Fatty Acids in Plasma Lipids of Newborn Infants and Their Mothers," *Biology of the Neonate* 57(1990): 172–78.

60. Hanis, T., V. Zidek, et al., "Effects of Dietary *Trans-*Fatty Acids on Reproductive Performance of Wistar Rats," *British Journal of Nutrition* 61(1989): 519–29.

61. Enig, Mary G., PhD, *Trans Fatty Acids in the Food Supply: A Comprehensive Report Covering 60 Years of Research,* 2nd ed., Enig Associates, Inc., 1995, p. 81.

62. Teter, B. B., J. Sampugna, et al., "Milk Fat Depression in C57B1/6J Mice Consuming Partially Hydrogenated Fat," *Journal of Nutrition* 120(1990): 818–24.

63. Mercola, Joseph, "No safe levels of trans fat," www.mercola.com/2002/jul/27/trans_fat.htm.

64. Beasley, Joseph D., MD, and Jerry Swift, MA, *The Kellog Report,* 1989, The Institute of Health Policy and Practice, Annandale-on-Hudson, NY, pp. 144–45.

65. Nestler, John E., Daniela J. Jakubowicz, et al., "Insulin Stimulates Testosterone Biosynthesis by Human Thecal Cells from Women with Polycystic Ovarian Syndrome by Activating Its Own Receptors and Using Inositolglycan Mediators as the Signal Transduction System," *Journal of Clinical Endocrinology and Metabolism* 83(6)(1998).

66. Lipinski, Lori, CNC, "Making the Transition: Replacing Refined Sugars with Natural Sugars, One Step at a Time," *Wise Traditions,* Summer 2002.

67. Divi, R. L., et al., "Anti-thyroid isoflavones from the soybean," *Biochem Pharmacol* 54(1997): 1087–96.

68. Setchell, K. D. R., et al., "Exposure of infants to phytoestrogens from soy-based infant formula," *Lancet* 350(1997): 23–27.

69. Freni-Titulaer, L. W., et al., "Premature thelarche in Puerto Rico: A search for environmental factors," *American Journal of Diseases of Children* 140(12)(1986): 1263–67.

70. Wisniewski, Amy B., Sabra L. Klein, et al., "Exposure to Genistein During Gestation and Lactation Demasculinizes the Reproductive System in Rats," *Journal of Urology* 169(April 2003): 1582–86.

71. Katz, S. H., "Food and Biocultural Evolution: A Model for the Investigation of Modern Nutritional Problems," *Nutritional Anthropology,* Alan Liss Inc., 1987.

72. Jennings, I. W., *Vitamins in Endocrine Metabolism,* Heineman, 1970.

73. Wilcox, A., et al., "Caffeinated beverages and decreased fertility," *Lancet* 2(1988): 1453–55.

74. Stanton, C., and R. Gray, "Effects of caffeine consumption on delayed conception," *American Journal of Epidemiology* 142(12)(1995): 1322–29.

75. Boulmar, F., et al., "Caffeine intake and delayed conception: A European multicentre study on infertility and subfecundity," *American Journal of Epidemiology* 145(4)(1997): 324–34.

76. Parazzini, F., et al., "Risk factors for unexplained dyspermia in infertile men: A case-control study," *Archives of Andrology* 31(2)(1993): 105–13.

77. *Nutrition News and Views* (6)(Nov. 1999).

78. Wiles, Richard, Kert Davies, et al., "A Shopper's Guide to Pesticides in Produce," Environmental Working Group, 1995; www.ewg.org/reports/Baby_food/baby_home.html.

Appendix

1. Kambic, R. T., and V. Lamprecht, "Calendar rhythm effecacy: A review," *Adv. Contracept* 12(1996): 123–28.

2. Trussel, J., and L. Grummer-Strawn, "Contraceptive failure of the ovulation method of periodic abstinence," *Fam Plann Perspect* 22(1990): 65–75.

3. Witkam, W. G. M., MD, "Holland and the History of Natural Family Planning," *CCL Family Foundations,* May 2000.

4. Hatcher, Robert A., MD, MPH, et al., *Contraceptive Technology* 17th rev. ed., Ardent Media, 1998, p. 312.

Index

Page numbers in italics indicate illustrations and charts.

Hazardous products (*cont.*)
  phthalates, 128–129
  the Pill, 129–132
  progesterone creams and gels, 132–133
  resources, 262–263
  tampons, 133–134
Healing, 135–136
  childbearing losses, 143–157
  six steps of, 136–137
    Step 0: Do nothing, 137
    Step 1: Collect information, 137
    Step 2: Engage the energy, 137–138
    Step 3: Nourish and tonify, 138
    Step 4: Sedate and stimulate, 138
    Step 5a: Use supplements, 138
    Step 5b: Use drugs, 138
    Step 6: Break and enter, 139
  women's stories of, 139–142
Health-care systems, 186–191
Health Care Without Harm (HCWH), 128
Hellinger, Bert, 151
Herbalism, 188
High-protein diet, 178
Homeopathy, 188–189
Hormones, 6, 100
  of breast-feeding, 64–65
Huggins, Hal, Dr., 127
Human chorionic gonadotropin (HCG), 9, 49
Human papillomavirus (HPV), 130
Hyde, Lewis, 84–87, 93
Hydrogenation, 174–175
Hyperthyroidism, 108, 194
Hypothalamus gland, 159
Hypothyroidism, 108, 113–114, *114–115*, 193–194
  charting, 203, *204–205*
Hypothyroidism: The Unsuspected Illness (Barnes), 108

Ibuprofen, 192
Ilyia, Elias, Dr., 132–133
Infertility, 154–157
  unambiguous, 66, 70
Iodine, 172

Johns Hopkins University, 177
Jung, Carl, 144
Justisse, 230

Katie, Byron, 154–156
Kegel exercises, 22, 39, 196
Keller, Deborah, 193
Kennard, Beth, Dr., 107–108
Kid's Herb Book, A (Tierra), 197

Kippley, Sheila, 64, 67–68, 70
Know Your Fats (Enig), 174
!Kung San, 66

Labia, 5
Lacey, Louise, 159–160
Lactational amenorrhea, 66
Langer, Stephen, Dr., 109, 131, 195
Lee, Mercedes, 180
Let's Have Healthy Children (Davis), 171
Levy, Thomas, Dr., 127
Lipinski, Lori, 176
Living Well with Hypothyroidism (Shomon), 109, 194
Lovemaking, and breast-feeding, 70–71
Lubricants, 196
Lunaception, 92, 159–163
Luteal phase, 7, 48, 69, 89, 101–102
  deficiency, 112
Luteinizing hormone (LH), 6, 105–106

Male reproductive system, 10–13, *12*
Matus, Geraldine, 233
McGill University, 178–179
Meditation, after miscarriage, 148–150
Melatonin, 92, 159
Menopause, 220, *221*
Menstrual cycle, 6–9, *10*
  charting, 102–105, *103–104*
  fertility determination during, 37
Menstruation, 14, 57
Mercury, 127
Midcycle spotting, 27
Mini-Pill, 130
Miscarriage, *117*, 117–118, 147–150
Mittelschmerz, 27
Moore, Johana, 153–154
Morton, Leah, Dr., 124, 131–132, 169, 176
Mothering Magazine, 127
Mucus, 4, 17–19
  dry, 71
  fertility determination by, 37–43
  slippery, 71

Naked at Noon: Understanding Sunlight and Vitamin D (Sullivan), 182
Naps, 70
National Academy of Science, 175
National Women's Health Report, 108
Natural cycles, 57, 72–73
Natural Family Planning, 64, 228–229
Natural remedies, 185–186
  for anovulation, 191–192
  for coming off the Pill, 194–195